Nutrition Essentials for Type 2 Diabetes

Nutrition Essentials for Type 2 Diabetes

Editor: Vanessa Artiga

AMERICAN
MEDICAL PUBLISHERS
www.americanmedicalpublishers.com

AMERICAN
MEDICAL PUBLISHERS
www.americanmedicalpublishers.com

Cataloging-in-Publication Data

Nutrition essentials for type 2 diabetes / edited by Vanessa Artiga.
p. cm.
Includes bibliographical references and index.
ISBN 978-1-63927-760-5
1. Type 2 diabetes. 2. Type 2 diabetes--Nutritional aspects.
3. Type 2 diabetes--Patients--Nutrition--Requirements.
4. Type 2 diabetes--Diet therapy. 5. Diet in disease.
6. Insulin--Metabolism--Regulation. 7. Nutrition. I. Artiga, Vanessa.
RC662.18 .N88 2023

American Medical Publishers,
41 Flatbush Avenue,
1st Floor, New York,
NY 11217, USA

ISBN 978-1-63927-760-5 (Hardback)

Contents

Preface VII

Chapter 1 **High Fat Rodent Models of Type 2 Diabetes: From Rodent to Human** 1
Nicole L. Stott and Joseph S. Marino

Chapter 2 **Low Reported Adherence to the 2019 American Diabetes Association Nutrition Recommendations among Patients with Type 2 Diabetes Mellitus, Indicating the Need for Improved Nutrition Education and Diet Care** 20
Savvas Katsaridis, Maria G. Grammatikopoulou, Konstantinos Gkiouras, Christos Tzimos, Stefanos T. Papageorgiou, Anastasia G. Markaki, Triada Exiara, Dimitrios G. Goulis and Theodora Papamitsou

Chapter 3 **Early-Life Nutritional Programming of Type 2 Diabetes: Experimental and Quasi-Experimental Evidence** 37
Alexander M. Vaiserman

Chapter 4 **Vitamin D Status, Calcium Intake and Risk of Developing Type 2 Diabetes: An Unresolved Issue** 53
Araceli Muñoz-Garach, Beatriz García-Fontana and Manuel Muñoz-Torres

Chapter 5 **Dietary Approaches for Japanese Patients with Diabetes** 70
Satoru Yamada, Yusuke Kabeya and Hiroshi Noto

Chapter 6 **Leucine Supplementation Differently Modulates Branched-Chain Amino Acid Catabolism, Mitochondrial Function and Metabolic Profiles at the Different Stage of Insulin Resistance in Rats on High-Fat Diet** 79
Rui Liu, Hui Li, Wenjuan Fan, Qiu Jin, Tingting Chao, Yuanjue Wu, Junmei Huang, Liping Hao and Xuefeng Yang

Chapter 7 **Glycemia Lowering Effect of an Aqueous Extract of *Hedychium coronarium* Leaves in Diabetic Rodent Models** 99
Ling-Shan Tse, Po-Lin Liao, Chi-Hao Tsai, Ching-Hao Li, Jiunn-Wang Liao, Jaw-Jou Kang and Yu-Wen Cheng

Chapter 8 **Butyrate Reduces HFD-Induced Adipocyte Hypertrophy and Metabolic Risk Factors in Obese LDLr-/-.Leiden Mice** 111
Charlotte E. Pelgrim, Bart A. A. Franx, Jessica Snabel, Robert Kleemann, Ilse A. C. Arnoldussen and Amanda J. Kiliaan

Chapter 9 **Glucose and Lipid Dysmetabolism in a Rat Model of Prediabetes Induced by a High-Sucrose Diet** 126
Ana Burgeiro, Manuela G. Cerqueira, Bárbara M. Varela-Rodríguez, Sara Nunes, Paula Neto, Frederico C. Pereira, Flávio Reis and Eugénia Carvalho

Chapter 10 **Integrated Assessment of Pharmacological and Nutritional Cardiovascular Risk Management: Blood Pressure Control in the DIAbetes and LifEstyle Cohort Twente (DIALECT)** **142**
Christina M. Gant, S. Heleen Binnenmars, Else van den Berg, Stephan J. L. Bakker, Gerjan Navis and Gozewijn D. Laverman

Chapter 11 **Carbohydrates from Sources with a Higher Glycemic Index during Adolescence: Is Evening Rather than Morning Intake Relevant for Risk Markers of Type 2 Diabetes in Young Adulthood?** **158**
Tanja Diederichs, Christian Herder, Sarah Roßbach, Michael Roden, Stefan A. Wudy, Ute Nöthlings, Ute Alexy and Anette E. Buyken

Chapter 12 **Effect of *n*-3 Polyunsaturated Fatty Acid Supplementation on Metabolic and Inflammatory Biomarkers in Type 2 Diabetes Mellitus Patients** **174**
M. Gorety Jacobo-Cejudo, Roxana Valdés-Ramos, Ana L. Guadarrama-López, Rosa-Virgen Pardo-Morales, Beatriz E. Martínez-Carrillo and Laurence S. Harbige

Chapter 13 **PREVIEW: Prevention of Diabetes through Lifestyle Intervention and Population Studies in Europe and around the World: Design, Methods and Baseline Participant Description of an Adult Cohort Enrolled into a Three-Year Randomised Clinical Trial** **185**
Mikael Fogelholm, Thomas Meinert Larsen, Margriet Westerterp-Plantenga, Ian Macdonald, J. Alfredo Martinez, Nadka Boyadjieva, Sally Poppitt, Wolfgang Schlicht, Gareth Stratton, Jouko Sundvall, Tony Lam, Elli Jalo, Pia Christensen, Mathijs Drummen, Elizabeth Simpson, Santiago Navas-Carretero, Teodora Handjieva-Darlenska, Roslyn Muirhead, Marta P. Silvestre, Daniela Kahlert, Laura Pastor-Sanz, Jennie Brand-Miller and Anne Raben

Chapter 14 **Nuts and Dried Fruits: An Update of their Beneficial Effects on Type 2 Diabetes** **201**
Pablo Hernández-Alonso, Lucía Camacho-Barcia, Mònica Bulló and Jordi Salas-Salvadó

Permissions

List of Contributors

Index

Preface

The world is advancing at a fast pace like never before. Therefore, the need is to keep up with the latest developments. This book was an idea that came to fruition when the specialists in the area realized the need to coordinate together and document essential themes in the subject. That's when I was requested to be the editor. Editing this book has been an honour as it brings together diverse authors researching on different streams of the field. The book collates essential materials contributed by veterans in the area which can be utilized by students and researchers alike.

Type-2 diabetes is the most common type of diabetes characterized by an increased blood sugar level in the body. The management of type-2 diabetes involves a diet rich in nutrient-dense foods. Fiber, proteins, vitamins, complex carbohydrates, and minerals are good sources of nutrients for type-2 diabetics. Diabetic diet should consist of nutritious food items including fruits such as peaches, berries, oranges, apples, melons, pears, and vegetables such as cucumbers, spinach, cauliflower, zucchini, broccoli, etc. Some foods such as full-fat dairy, sweets, sugar-sweetened beverages, processed foods, high fat meat, and trans-fats should be avoided. Protein-rich foods such as eggs, seafood, peas, tofu, lean meats, and poultry provide energy and keep the blood sugar level stable. This book provides a detailed explanation with respect to the nutrients essential for managing type-2 diabetes. A number of latest researches have been included to keep the readers updated with the recent concepts in this area of study. The book will serve as a reference to a broad spectrum of readers.

Each chapter is a sole-standing publication that reflects each author´s interpretation. Thus, the book displays a multi-facetted picture of our current understanding of application, resources and aspects of the field. I would like to thank the contributors of this book and my family for their endless support.

Editor

High Fat Rodent Models of Type 2 Diabetes: From Rodent to Human

Nicole L. Stott and Joseph S. Marino *

Laboratory of Systems Physiology, Department of Kinesiology, The University of North Carolina at Charlotte, Charlotte, NC 28223, USA; Nstott1@uncc.edu

* Correspondence: jmarin10@uncc.edu

Abstract: Poor dietary habits contribute to increased incidences of obesity and related co-morbidities, such as type 2 diabetes (T2D). The biological, genetic, and pathological implications of T2D, are commonly investigated using animal models induced by a dietary intervention. In spite of significant research contributions, animal models have limitations regarding the translation to human pathology, which leads to questioning their clinical relevance. Important considerations include diet-specific effects on whole organism energy balance and glucose and insulin homeostasis, as well as tissue-specific changes in insulin and glucose tolerance. This review will examine the T2D-like phenotype in rodents resulting from common diet-induced models and their relevance to the human disease state. Emphasis will be placed on the disparity in percentages and type of dietary fat, the duration of intervention, and whole organism and tissue-specific changes in rodents. An evaluation of these models will help to identify a diet-induced rodent model with the greatest clinical relevance to the human T2D pathology. We propose that a 45% high-fat diet composed of approximately one-third saturated fats and two-thirds unsaturated fats may provide a diet composition that aligns closely to average Western diet macronutrient composition, and induces metabolic alterations mirrored by clinical populations.

Keywords: high-fat diet; metabolism; type 2 diabetes; insulin resistance; obesity; rodent models of type 2 diabetes

1. Introduction

High fat diet (HFD) animal models utilize a variety of fat sources to mimic the typical Western diet, which in the U.S. population consists of ~70% more saturated fat than the recommended dietary guidelines [1]. A twelve-year National Health and Nutrition Examination Study (NHANES) study demonstrated that individuals consuming high amounts of carbohydrates, cholesterol, saturated fatty acids, polyunsaturated fats, monounsaturated fats, and protein have a greater propensity to develop glucose intolerance when compared to individuals with dietary patterns high in vitamin, mineral, and fiber content [2]. Saturated fatty acids (SFA), which are stored more readily in rodents and humans compared to monounsaturated and polyunsaturated fats, increase the risk of obesity [3]. Therefore, it is important to work towards the uniform formulation of a rodent diet that best represents human consumption, while promoting a similar type 2 diabetes (T2D) phenotype.

HFD consumed *ab libitum* results in rodents exceeding typical daily caloric intake [4], and animal-based fats promote diet-induced obesity and insulin resistance better than vegetable-based fats in rats [5]. Commonly used saturated fatty acid sources include hydrogenated coconut oil, corn oil, lard, palmitic acid, and stearic acid [6,7]. Unsaturated fats, such as oleic acid and linoleic acid, are also utilized in some nutritional animal models [8]. HFD, even when isocalorically matched with a standard purified control diet, induces obesity in rodents through alterations in metabolic homeostasis and reduced physical activity levels [9]. HFD-induced phenotypes of T2D in rodents and humans share weight gain, hyperglycemia, hyperinsulinemia, insulin resistance, inflammatory cytokine secretion, and ectopic lipid accumulation [10]. However, diet-induced animal models employ marked differences in micronutrient and macronutrient composition, including a variety of saturated fats, resulting in significant inter-study variability [11–13].

Despite these variables, the chronic consumption of a HFD by rodents alters a variety of genes and/or receptors involved in metabolism, inflammation, oxidative stress, substrate transport, protein synthesis and modification, and transcriptional regulation [6,7,14–16]. Notably, the modification of such genes is tissue-specific [6]. A better understanding of tissue specific effects in response to dietary composition will provide guidance into the most appropriate HFD-induced animal model(s) to study the pathogenesis of T2D and associated phenotypic changes.

Thorough review articles addressing the value and limitations of T2D animal models have been published [10,17,18]. Variable diet composition, rodent strain, intervention time-points, and duration of protocols further complicate the translatability of animal-based findings to the human disease state. Here, we summarize how the combination of percentage and type of fat with varying durations of intervention, affect the major insulin responsive tissues. These are important considerations to get closer to an animal model with high clinical relevance to the human disease.

2. Tissue-Specific Effects of HFD Models

2.1. Liver

Mice. The composition of saturated fatty acids in a HFD differentially affects adipose deposition within the liver and subsequently cellular and molecular signaling. Examples of saturated fats that adversely affect the liver of C57BL/6 male mice include corn oil, lard, and hydrogenated coconut oil (Table 1). The composition of HFD is responsible for the different effects in hepatic lipid storage. For example, a 45% HFD containing palm oil (high in saturated fat) or olive oil (low in saturated fat) increased hepatic triacylglycerol (TAG) content following an 8-week intervention in C57BL/6 mice [19]. In male and female C57BL/6 mice, 18 to 20 weeks of a 60% lard-based diet increased lipid accumulation and steatosis in the liver [20–22]. Other studies showed hepatic inflammation and fibrosis following only 8 weeks of a similar diet [23].

On a whole organism level, male and female mice developed insulin resistance and glucose intolerance in response to 45% [19] and 60% HFD [20–22]. However, the source of the fat must be considered [19] (Table 1).

Table 1. Liver.

Source	Fat Source	Macronutrients (% kcal)	Duration	Strain; Sex	Tissue Findings	T2D Status
[19]	(a) Cocoa butter (b) Palm oil (c) Olive oil (d) Safflower oil	45% fat 20% protein 35% carbohydrate All diet formulations maintained same ratio	8 weeks	C57BL/6 mice; Male	↑ Liver TAG in palm and olive oil groups	↑ Body weight in palm oil compared to cocoa butter. ↓ Glucose tolerance: cocoa, palm and safflower oils
[6]	Hydrogenated coconut oil	59% fat 15% protein 26% carbohydrate	20 weeks	C57BL/6 mice; Male	↑ FABP mRNA ↑ Inflammation ↑ Increased BTNL2	↑ Fat mass ↓ Insulin sensitivity ↑ Plasma insulin
[22]	Lard and Soybean oil	60% fat 20% protein 20% carbohydrate	20 weeks	C57BL/6 mice; Female	↑ Lipid accumulation ↑ Hepatic steatosis	↑ Body weight ↓ Glucose tolerance ↑Serum insulin ↑ Serum glucose
[20,21,23,24]	Lard and Soybean oil	60% fat ~20% protein ~20% carbohydrate	8 weeks [23] 15 weeks [24] 18 weeks [20] 20 weeks [21]	C57BL/6 mice; Male	↑ Inflammation ↑ Lipid accumulation ↑ Fibrosis	↑ Body weight ↑ Serum glucose ↑ Serum insulin ↑ HOMA-IR
[25]	Lard	45% fat 30% protein 25% carbohydrate	4 weeks	Wister rats; Male	↑ Liver mass ↑ Liver TAG ↑ Hepatic steatosis	↑ Body weight ↓Insulin sensitivity ←→ Plasma glucose
[26]	Lard and Soybean oil	45% fat 20% protein 35% carbohydrate	12 weeks	Sprague-Dawley rats; Male	↑ Lipid accumulation ↑ Lipogenic gene and protein expression	↑ Body weight
[27]	Butter	58% fat 25% protein 17% carbohydrate	18 weeks	Sprague-Dawley rats; Male	↑ Inflammation ↑ Lipid accumulation ↓ Insulin signaling ↑ Hepatic necrosis ↑ Oxidative stress	↑ Body weight ↑ Serum glucose ↑ Serum insulin ↑ HOMA-IR

Studies cited in this table were limited to those that included macronutrient composition. The direction of arrows indicate change when compared to a standard diet control group within that study. Triacylglycerol (TAG), butyrophilin-like Protein 2 (BTNL2), fatty acid binding protein (FABP), major histocompatibility complex I and II (MHC I and II), and homeostatic model assessment of insulin resistance (HOMA-IR).

Inflammatory responses and β-oxidation gene changes in mice have been reported, particularly as a result of a HFD containing more than 45% fat. Inflammatory responses are a known etiology of T2D development in rodents and humans [16,28]. However, establishing similarities between species is difficult when models vary in the percentage of fat, 59% to 82%, and duration, 12 to 36 weeks [6,29]. Eighteen to 20 weeks of a 60% lard-based diet increased cellular and biochemical markers of hepatic inflammation in male [20,21], but not female mice [22]. As the percentage of saturated fat increases, so does liver dysfunction. Interestingly an extremely HFD, 82% lard, caused hepatic lipid deposition accompanied by a transient increase in the expression of genes regulating fatty acid oxidation and synthesis after just 2 weeks [29]. By 4 weeks of consuming such a diet, gene expression patterns changed to reflect 2 to 4-fold increases adipogenesis (PPARγ and fatty acid binding protein) and lipid deposition (CD36) [29]. Not surprisingly, as the percentage of HFD increased, the inflammatory response followed the same trend. These studies suggest that excessive high fat content may cause a rapid transient pattern in hepatic fatty acid metabolism. Due to the rapid changes, it is plausible that many of the cellular and molecular events that alter hepatic lipid accumulation may be missed by studies focusing on prolonged consumption, especially when employing very high fat content. Due to the more progressive phenotype of lipid accumulation in human liver, such studies may contribute little to the understanding of the human phenotype.

Rats. Four weeks of a 45% lard-based diet caused hepatic steatosis, increased liver mass and increased hepatic TAG content in Wister rats [25] (Table 1). Changes in liver characteristics were accompanied by obesity and reduced insulin sensitivity, despite no evidence of hyperglycemia [25]. This more mild phenotype may be the result of a short diet intervention period and/or modest concentration of fat. In response to diets containing higher concentrations of SFA, a more severe phenotype emerges. Sprague–Dawley rats developed hepatic insulin resistance, fatty liver, inflammation, and necrosis following consumption of a 58% butter [27] or 65% lard-based diet [30]. Under both dietary conditions, a severer whole body T2D phenotype emerged [27,30] (Table 1).

The composition of fat within a diet may be just as important as the percentage and treatment duration. While a 45.5% HFD composed of SFA, monounsaturated fatty acids (MUFA), and polyunsaturated fatty acids (PUFA) did not cause an increase in body mass compared to control fed animals, liver mass and blood glucose were elevated after 15 weeks [31]. Such findings are similar to those reported in mice, such that higher concentrations of MUFA and PUFA mixtures produce a more mild phenotype [19] (Table 1).

2.2. Adipose

Mice. Insulin promotes lipogenesis in adipose tissue, reducing glycerol and fatty acid availability. Insulin resistant adipose tissue impairs glucose disposal and increases lipolysis, promoting fatty acid and glycerol availability for hepatic gluconeogenesis [32]. When unable to regulate hepatic glucose production properly, hyperglycemia coincides with lipid accumulation in adipose depots and peripheral tissues.

Saturated and unsaturated fat differentially effect the metabolic and immune responses in adipose tissue. A 45% HFD enriched with palmitic acid (SFA) induced adipose tissue hypertrophy, but a 45% HFD, enriched with oleic acid (MUFA), caused adipose tissue hyperplasia [33] (Table 2). Insulin sensitivity was improved, but not normalized, in mice fed monounsaturated fat [34]. Improved insulin sensitivity was partially a result of adipose-mediated inflammatory signaling. Adipose tissue macrophages secrete pro-inflammatory mediators, such as tumor necrosis factor-alpha (TNF-α), interleukin-6 (IL-6), and monocyte chemoattractant protein-1 (MCP-1), which correlate with adipocyte cell death [35] (Table 2). A 45% HFD enriched with saturated fats exacerbated the inflammatory response within adipose tissue, evidenced by increased TNF-α and IL-6 gene expression and reduced insulin sensitivity [36]. Furthermore, 31 weeks of a 42% HFD composed of SFA and MUFA caused white adipose tissue inflammation, reduced insulin signaling, and reduced the capacity for mitochondrial biogenesis and function in male mice [34]. However, when the fat source was based on mono or polyunsaturated fats, the inflammatory response was mitigated, and insulin responsiveness restored [36].

Table 2. Adipose.

Source	Fat Source	Macronutrients (% kcal)	Duration	Strain; Sex	Findings	T2D Status
[38]	Lard and Soybean oil	45% fat 20% protein 35% carbohydrate	12 weeks	C57BL/6; Male	↑ Body weight ↑ Epididymal fat mass and adipocyte size ↑ Inflammation	↑ Body weight ↑ Blood glucose
[33]	(1) Palm oil (2) Sunflower oil	(1) 45% fat 20% protein 35% carbohydrate (2) 45% fat 20% protein35% carbohydrate	24 weeks	C57BL/6; Male	↓ SFA: Adipose insulin signaling ↑ SFA: Inflammation ↑ SFA: Adipocyte size ↑ SFA and MUFA: Epididymal, visceral, subcutaneous, and perirenal fat pad mass	↓ Palm and sunflower oils: Glucose tolerance ↑ Sunflower oil: Hyperinsulinemia ↑ Palm oil: Hyperinsulinemia above sunflower oil
[37,39]	Lard and Soybean oil	60% fat 20% protein 20% carbohydrate	7 to 8 weeks	C57BL/6; Male	↑ Subcutaneous fat ↑ Visceral fat ↑ Adipocyte size ↑ Lipogenic gene expression	↑ Body weight ↑ Serum glucose
[40]	Lard and Soybean oil	60% fat 20% protein 20% carbohydrate	12 weeks	C57BL/6; female	↑ Perirenal fat ↑ Gonadal fat ↑ Mesenteric fat	↑ Body weight ←→ Glucose tolerance
[35]	Lard and Soybean oil	60% fat 20% protein20% carbohydrate	20 weeks	C57BL/6; Male	↑ Adipose weight ↑ Adipocyte size peaks at 12 weeks ↑ Adipocyte death peaks at 16 weeks ↑ Inflammation	↑ Body weight ↑ Serum insulin by 8 weeks ↑ Insulin resistance by 8 weeks ↑ HOMA-IR by 8 weeks
[41]	Lard and Soybean oil	45% fat 20% protein 35% carbohydrate	13 weeks	Sprague-Dawley rats; Male	↑ Retroperitoneal and epididymal fat mass ↑ Adipocyte size ↑ Adipogenic gene expression ↑ Macrophage accumulation ↑ Inflammation	↑ Body weight
[42]	Unknown	57% fat 10% protein 31% carbohydrate	11 weeks	Wister rats; Male and Female	↑ Subcutaneous and retroperitoneal fat mass and adipocyte diameter in males and females ↑ Oxidative stress in males only ↑ Subcutaneous fat inflammation in males only	↑ Body weight males only
[43]	Lard and Soybean oil	60% fat 20% protein 20% carbohydrate	8 weeks	Wister rats; Male	↑ Ceramide content ↑ DAG content ↑ Plasma free fatty acids	←→ Body weight ↑ Plasma glucose ↑ Plasma insulin ↑ HOMA-IR
[44]	UFA Mix: Sheep rump fat	62.1% fat 16% protein 28.2% fat	20 weeks	Wister rats; Males	↑ Inguinal, mesenteric, epididymal, retroperitoneal, and perirenal fat mass ↓ Capillary density ↑ Increased macrophage crown-like structures	↑ Body weight ↑ Blood glucose ↑ HOMA-IR ←→ Insulin

Studies cited in this table were limited to those that included macronutrient composition. The direction of arrows indicate change when compared to a standard diet control group within that study. Homeostatic model assessment of insulin resistance (HOMA-IR), saturated fatty acid (SFA), monounsaturated fatty acid (MUFA, and diacylglycerol (DAG).

An HFD of 60% caused a more severe inflammatory response [35]. Progressive increases in adipocyte size were followed by cell death with increased fat pad weight through 20 weeks [35]. This phase of adipose tissue remolding was largely driven by macrophage infiltration [35] and may be associated with adipose hyperplasia to account for adipocyte death. Following as little as 1 week of a 60% lard-based HFD, pro-inflammatory macrophages (M1-like macrophages) were significantly increased and remained elevated through 7 weeks [37]. However, consumption of a 45% HFD for 12 weeks led to a similar phenotype [38] (Table 2).

Rats. Diets ranging from 45% to 62% fat caused adipocyte dysfunction and a T2D-like phenotype [41,43,44] (Table 2). Thirteen weeks of a 45% lard-based diet increased fat pad mass, adipocyte size and inflammation, but markers of T2D were not reported [41]. Diets of ~60% fat induced similar characteristics of adipose dysfunction with insulin and glucose intolerance, despite different fat sources [43,44]. Specifically, 62% mixed unsaturated fat caused significant adipose inflammation, accompanied by increased fasting glucose and homeostatic model assessment of insulin resistance (HOMA-IR) [44]. Diets composed of lower [41] and similar [43] percentages of fat from lard, reported comparable cellular and phenotypic changes in adipose. However, the duration of HFD consumption varied greatly in such studies, making it difficult to distinguish the importance of the fat concentration or source, from the duration of consumption (Table 2).

Changes in adipose integrity are influenced by sex, supporting the necessity for inclusion of female subjects. Following 11 weeks of a 57% HFD, only male rats developed oxidative stress and inflammation in subcutaneous adipose [42]. In female rats, increased subcutaneous and retroperitoneal fat mass was not associated with increased inflammatory cytokines or evidence of immune cell accumulation [42]. Notably, the source of fat and markers of T2D were not reported. However, in female mice, a similar diet increased adiposity without a change in glucose tolerance [40].

2.3. Pancreas

Mice. The pancreas serves as a critical regulator of insulin and glucose homeostasis. Under low energy availability, glucagon could stimulate hepatic glucose production, while under energy surplus, insulin could facilitate glucose uptake. A better understanding of how different dietary models affect the pancreas will facilitate the development of a model that aligns with alterations in pancreatic function in the progression of human T2D.

Six weeks of a 45% lard-based diet increased β-cell proliferation and mass, in the splenic region, contributing to the onset of insulin resistance in C57BL/6 male mice [45]. Following 12 weeks of the same diet, β-cell expression of adipose differentiation-related protein (ADFP) was increased, and pancreatic lipid accumulation was evident [46]. As a result, mice were hyperglycemic and hyperinsulinic. Human pancreatic β-cells treated with fatty acids showed a similar trend in ADFP expression [46].

In response to a 60% lard-based diet, reduced glucose tolerance and hyperinsulinemia were evident within 1 week, but insulin resistance did not manifest until 11 weeks [47]. At the onset, pancreatic cells compensated for increased glucose levels by doubling insulin secretion (detectable within 2 weeks), but insulin secretion became significantly impaired as insulin resistance developed and β-cell mass continued to increase [47]. Genes associated with hyperinsulinemia and β-cell proliferation were significantly elevated by week 8, which was 3 weeks prior to measurable insulin resistance [47]. More recently, a 60% HFD for 8 weeks, caused obesity, hyperglycemia, hyperlipidemia, and pancreatic β-cell hypertrophy in C57BL/6 mice [48] (Table 3). Metabolic profiling revealed that global metabolite changes of bioactive lipids associated with β-cell expansion and β-cell proliferation increased 1.75-fold [49].

Rats. Pancreatic inflammation in 60% HFD fed male Sprague–Dawley rats was associated with pancreatic atrophy, hyperinsulinemia, hyperglycemia, increased HOMA-IR, and pancreatic triglyceride (TG) accumulation following 24 weeks [50]. A similar dietary composition (66% fat), increased β-cell autophagy and glucagon production after 16 weeks [51] (Table 3). Elevated glucagon production is likely the cause for hyperglycemia reported at 16 weeks and at later time points in other studies [51,52]. However, 46% HFD for 12 weeks reduced glucose tolerance, indicating progression of the diabetic phenotype with a lower fat load [53]. Taken together, 46% and 66% HFD elicit β and α cell expansion, hyperinsulinemia, and reduced glucose tolerance [51,53]. Importantly, the source of fat in the aforementioned studies was not reported. Nonetheless, these similarities suggest that a fat content closer to a Western-based diet provides a sufficient stimulus to study HFD-induced pancreatic dysfunction.

Identifying the concentration and composition that best relates to pancreatic alterations in the human T2D population should be the priority, rather than adjusting the percentage of fat for the greatest tissue insult. Indeed, species-specific differences exist, such as primarily β-cell proliferation in rodents and β-cell apoptosis in humans prior to insulin resistance [49,54]. Therefore, if the pancreas is the tissue of interest, it may be beneficial to combine a moderate HFD model with low dose streptozotocin to reduce β-cell mass and allow for insulin levels to decline throughout T2D progression [55].

Table 3. Pancreas.

Source	Fat Source	Macronutrients (% kcal)	Duration	Strain; Sex	Findings	T2D Status
[45]	Lard and Soybean oil	45% fat 20% protein 35% carbohydrate	6 weeks	C57BL/6; Male	↑ Beta cell proliferation in splenic region ↑ Increased insulin secretion from isolated islets	↑ Body weight ↑ Plasma insulin ↓ Glucose tolerance ↓ Insulin tolerance
[46]	Lard and Soybean oil	45% fat 20% protein 35% carbohydrate	12 weeks	C57BL/6; Male	↑ Lipid accumulation in acinar cells ↑ Adipose differentiation-related protein (ADFP)	↑ Body weight ↑ Serum insulin ↑ Blood glucose
[48]	Lard and Soybean oil	60% fat 20% protein 20% carbohydrate	8 weeks	C57BL/6; Male	↑ Islet size ↑ Islet Insulin	↑ Body weight ↑ Blood glucose ↑ HbA1c ↑ Serum Insulin ↑ HOMA-IR
[53]	Not reported	46% fat 20.3% protein 24% carbohydrate	12 weeks	Sprague-Dawley rats; Male	↑ Mast cell accumulation ↑ Islet area and proliferation ↑ β and α cell area	↑ Plasma insulin ↓ Glucose tolerance
[56]	Not reported	60% fat 18% protein 22% carbohydrate	8 weeks	Sprague-Dawley rats; Male	Glucose-stimulated islet insulin secretion	Glucose tolerance
[51]	Not reported	66.43% fat 18.08% protein 15.48% carbohydrate	8 and 16 weeks	Sprague-Dawley rats; Male	↑ Islet cell insulin at 8 and 16 weeks ↑ Glucagon at 16 weeks ↑ β and α cell area at 16 weeks ↑ β cell autophagy at 16 weeks	↑ Body weight at 16 weeks ↑ Plasma glucose at 16 weeks ↑ Serum insulin at 8 and 16 weeks ↑ HOMA-IR at 8 and 16 weeks

Studies cited in the table were limited to those that included macronutrient composition. The direction of arrows indicate change when compared to a standard diet control group within that study. Homeostatic model assessment of insulin resistance (HOMA-IR) and hemoglobin A1c (HbA1c).

2.4. Brain

Mice. Chronic consumption of a HFD significantly impairs cognitive function by altering neuronal activity in the hippocampus of humans and rodents [57–59]. Altered hippocampal function is likely a result of chronic inflammation associated with obesity, with more severe outcomes from saturated fatty acids [59–61]. Furthermore, peripheral insulin and glucose homeostasis is largely regulated by hypothalamic insulin responsiveness [62]. Therefore, HFD-induced neuroinflammation, mitochondrial dysfunction, cognitive impairment, and whole-body glucose and insulin resistance highlight the brain as a critical organ in the pathogenesis of the T2D phenotype.

Lard-based diets of 45% and 60% increased the microglial and astrocyte activity in the hypothalamus, the primary regulatory region of energy balance [63,64]. Furthermore, both fat concentrations caused hyperinsulinemia, hyperglycemia, and reduced glucose tolerance, though this was more severe in response to 60% fat [63] (Table 4). Only the 60% HFD altered the hypothalamic, hippocampal, and cortex metabolite profile, showing a shift in cellular energy and metabolism. Similar metabolic dysfunction was reported following 4 weeks of HFD, accompanied by reduced insulin signaling in hypothalamic and hippocampal neurons [65] (Table 4). HFD also induces changes in the neuropeptide milieu to account for high nutrient density. In response to 60% HFD, the population of anorexigenic proopiomelanocortin (POMC) increased [64], and the expression of orexigenic neuropeptide-Y (NPY) decreased [66] (Table 4).

Table 4. Brain.

Source	Fat Source	Macronutrients (% kcal)	Duration	Strain; Sex	Findings	T2D Status
[63]	Lard and soybean oil	10, 45, or 60% fat 20% protein 70, 35, or 20 % carbohydrates	24 weeks	C57BL/6; Male	45% and 60% fat ↓ Spontaneous activity ↓ Locomotion ↑ Neuroinflammation 60% fatAltered metabolite profile	45% and 60% fat ↑ Body weight: 60% > 45% ↑ Plasma glucose: 60% > 45% ↑ Plasma insulin ↑ Plasma Leptin ↓ Glucose tolerance: 60% > 45% at 2 h
[65]	Lard and soybean oil	60% fat 20% protein 20% carbohydrates	4 weeks	C57BL/6; Male	↓ Insulin signaling in isolated hypothalamic and hippocampal neurons ↓ Mitochondrial function ↑ Oxidative stress	↑ Body weight ↑ Fat mass ↑ Plasma glucose ↑ Plasma insulin ↑ HOMA-IR
[66]	Palm oil	60% fat 16% protein 24% carbohydrates	8 weeks	C57BL/6; Male	↓ Socialization behavior ↑ Disruption of normal circadian feeding Hypothalamic NPY expression	↑ Body weight
[64]	Lard and soybean oil	60% fat 20% protein 20% carbohydrates	12 weeks	C57BL/6; Female	↑ Microglia in hypothalamic arcuate nucleus ↑ Trend in neurogenesis of POMC neurons	↑ Body weight ↑ Fat mass
[67]	Lard	10 % added to standard diet	3 days	Sprague-Dawley Rats; Male	↓ Hypothalamic insulin sensitivity ↓ Hypothalamic insulin-stimulated adipose lipolysis ↓ Hypothalamic insulin-stimulated hepatic glucose production	←→ Body weight ←→ Plasma glucose ←→ Plasma insulin
[68]	Not reported	45% fat 20% protein 35% carbohydrates	20 weeks	Wistar-Han Rats; Male	←→ CSF glucose ↓ CSF glucose tolerance	↑ Body weight Plasma glucose ↓ Glucose tolerance
[69]	Lard and soybean oil	60% fat 20% protein 20% carbohydrates	24 weeks	Sprague-Dawley Rats; Male	↓ Cognitive function ↓ Insulin-stimulated hippocampal perfusion ↓ Hippocampal insulin signaling ↓ Hippocampal eNOS	↓ Whole body glucose disposal ↑ Plasma insulin

Studies cited in the table were limited to those that included macronutrient composition. The direction of arrows indicate change when compared to a standard diet control group within that study. Cerebrospinal fluid (CSF), proopiomelanocortin (POMC), endothelial nitric oxide synthase (eNOS), and homeostatic model assessment of insulin resistance (HOMA-IR).

Rats. Impaired hypothalamic insulin signaling occurred following just three days of a low saturated fat diet (10% lard) in male Sprague–Dawley rats [67] (Table 4). The ability for hypothalamic insulin signaling to suppress white adipose lipolysis and hepatic glucose production was significantly impaired. Such hypothalamic insulin resistance was likely the cause of acute increases in plasma free fatty acids [67]. Diets slightly higher in saturated fats (20%) impaired learning and memory function when compared to standard diet (~4.5% fat) and diets higher in polyunsaturated fat (soybean oil) [70]. Following 18 weeks of a 39% HFD, Wistar rats developed glucose intolerance and increased body weight without hyperglycemia, hyperinsulinemia, or insulin resistance [71]. These rats displayed distinct neurometabolic alterations in the hippocampus and caudate-putamen, including glutamine and N-acetylaspartate (NAA), two prominent amino acids in the brain that play a role in energy metabolism via lipid turnover and the citric acid cycle [52,71,72]. These data do contradict previous studies that showed no alterations in hippocampus metabolic profiles, particularly in genetically modified obese rats [73]. Male Wistar–Han rats fed a 40% HFD for 20 weeks demonstrated reductions in glucose tolerance in both plasma and cerebrospinal fluid following glucose challenge, suggesting that HFD induced changes in both central and peripheral glucose tolerance [68] (Table 4).

Six months of a 60% lard and soybean oil-based HFD impaired insulin-mediated microvascular perfusion and hippocampal cognitive function in Sprague–Dawley rats [74]. A similar response was reported in C57BL/6J mice [63,66,75].

Collectively, the literature supports moderate (45%) and high (60%) saturated fat concentrations as perturbing central and peripheral glucose and insulin sensitivity. While a 60% diet produces a more severe phenotype [63], we must consider whether the increased severity in a rodent model recapitulates the pathogenesis of T2D in humans. A 45% HFD, more in line with a Western-based diet, produces similar central and peripheral metabolic dysfunction, and may align more with the progressive development of human T2D.

2.5. Skeletal Muscle

Mice. Chronic HFD consumption results in intramyocellular lipid storage in skeletal muscle, one of the largest contributors to glucose disposal in the body [24,74,76]. Excess intramyocellular lipid storage, particularly in sedentary populations promotes DAG accretion, protein kinase C activity, AMP-activated protein kinase (AMPK) inhibition, and attenuated glucose uptake [77,78]. The amount of saturated fatty acid in HFD differentially effects lipid deposition within skeletal muscle, potentially promoting differences in metabolism and oxidative capacity.

When consumed for 8 weeks, a 45% cocoa butter (saturated fat), olive oil (monounsaturated fat), or palm oil (a combination of fats), but not safflower oil (polyunsaturated fat)-based HFD, increased TAG and DAG content in skeletal muscle of C57BL/6J mice [19] (Table 5). All cohorts, except the 45% olive oil, demonstrated similar reductions in systemic glucose clearance, despite no changes in insulin-glucose transporter type 4 (GLUT4) expression [19]. β-oxidative remained unchanged, suggesting lipid accumulation occurred without a compensatory increase in oxidation [19].

One week of a 60% lard-based HFD reduced carbohydrate metabolism within skeletal muscle without insulin resistance [49]. When consumed for 15 to 20 weeks, a 60% lard-based diet causes significant dysfunction within skeletal muscle [6,14,30]. Such a diet caused skeletal muscle lipid accumulation, increased fasting glucose levels, and increased peroxisome proliferator-activated receptor gramma coactivator 1alpha (PGC-1α) protein expression [24]. Elevated PGC-1α expression is a characteristic of lipid accumulation in human muscle cells [79]. Furthermore, 191 skeletal muscle genes were altered following 20 weeks of the 60% lard-based HFD, favoring adipogenesis [6]. In agreement, 8 weeks of a similar diet reduced fatty acid oxidation and mitochondrial function [80] (Table 5). In human skeletal muscle, ectopic lipid accumulation, led to insulin resistance [81,82], similarly to that observed in rodent studies [19,24,83]. Subcellular localization of DAG in human skeletal muscle suggests that mitochondrial DAG is elevated in individuals with low insulin sensitivity and may be contributing to alterations in mitochondrial function [84].

Female mice are seldom studied in metabolic research; however, it is naive to assume that male and female rodents respond similarly to HFD models. A 58% coconut oil-based diet caused obesity only in male mice [85]. While muscle insulin sensitivity was reduced in both sexes, only males showed reduced whole-body glucose and insulin tolerance [85] (Table 5).

Table 5. Skeletal Muscle.

Source	Fat Source	Macronutrients (%kcal)	Duration	Strain; Sex	Findings	T2D Status
[19]	(a) Cocoa butter (b) Palm oil (c) Olive oil (d) Safflower oil	45% fat 20% protein 35% carbohydrateAll diet formulations maintained same ratio	8 weeks	C57BL/6; Male	↑ Gastrocnemius TAG and DAG: cocoa butter, palm oil, and olive oil	↑ Body weight in palm oil compared to cocoa butter. ↑ Glucose tolerance: cocoa, palm and safflower oils
[85]	Coconut oil and soybean oil	58% fat 17% protein 25% carbohydrate	16 weeks	FVB; B6;Male and Female	↓ Muscle insulin sensitivity: Males and Females	↑ Body weight: Males only ↑ Plasma glucose: Males only ↓ Glucose and insulin tolerance: Males only
[6,80]	Hydrogenated coconut oil	59% fat 15% protein 26% carbohydrate	8 weeks [83] 20 weeks [6]	C57BL/6; Male	↑ Fatty acid transport ↑ Lipogenesis ↑ Muscle Adipocyte differentiation ↓ Fatty acid oxidation ↓ Mitochondrial function	↑ Body weight ↑ Blood glucose ↑ Plasma insulin ↓ Insulin sensitivity
[86]	Lard and soybean oil	60% fat 20% protein 20% carbohydrate	15 weeks	C57BL/6; Male	↓ Insulin sensitivity ↑ Muscle weight ↑ Inflammatory mRNA profile	↑ Body weight ↑ Serum insulin ↕ Glucose tolerance
[87]	Lard	45% fat 20% protein 35% carbohydrate	15 weeks	Sprague-Dawley rats; Male	↑ Soleus lipid accumulation ↑ Protein and mRNA supporting fatty acid transport and lipogenesis	↑ Body weight ↑ Plasma glucose ↑ Serum insulin ↑ HOMA-IR ↓ Insulin sensitivity
[88,89]	Lard and soybean oil	60% fat 20% protein 20% carbohydrate	2 weeks	Wister rats; Male	←→ Soleus and extensor digitorum longus weight ←→ Soleus and extensor digitorum longus insulin signaling ↓ Soleus force production ↓ Soleus glutathione ↑ Soleus IL-6 mRNA ↑ Lipid droplet size in soleus ↑ Percentage of large lipid droplets in soleus ↑ Lipogenic mRNA in soleus	←→ Body weight
[90,91]	Lard and soybean oil	60% fat 20% protein 20% carbohydrate	2 weeks	Wister rats; Male	↓ Glucose uptake by isolated type IIAX, IIX, IIBX, and IIB fibers ↑ Lipid droplet density in type I, IIA, and IIAX fibers ↑ Lipid droplet size in type I and IIA fibers ↓ Insulin-stimulated glucose uptake in whole muscle ↓ Insulin-stimulated glucose uptake in isolated type IIA, IIAX, and IIB fibers	←→ Body weight

Studies cited in the table were limited to those that included macronutrient composition. The direction of arrows indicate change when compared to a standard diet control group within that study. Diacylglycerol (DAG), triacylglycerol (TAG), interleukin 6 (IL-6), and homeostatic model assessment of insulin resistance (HOMA-IR).

Rats. Within a short exposure to 60% HFD, skeletal muscle metabolism and function are altered. These effects are fiber-type specific with increased lipid accumulation in type I and II intermediate fibers and reduced insulin-stimulated glucose uptake in a spectrum of type II fibers [88–91] (Table 5). Increased lipid accumulation in the soleus is associated with increase inflammatory signaling, evidenced by changes in IL-6 mRNA, and decreased control of oxidative stress [88].

A moderate 45% HFD also increased soleus lipid accumulation, as determined after 15 weeks [87]. Lipid accumulation was supported by increases in plasma membrane fatty acid binding protein (FABPpm), fatty acid transporter protein 1 (FATP1), fatty acid transporter protein 4 (FATP4), and CD36 [87] (Table 5). This diet was also associated with significant changes in whole-body insulin and glucose homeostasis. Hyperglycemia, hyperinsulinemia, and increased HOMA-IR were evident by 8 weeks of dietary consumption and persisted for 15 weeks [87]. Therefore, these data support the suitability of a macronutrient composition more closely aligned to a Western-based diet for studying the effects of HFD on skeletal muscle metabolism.

3. Choosing the Most Appropriate Model

As the percentage of fat in a diet increases, the metabolic changes become more significant, demonstrated by a 60% HFD animal model decreasing glucose sensitivity more rapidly (within one week) than a 45% HFD [92]. Furthermore, using a fat percentage that is 1.7-fold greater than a typical Western diet (~35% HFD) may induce pathology that is not characteristic of the T2D-like phenotype found in humans. Challenges with data interpretation and translatability to human studies include animal strain-specific responses, dietary variation, and the metabolic differences between humans and murine models [93]. A rodent's heart rate ranges from 350–550 beats·min^{-1}, but a human's resting heart is approximately 70 beats·min^{-1} [93]. A mouse's basal metabolic rate is ~7.5-fold greater than a human's, suggesting the metabolic demand on a mouse is significantly greater [94]. Hepatic glycogen storage in a mouse is depleted every 16–24 h, and gluconeogenesis provides the majority of endogenous glucose, demonstrated by over 80% of glucose supplied via gluconeogenesis following a 4-h fasting period [94,95]. In contrast, humans utilize hepatic glycogen at approximately half that rate, even after an overnight (~12 h) fasting period [94]. Due to the faster depletion of glycogen stores and increased metabolic rate, mice consumed food and water more frequently throughout a 24-h period than humans. On average, mice consumed ~4.5 g food across 36 feedings and ~5.8 mL of water across 32 drinking times per day [96]. Feeding habit variability between rodents and humans may also contribute to dissimilarities in metabolism. As nocturnal animals, rodents consume the majority of their food in the evenings, but humans primarily eat during the day [97]. Further complicating this comparison is the treatment of rodents as diurnal rather than using a reverse light cycle to create a more natural rodent living environment. Circadian clocks are involved in many biological processes, including glucose metabolism and insulin secretion, particularly within pancreatic β-cells [98–100]. Disruptions in circadian rhythms could alter disease pathology or data interpretation, making translatability further challenging. Obesity and insulin resistance induced by a 60% high-fat diet caused alterations in circadian rhythm patterns in the hypothalamus [101]. Exogenous dopamine administration during appropriate peaks of circadian rhythm stimulated a physiological response mirroring a non-obese and an insulin sensitive rodent [101].

The full etiology of T2D cannot be accurately assessed and entirely translated to clinical practice because rodents experience β-cell proliferation or increased β-cell mass, rather than the loss of β-cell mass or β-cell failure [54]. To most effectively translate findings to the human population, an optimal animal model or a combination of a few select models may be most appropriate. Although the Western diet is known for excess fats, carbohydrates, and sugars, a longitudinal study over 17 years concluded that less than 35% of the average adult's diet actually comes from fats [102]. According to the National Health and Nutrition Examination Survey, the mean dietary intake for adults (≥20 years) is composed of ~16% protein, ~47% carbohydrates, and ~35% fat. Nearly one-third of the total fat intake is saturated fat, demonstrating that there is a combination of fat sources in the typical Western diet. This data suggests that including a variety of fat sources (saturated, monounsaturated and polyunsaturated fats) would more accurately mimic the diet macronutrient composition seen in the average population. Based on this literature review, a 45% HFD with a combination of fat sources (monounsaturated, polyunsaturated, and saturated fats) induces pathological changes in rodents that closely resembles the T2D-like phenotype etiology in human populations. For example, adipose tissue becomes inflamed with a 45% high-fat model, but adipose tissue undergoes severe inflammation, remodulation, and adipocytosis following a 60% high-fat diet [35,103]. Commonly used 60% HFDs also contain more than nine times the amount of saturated fat (lard) when compared to unsaturated fat (soybean oil), suggesting that there are fat composition variables that need continued refinement to improve mirroring the human diet composition and translatability to target populations. Based on the literature reviewed here, we propose a 45% HFD composed of one-third saturated fats and two-thirds unsaturated fat closely aligns with the typical human Western diet and disease progression (Figure 1). Utilizing such a composition may provide better alignment between rodent and human T2D phenotypes and more inter-study agreement.

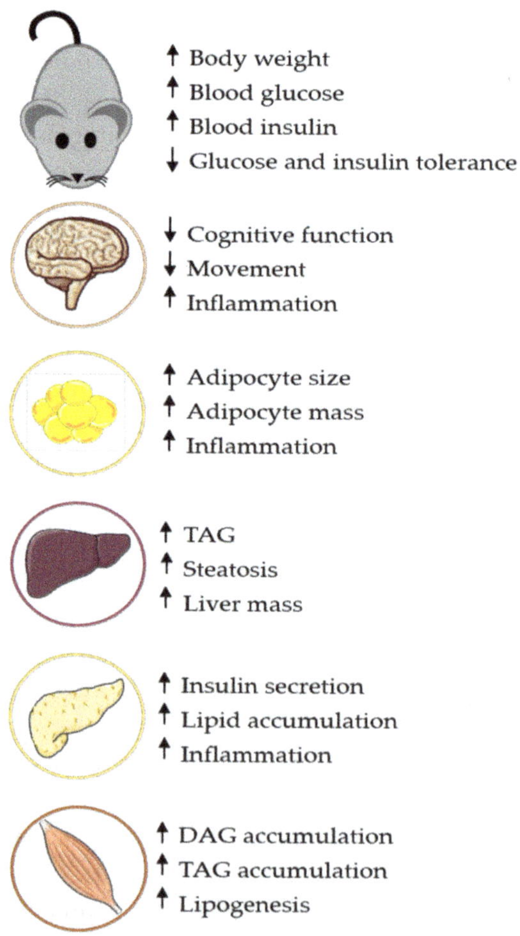

Figure 1. Rodent tissue responses to Western-like diet. A 45% HFD provides a progressive development of tissue and whole-body changes consistent with the T2D-like phenotype. Using higher fat percentages may create a greater magnitude of tissue dysfunction or accelerate the process, resulting in missed opportunity to study key aspects of disease progression. Detailed tissue responses could be found in Table 1 through Table 5. High-fat diet (HFD), Type 2 Diabetes (T2D), Triacylglycerol (TAG) and Diacylglycerol (DAG).

It is important to acknowledge limitations to this review. While we attempted to use an un-biased review of the literature that used non-genetically altered rodents, we were not able to include all relevant publications. Those chosen provided sufficient methodological detail regarding dietary composition, intervention duration, and comprehensive sets of data. Moreover, only studies that compared HFD to a standard diet groups were included. Those in which the HFD served as the control against a pharmacological treatment were excluded. Mouse studies were focused on the C57BL/6 background because it is the most common. However, because the inclusion for female mice was rare, we included studies that investigated sexual dimorphism using other strains. Sprague–Dawley and Wister strains were targeted for rat studies because of their predominance in the literature. We attempted to narrow our literature to the last 5 years, particularly for studies included in the tables; however, in some cases we had to expand our search to accommodate for our inclusion criteria. Furthermore, this review focuses exclusively on HFD composition and concentration. Other dietary concerns, such as sugar, cholesterol, fiber, vitamin, and mineral composition and their combination with pharmacological strategies should be considered but are beyond the scope of this review. Additionally, numerous transgenic models exist, such as Ob/Ob, db/db, and KKAy, which cause metabolic dysfunction. Likewise, genetic models alone and in combination with dietary and pharmacological intervention are commonly used, particularly in the study of central insulin and glucose homeostasis. Lastly, animal models often include one gender, typically males, to avoid complications with the estrous cycle in female rodents, but diet-induced animal models can exhibit sexual dimorphisms [104]. Future studies should make every effort to include male and female rodents to comprehensively enhance our understanding of HFD models of T2D and associated phenotypes.

Author Contributions: Conceptualization, N.L.S. and J.S.M.; writing—original draft preparation, N.L.S. and J.S.M.; writing—review and editing, J.S.M. All authors have read and agreed to the published version of the manuscript.

Acknowledgments: The authors would like to thank the Laboratory of Systems Physiology group for their support and feedback during the writing of this manuscript.

References

1. Agriculture, USA. *2015–2020 Dietary Guidelines for Americans*; U.S. Department of Health and Human Services and U.S. Department of Agriculture: Washington, DC, USA, 2015; pp. 1–144.
2. Mazidi, M.; Kengne, A.-P.; Mikhailidis, D.P.; Toth, P.P.; Ray, K.K.; Banach, M. Dietary food patterns and glucose/insulin homeostasis: A cross-sectional study involving 24,182 adult Americans. *Lipids Health Dis.* **2017**, *16*, 192. [CrossRef]
3. Hariri, N.; Gougeon, R.; Thibault, L. A highly saturated fat-rich diet is more obesogenic than diets with lower saturated fat content. *Nutr. Res.* **2010**, *30*, 632–643. [CrossRef]
4. Licholai, J.A.; Nguyen, K.P.; Fobbs, W.C.; Schuster, C.J.; Ali, M.A.; Kravitz, A.V. Why Do Mice Overeat High-Fat Diets? How High-Fat Diet Alters the Regulation of Daily Caloric Intake in Mice. *Obesity (Silver Spring)* **2018**, *26*, 1026–1033. [CrossRef]
5. Kubant, R.; Poon, A.N.; Sanchezhernandez, D.; Domenichiello, A.F.; Huot, P.S.P.; Pannia, E.; Cho, C.E.; Hunschede, S.; Bazinet, R.P.; Anderson, G.H. A comparison of effects of lard and hydrogenated vegetable shortening on the development of high-fat diet-induced obesity in rats. *Nutr. Diabetes* **2015**, *5*, e188. [CrossRef]
6. Lee, R.K.; Hittel, D.S.; Nyamandi, V.Z.; Kang, L.; Soh, J.; Sensen, C.W.; Shearer, J. Unconventional microarray design reveals the response to obesity is largely tissue specific: Analysis of common and divergent responses to diet-induced obesity in insulin-sensitive tissues. *Appl. Physiol. Nutr. Metab.* **2012**, *37*, 257–268. [CrossRef]
7. De Fourmestraux, V.; Neubauer, H.; Poussin, C.; Farmer, P.; Falquet, L.; Burcelin, R.; Delorenzi, M.; Thorens, B. Transcript Profiling Suggests That Differential Metabolic Adaptation of Mice to a High Fat Diet Is Associated with Changes in Liver to Muscle Lipid Fluxes. *J. Biol. Chem.* **2004**, *279*, 50743–50753. [CrossRef]
8. Tajima, K.; Shirakawa, J.; Okuyama, T.; Kyohara, M.; Yamazaki, S.; Togashi, Y.; Terauchi, Y. Effects of metformin on compensatory pancreatic β-cell hyperplasia in mice fed a high-fat diet. *Am. J. Physiol. Endocrinol. Metab.* **2017**, *313*, E367–E380. [CrossRef]
9. Moretto, T.L.; Benfato, I.D.; De Carvalho, F.P.; Barthichoto, M.; Le Sueur-Maluf, L.; De Oliveira, C.A.M. The effects of calorie-matched high-fat diet consumption on spontaneous physical activity and development of obesity. *Life Sci.* **2017**, *179*, 30–36. [CrossRef]

10. Kleinert, M.; Clemmensen, C.; Hofmann, S.M.; Moore, M.C.; Renner, S.; Woods, S.C.; Huypens, P.; Beckers, J.; De Angelis, M.H.; Schürmann, A.; et al. Animal models of obesity and diabetes mellitus. *Nat. Rev. Endocrinol.* **2018**, *14*, 140–162. [CrossRef]
11. Islam, S.; Wilson, R.D. Experimentally Induced Rodent Models of Type 2 Diabetes. *Animal Models Diabetes Res.* **2012**, *933*, 161–174. [CrossRef]
12. Kanuri, G.; Bergheim, I. In Vitro and in Vivo Models of Non-Alcoholic Fatty Liver Disease (NAFLD). *Int. J. Mol. Sci.* **2013**, *14*, 11963–11980. [CrossRef]
13. Warden, C.H.; Fisler, J.S. Comparisons of Diets Used in Animal Models of High-Fat Feeding. *Cell Metab.* **2008**, *7*, 277. [CrossRef]
14. Bullen, J.W.; Bluher, S.; Kelesidis, T.; Mantzoros, C.S. Regulation of adiponectin and its receptors in response to development of diet-induced obesity in mice. *Am. J. Physiol. Endocrinol. Metab.* **2007**, *292*, E1079–E1086. [CrossRef]
15. Kim, S.; Sohn, I.; Ahn, J.-I.; Lee, K.-H.; Lee, Y.S.; Lee, Y.S. Hepatic gene expression profiles in a long-term high-fat diet-induced obesity mouse model. *Gene* **2004**, *340*, 99–109. [CrossRef]
16. Flanagan, A.M.; Brown, J.L.; Santiago, C.A.; Aad, P.Y.; Spicer, L.J.; Spicer, M.T. High-fat diets promote insulin resistance through cytokine gene expression in growing female rats. *J. Nutr. Biochem.* **2008**, *19*, 505–513. [CrossRef]
17. Xavier, G.D.S.; Hodson, D.J. Mouse models of peripheral metabolic disease. *Best Pr. Res. Clin. Endocrinol. Metab.* **2018**, *32*, 299–315. [CrossRef]
18. Hintze, K.J.; Benninghoff, A.D.; Cho, C.E.; Ward, R.E. Modeling the Western Diet for Preclinical Investigations. *Adv. Nutr.* **2018**, *9*, 263–271. [CrossRef]
19. Timmers, S.; Bosch, J.D.V.-V.D.; De Wit, N.; Schaart, G.; Van Beurden, D.; Hesselink, M.K.C.; Van Der Meer, R.; Schrauwen, P. Differential effects of saturated versus unsaturated dietary fatty acids on weight gain and myocellular lipid profiles in mice. *Nutr. Diabetes* **2011**, *1*, e11. [CrossRef]
20. An, X.; Liu, J.; Li, Y.; Dou, Z.; Li, N.; Suo, Y.; Ma, Y.; Sun, M.; Tian, Z.; Xu, L. Chemerin/CMKLR1 ameliorates nonalcoholic steatohepatitis by promoting autophagy and alleviating oxidative stress through the JAK2-STAT3 pathway. *Peptides* **2020**, *135*, 170422. [CrossRef]
21. Lu, Z.; Li, Y.; Syn, W.-K.; Li, A.-J.; Ritter, S.; Wank, S.A.; Lopes-Virella, M.F.; Huang, Y. GPR40-Deficiency Is Associated with Hepatic FAT/CD36 Upregulation, Steatosis, Inflammation and Cell Injury in C57BL/6 Mice. *Am. J. Physiol. Endocrinol. Metab.* **2020**. [CrossRef]
22. Sardi, C.; Martini, E.; Mello, T.; Camelliti, S.; Sfondrini, L.; Marcucci, F.; Kallikourdis, M.; Sommariva, M.; Rumio, C. Effect of acetylsalicylic acid on inflamed adipose tissue. Insulin resistance and hepatic steatosis in a mouse model of diet-induced obesity. *Life Sci.* **2020**, 118618. [CrossRef]
23. Shen, H.H.; Alex, R.; Bellner, L.; Raffaele, M.; Licari, M.; Vanella, L.; Stec, D.E.; Abraham, N.G. Milk thistle seed cold press oil attenuates markers of the metabolic syndrome in a mouse model of dietary-induced obesity. *J. Food Biochem.* **2020**, e13522. [CrossRef] [PubMed]
24. Peck, B.; Huot, J.; Renzi, T.; Arthur, S.; Turner, M.J.; Marino, J.S. Mice Lacking PKCtheta in Skeletal Muscle Have Reduced Intramyocellular Lipid Accumulation and Increased Insulin Responsiveness in Skeletal Muscle. *Am. J. Physiol. Regul. Integr. Comp. Physiol.* **2017**, *314*, 468–477. [CrossRef]
25. Bezan, P.; Holland, H.; De Castro, G.S.; Cardoso, J.; Ovidio, P.; Calder, P.C.; Jordão, A. High Dose of A Conjugated Linoleic Acid Mixture Increases Insulin Resistance in Rats Fed Either A Low Fat or A High Fat Diet. *Exp. Clin. Endocrinol. Diabetes* **2018**, *126*, 379–386. [CrossRef]
26. Baek, K.-W.; Gim, J.-A.; Park, J.-J. Regular moderate aerobic exercise improves high-fat diet-induced nonalcoholic fatty liver disease via monoacylglycerol O-acyltransferase 1 pathway suppression. *J. Sport Health Sci.* **2020**, *9*, 472–478. [CrossRef]
27. Abdulmalek, S.A.; Fessal, M.; El-Sayed, M. Effective amelioration of hepatic inflammation and insulin response in high fat diet-fed rats via regulating AKT/mTOR signaling: Role of Lepidium sativum seed extracts. *J. Ethnopharmacol.* **2021**, *266*, 113439. [CrossRef] [PubMed]
28. Saltiel, A.R.; Olefsky, J.M. Inflammatory mechanisms linking obesity and metabolic disease. *J. Clin. Investig.* **2017**, *127*, 1–4. [CrossRef]

29. Inoue, M.; Ohtake, T.; Motomura, W.; Takahashi, N.; Hosoki, Y.; Miyoshi, S.; Suzuki, Y.; Saito, H.; Kohgo, Y.; Okumura, T. Increased expression of PPARgamma in high fat diet-induced liver steatosis in mice. *Biochem. Biophys. Res. Commun.* **2005**, *336*, 215–222. [CrossRef]
30. Wikan, N.; Tocharus, J.; Sivasinprasasn, S.; Kongkaew, A.; Chaichompoo, W.; Suksamrarn, A.; Tocharus, C. Capsaicinoid nonivamide improves nonalcoholic fatty liver disease in rats fed a high-fat diet. *J. Pharmacol. Sci.* **2020**, *143*, 188–198. [CrossRef]
31. Ramalho, L.; Da Jornada, M.N.; Antunes, L.D.C.; Hidalgo, M.P.L. Metabolic disturbances due to a high-fat diet in a non-insulin-resistant animal model. *Nutr. Diabetes* **2017**, *7*, e245. [CrossRef]
32. Erion, D.M.; Park, H.-J.; Lee, H.-Y. The role of lipids in the pathogenesis and treatment of type 2 diabetes and associated co-morbidities. *BMB Rep.* **2016**, *49*, 139–148. [CrossRef] [PubMed]
33. Finucane, O.M.; Lyons, C.L.; Murphy, A.M.; Reynolds, C.M.; Klinger, R.; Healy, N.P.; Cooke, A.A.; Coll, R.C.; McAllan, L.; Nilaweera, K.N.; et al. Monounsaturated Fatty Acid–Enriched High-Fat Diets Impede Adipose NLRP3 Inflammasome–Mediated IL-1β Secretion and Insulin Resistance Despite Obesity. *Diabetes* **2015**, *64*, 2116–2128. [CrossRef] [PubMed]
34. Shen, H.H.; Peterson, S.J.; Bellner, L.; Choudhary, A.; Levy, L.; Gancz, L.; Sasson, A.; Trainer, J.; Rezzani, R.; Resnick, A.; et al. Cold-Pressed Nigella Sativa Oil Standardized to 3% Thymoquinone Potentiates Omega-3 Protection against Obesity-Induced Oxidative Stress, Inflammation, and Markers of Insulin Resistance Accompanied with Conversion of White to Beige Fat in Mice. *Antioxidants* **2020**, *9*, 489. [CrossRef]
35. Strissel, K.J.; Stancheva, Z.; Miyoshi, H.; Perfield, J.W.; DeFuria, J.; Jick, Z.; Greenberg, A.S.; Obin, M.S. Adipocyte death, adipose tissue remodeling, and obesity complications. *Diabetes* **2007**, *56*, 2910–2918. [CrossRef] [PubMed]
36. Lyons, C.L.; Kennedy, E.B.; Roche, H.M. Metabolic Inflammation-Differential Modulation by Dietary Constituents. *Nutrition* **2016**, *8*, 247. [CrossRef] [PubMed]
37. Liu, Y.; Lu, X.; Li, X.; Du, P.; Qin, G. High-fat diet triggers obesity-related early infiltration of macrophages into adipose tissue and transient reduction of blood monocyte count. *Mol. Immunol.* **2020**, *117*, 139–146. [CrossRef] [PubMed]
38. Hu, Q.; Lu, Y.; Hu, F.; He, S.; Xu, X.; Niu, Y.; Zhang, H.; Li, X.; Su, Q. Resistant dextrin reduces obesity and attenuates adipose tissue inflammation in high-fat diet-fed mice. *Int. J. Med Sci.* **2020**, *17*, 2611–2621. [CrossRef]
39. Eom, J.; Thomas, S.S.; Sung, N.-Y.; Kim, D.-S.; Cha, Y.-S.; Kim, K.-A. *Abeliophyllum distichum* Ameliorates High-Fat Diet-Induced Obesity in C57BL/6J Mice by Upregulating the AMPK Pathway. *Nutrients* **2020**, *12*, 3320. [CrossRef]
40. Liang, H.; Jiang, F.; Cheng, R.; Luo, Y.; Wang, J.; Luo, Z.; Li, M.; Shen, X.; He, F. A high-fat diet and high-fat and high-cholesterol diet may affect glucose and lipid metabolism differentially through gut microbiota in mice. *Exp. Anim.* **2020**, 20. [CrossRef]
41. Kim, S.-Y.; Lee, M.-S.; Chang, E.; Jung, S.; Ko, H.; Lee, E.; Lee, S.; Kim, C.-T.; Kim, I.-H.; Kim, Y. Tartary Buckwheat Extract Attenuated the Obesity-Induced Inflammation and Increased Muscle PGC-1a/SIRT1 Expression in High Fat Diet-Induced Obese Rats. *Nutrition* **2019**, *11*, 654. [CrossRef]
42. Vasconcelos, R.P.; Peixoto, M.S.; De Oliveira, K.A.; Ferreira, A.C.F.; Coelho-De-Souza, A.N.; Carvalho, D.P.; De Oliveira, A.C.; Fortunato, R.S. Sex differences in subcutaneous adipose tissue redox homeostasis and inflammation markers in control and high-fat diet fed rats. *Appl. Physiol. Nutr. Metab.* **2019**, *44*, 720–726. [CrossRef] [PubMed]
43. Grycel, S.; Markowski, A.R.; Hady, H.R.; Zabielski, P.; Kojta, I.; Imierska, M.; Górski, J.; Błachnio-Zabielska, A. Metformin treatment affects adipocytokine secretion and lipid composition in adipose tissues of diet-induced insulin-resistant rats. *Nutrition* **2019**, *63*, 126–133. [CrossRef] [PubMed]
44. Kolahdouzi, S.; Talebi-Garakani, E.; Hamidian, G.; Safarzade, A. Exercise training prevents high-fat diet-induced adipose tissue remodeling by promoting capillary density and macrophage polarization. *Life Sci.* **2019**, *220*, 32–43. [CrossRef]
45. Ellenbroek, J.H.; Töns, H.A.; De Graaf, N.; Loomans, C.J.; Engelse, M.A.; Vrolijk, H.; Voshol, P.J.; Rabelink, T.J.; Carlotti, F.; De Koning, E.J.P. Topologically Heterogeneous Beta Cell Adaptation in Response to High-Fat Diet in Mice. *PLoS ONE* **2013**, *8*, e56922. [CrossRef]

46. Faleck, D.M.; Ali, K.; Roat, R.; Graham, M.J.; Crooke, R.M.; Battisti, R.; Garcia, E.; Ahima, R.S.; Imai, Y. Adipose differentiation-related protein regulates lipids and insulin in pancreatic islets. *Am. J. Physiol. Endocrinol. Metab.* **2010**, *299*, E249–E257. [CrossRef] [PubMed]
47. Gupta, D.; Jetton, T.L.; LaRock, K.; Monga, N.; Satish, B.; Lausier, J.; Peshavaria, M.; Leahy, J.L. Temporal characterization of beta cell-adaptive and -maladaptive mechanisms during chronic high-fat feeding in C57BL/6NTac mice. *J. Biol. Chem.* **2017**, *292*, 12449–12459. [CrossRef]
48. Li, H.; Park, H.-M.; Ji, H.-S.; Han, J.; Kim, S.K.; Park, H.-Y.; Jeong, T.-S. Phenolic-enriched blueberry-leaf extract attenuates glucose homeostasis, pancreatic β-cell function, and insulin sensitivity in high-fat diet–induced diabetic mice. *Nutr. Res.* **2020**, *73*, 83–96. [CrossRef]
49. Seferovic, M.D.; Beamish, C.A.; Mosser, R.E.; Townsend, S.; Pappan, K.; Poitout, V.; Aagaard, K.M.; Gannon, M.A. Increases in bioactive lipids accompany early metabolic changes associated with β-cell expansion in response to short-term high-fat diet. *Am. J. Physiol. Endocrinol. Metab.* **2018**, *315*, E1251–E1263. [CrossRef]
50. Ye, T.; Chen, Y.-H.; Gao, J.-H.; Wang, X.-X.; Qiang, O.; Tang, C.-W.; Liu, R. Effect of octreotide on pancreatic fibrosis in rats with high-fat diet-induced obesity. *Int. J. Clin. Exp. Pathol.* **2018**, *11*, 4784–4794. [CrossRef]
51. Sun, Q.; Nie, S.; Wang, L.; Yang, F.; Meng, Z.; Xiao, H.; Xiang, B.; Li, X.; Fu, X.; Wang, S. Factors that Affect Pancreatic Islet Cell Autophagy in Adult Rats: Evaluation of a Calorie-Restricted Diet and a High-Fat Diet. *PLoS ONE* **2016**, *11*, e0151104. [CrossRef]
52. Teleman, A. Faculty Opinions recommendation of Glutamine oxidation maintains the TCA cycle and cell survival during impaired mitochondrial pyruvate transport. *Fac. Opin.* **2015**, *56*, 414–424. [CrossRef]
53. Abdel-Hamid, A.A.M.; Firgany, A.E.-D.L. Correlation between pancreatic mast cells and the low grade inflammation in adipose tissue of experimental prediabetes. *Acta Histochem.* **2019**, *121*, 35–42. [CrossRef] [PubMed]
54. Butler, A.E.; Janson, J.; Bonner-Weir, S.; Ritzel, R.A.; Rizza, R.A.; Butler, P.C. Cell Deficit and Increased -Cell Apoptosis in Humans With Type 2 Diabetes. *Diabetes* **2003**, *52*, 102–110. [CrossRef] [PubMed]
55. Parilla, J.H.; Willard, J.R.; Barrow, B.M.; Zraika, S. A Mouse Model of Beta-Cell Dysfunction as Seen in Human Type 2 Diabetes. *J. Diabetes Res.* **2018**, *2018*, 6106051. [CrossRef]
56. Lu, B.; Wu, H.; Gu, P.; Du, H.; Shao, J.; Wang, J.; Zou, D. Improved glucose-stimulated insulin secretion by intra-islet inhibition of protein-tyrosine phosphatase 1B expression in rats fed a high-fat diet. *J. Endocrinol. Investig.* **2011**, *35*, 63–70.
57. Cordner, Z.A.; Tamashiro, K.L. Effects of high-fat diet exposure on learning & memory. *Physiol. Behav.* **2015**, *152 Pt B*, 363–371. [CrossRef]
58. Kanoski, S.E.; Davidson, T.L. Western diet consumption and cognitive impairment: Links to hippocampal dysfunction and obesity. *Physiol. Behav.* **2011**, *103*, 59–68. [CrossRef]
59. Beilharz, J.E.; Maniam, J.; Morris, M.J. Diet-Induced Cognitive Deficits: The Role of Fat and Sugar, Potential Mechanisms and Nutritional Interventions. *Nutrients* **2015**, *7*, 6719–6738. [CrossRef]
60. Chesnokova, V.; Pechnick, R.N.; Wawrowsky, K. Chronic peripheral inflammation, hippocampal neurogenesis, and behavior. *Brain Behav. Immun.* **2016**, *58*, 1–8. [CrossRef]
61. Kowiański, P.; Lietzau, G.; Czuba, E.; Waśkow, M.; Steliga, A.; Moryś, J. BDNF: A Key Factor with Multipotent Impact on Brain Signaling and Synaptic Plasticity. *Cell. Mol. Neurobiol.* **2018**, *38*, 579–593. [CrossRef]
62. Marino, J.S.; Xu, Y.; Hill, J.W. Central insulin and leptin-mediated autonomic control of glucose homeostasis. *Trends Endocrinol. Metab.* **2011**, *22*, 275–285. [CrossRef] [PubMed]
63. Lizarbe, B.; Soares, A.F.; Larsson, S.; Duarte, J.M.N.; Lizarbe, B.; Soares, A.F.; Larsson, S.; Duarte, J.M.N. Neurochemical Modifications in the Hippocampus, Cortex and Hypothalamus of Mice Exposed to Long-Term High-Fat Diet. *Front. Neurosci.* **2019**, *12*, 985. [CrossRef] [PubMed]
64. Klein, C.; Jonas, W.; Wiedmer, P.; Schreyer, S.; Akyüz, L.; Spranger, J.; Hellweg, R.; Steiner, B. High-fat Diet and Physical Exercise Differentially Modulate Adult Neurogenesis in the Mouse Hypothalamus. *Neuroscience* **2019**, *400*, 146–156. [CrossRef]
65. Ruegsegger, G.N.; Vanderboom, P.M.; Dasari, S.; Klaus, K.A.; Kabiraj, P.; McCarthy, C.B.; Lucchinetti, C.F.; Nair, K.S. Exercise and metformin counteract altered mitochondrial function in the insulin-resistant brain. *JCI Insight* **2019**, *4*. [CrossRef] [PubMed]

66. Hassan, A.M.; Mancano, G.; Kashofer, K.; Fröhlich, E.E.; Matak, A.; Mayerhofer, R.; Reichmann, F.; Olivares, M.; Neyrinck, A.M.; Delzenne, N.M.; et al. High-fat diet induces depression-like behaviour in mice associated with changes in microbiome, neuropeptide Y, and brain metabolome. *Nutr. Neurosci.* **2019**, *22*, 877–893. [CrossRef]
67. Scherer, T.; Lindtner, C.; Zielinski, E.; O'Hare, J.; Filatova, N.; Buettner, C. Short Term Voluntary Overfeeding Disrupts Brain Insulin Control of Adipose Tissue Lipolysis*. *J. Biol. Chem.* **2012**, *287*, 33061–33069. [CrossRef]
68. Top, M.V.D.; Zhao, F.-Y.; Viriyapong, R.; Michael, N.J.; Munder, A.C.; Pryor, J.T.; Renaud, L.P.; Spanswick, D. The impact of ageing, fasting and high-fat diet on central and peripheral glucose tolerance and glucose-sensing neural networks in the arcuate nucleus. *J. Neuroendocr.* **2017**, *29*, e12528. [CrossRef]
69. Fu, Z.; Wu, J.; Nesil, T.; Li, M.D.; Aylor, K.W.; Liu, Z. Long-term high-fat diet induces hippocampal microvascular insulin resistance and cognitive dysfunction. *Am. J. Physiol. Endocrinol. Metab.* **2017**, *312*, E89–E97. [CrossRef]
70. Greenwood, E.C.; Winocur, G. Cognitive impairment in rats fed high-fat diets: A specific effect of saturated fatty-acid intake. *Behav. Neurosci.* **1996**, *110*, 451–459. [CrossRef]
71. Ribeiro, M.; Castelhano, J.; Petrella, L.; Sereno, J.; Rodrigues, T.; Neves, C.; Letra, L.; Baptista, F.I.; Seiça, R.; Matafome, P.; et al. High-fat diet induces a neurometabolic state characterized by changes in glutamate and N-acetylaspartate pools associated with early glucose intolerance: An in vivo multimodal MRI study. *J. Magn. Reson. Imaging* **2018**, *48*, 757–766. [CrossRef]
72. Moffett, J.R.; Arun, P.; Ariyannur, P.S.; Namboodiri, A.M.A. N-Acetylaspartate reductions in brain injury: Impact on post-injury neuroenergetics, lipid synthesis, and protein acetylation. *Front. Neuroenerg.* **2013**, *5*, 11. [CrossRef] [PubMed]
73. van der Graaf, M.; Janssen, S.W.; van Asten, J.J.; Hermus, A.R.; Sweep, C.G.; Pikkemaat, J.A.; Martens, G.J.; Heerschap, A. Metabolic profile of the hippocampus of Zucker Diabetic Fatty rats assessed by in vivo 1H magnetic resonance spectroscopy. *NMR Biomed.* **2004**, *17*, 405–410. [CrossRef] [PubMed]
74. Bouchard-Mercier, A.; Rudkowska, I.; Lemieux, S.; Couture, P.; Vohl, M.-C. The metabolic signature associated with the Western dietary pattern: A cross-sectional study. *Nutr. J.* **2013**, *12*, 158. [CrossRef] [PubMed]
75. Tsai, S.-F.; Chen, Y.-W.; Kuo, Y.-M. High-fat diet reduces the hippocampal content level of lactate which is correlated with the expression of glial glutamate transporters. *Neurosci. Lett.* **2018**, *662*, 142–146. [CrossRef]
76. Krssak, M.; Petersen, K.F.; Dresner, A.; DiPietro, L.; Vogel, S.M.; Rothman, D.L.; Shulman, G.I.; Roden, M. Intramyocellular lipid concentrations are correlated with insulin sensitivity in humans: A 1 H NMR spectroscopy study. *Diabetology* **1999**, *42*, 113–116. [CrossRef]
77. Jiang, L.Q.; de Castro Barbosa, T.; Massart, J.; Deshmukh, A.S.; Löfgren, L.; Duque-Guimaraes, D.E.; Ozilgen, A.; Osler, M.E.; Chibalin, A.V.; Zierath, J.R. Diacylglycerol kinase-delta regulates AMPK signaling, lipid metabolism, and skeletal muscle energetics. *Am. J. Physiol. Endocrinol. Metab.* **2016**, *310*, E51–E60. [CrossRef]
78. Gao, Z.; Wang, Z.; Zhang, X.; Butler, A.A.; Zuberi, A.; Gawronska-Kozak, B.; Lefevre, M.; York, D.; Ravussin, E.; Berthoud, H.R.; et al. Inactivation of PKCtheta leads to increased susceptibility to obesity and dietary insulin resistance in mice. *Am. J. Physiol. Endocrinol. Metab.* **2007**, *292*, E84–E91. [CrossRef]
79. Mormeneo, E.; Jimenez-Mallebrera, C.; Palomer, X.; De Nigris, V.; Vázquez-Carrera, M.; Orozco, A.; Nascimento, A.; Colomer, J.; Lerin, C.; Gómez-Foix, A.M. PGC-1α Induces Mitochondrial and Myokine Transcriptional Programs and Lipid Droplet and Glycogen Accumulation in Cultured Human Skeletal Muscle Cells. *PLoS ONE* **2012**, *7*, e29985. [CrossRef]
80. De Mendonça, M.; De Sousa, É.; Da Paixão, A.O.; Dos Santos, B.A.; Spagnol, A.R.; Murata, G.M.; Araújo, H.N.; De Lima, T.I.; Guimarães, D.S.P.S.F.; Silveira, L.R.; et al. MicroRNA miR-222 mediates pioglitazone beneficial effects on skeletal muscle of diet-induced obese mice. *Mol. Cell. Endocrinol.* **2019**, *501*, 110661. [CrossRef]
81. Gao, Z.; Wang, Z.; Zhang, X.; Butler, A.A.; Zuberi, A.; Gawronska-Kozak, B.; Lefevre, M.; York, D.; Ravussin, E.; Berthoud, H.R.; et al. Role of diacylglycerol activation of PKCtheta in lipid-induced muscle insulin resistance in humans. *Proc. Natl. Acad. Sci. USA* **2014**, *111*, 9597–9602.
82. Bergman, B.C.; Hunerdosse, D.M.; Kerege, A.; Playdon, M.C.; Perreault, L. Localisation and composition of skeletal muscle diacylglycerol predicts insulin resistance in humans. *Diabetology* **2012**, *55*, 1140–1150. [CrossRef] [PubMed]

83. Kim, J.K.; Fillmore, J.J.; Sunshine, M.J.; Albrecht, B.; Higashimori, T.; Kim, D.-W.; Liu, Z.-X.; Soos, T.J.; Cline, G.W.; O'Brien, W.R.; et al. PKC knockout mice are protected from fat-induced insulin resistance. *J. Clin. Investig.* **2004**, *114*, 823–827. [CrossRef] [PubMed]
84. Perreault, L.; Newsom, S.A.; Strauss, A.; Kerege, A.; Kahn, D.E.; Harrison, K.A.; Snell-Bergeon, J.K.; Nemkov, T.; D'Alessandro, A.; Jackman, M.R.; et al. Intracellular localization of diacylglycerols and sphingolipids influences insulin sensitivity and mitochondrial function in human skeletal muscle. *JCI Insight* **2018**, *3*. [CrossRef] [PubMed]
85. Rudnicki, M.; Abdifarkosh, G.; Rezvan, O.; Nwadozi, E.; Roudier, E.; Haas, T.L. Female Mice Have Higher Angiogenesis in Perigonadal Adipose Tissue Than Males in Response to High-Fat Diet. *Front. Physiol.* **2018**, *9*, 1452. [CrossRef] [PubMed]
86. Kim, B.; Kwon, J.; Kim, M.-S.; Park, H.; Ji, Y.; Holzapfel, W.; Hyun, C.-K. Protective effects of Bacillus probiotics against high-fat diet-induced metabolic disorders in mice. *PLoS ONE* **2018**, *13*, e0210120. [CrossRef] [PubMed]
87. Cao, Y.; Chang, S.; Dong, J.; Zhu, S.; Zheng, X.; Li, J.; Long, R.; Zhou, Y.; Cui, J.; Zhang, Y. Emodin ameliorates high-fat-diet induced insulin resistance in rats by reducing lipid accumulation in skeletal muscle. *Eur. J. Pharmacol.* **2016**, *780*, 194–201. [CrossRef]
88. Andrich, D.E.; Melbouci, L.; Ou, Y.; Auclair, N.; Mercier, J.; Grenier, J.-C.; Lira, F.S.; Barreiro, L.B.; Danialou, G.; Comtois, A.-S.; et al. A Short-Term High-Fat Diet Alters Glutathione Levels and IL-6 Gene Expression in Oxidative Skeletal Muscles of Young Rats. *Front. Physiol.* **2019**, *10*, 372. [CrossRef]
89. Andrich, D.E.; Ou, Y.; Melbouci, L.; Leduc-Gaudet, J.-P.; Auclair, N.; Mercier, J.; Secco, B.; Tomaz, L.M.; Gouspillou, G.; Danialou, G.; et al. Altered Lipid Metabolism Impairs Skeletal Muscle Force in Young Rats Submitted to a Short-Term High-Fat Diet. *Front. Physiol.* **2018**, *9*. [CrossRef]
90. Pataky, M.W.; Wang, H.; Yu, C.S.; Arias, E.B.; Ploutz-Snyder, R.J.; Zheng, X.; Cartee, G.D. High-Fat Diet-Induced Insulin Resistance in Single Skeletal Muscle Fibers is Fiber Type Selective. *Sci. Rep.* **2017**, *7*, 13642. [CrossRef]
91. Pataky, M.W.; Yu, C.S.; Nie, Y.; Arias, E.B.; Singh, M.; Mendias, C.L.; Ploutz-Snyder, R.J.; Cartee, G.D. Skeletal muscle fiber type-selective effects of acute exercise on insulin-stimulated glucose uptake in insulin-resistant, high-fat-fed rats. *Am. J. Physiol. Endocrinol. Metab.* **2019**, *316*, E695–E706. [CrossRef]
92. Soares, A.F.; Duarte, J.M.N.; Gruetter, R. Increased hepatic fatty acid polyunsaturation precedes ectopic lipid deposition in the liver in adaptation to high-fat diets in mice. *MAGMA* **2017**, *31*, 341–354. [CrossRef]
93. Lai, M.; Chandrasekera, P.C.; Barnard, N.D. You are what you eat, or are you? The challenges of translating high-fat-fed rodents to human obesity and diabetes. *Nutr. Diabetes* **2014**, *4*, e135. [CrossRef] [PubMed]
94. Kowalski, G.M.; Bruce, C.R. The regulation of glucose metabolism: Implications and considerations for the assessment of glucose homeostasis in rodents. *Am. J. Physiol. Endocrinol. Metab.* **2014**, *307*, E859–E871. [CrossRef] [PubMed]
95. Burgess, S.M.; Jeffrey, F.M.H.; Storey, C.; Milde, A.; Hausler, N.; Merritt, M.E.; Mulder, H.; Holm, C.; Sherry, A.D.; Malloy, C.R. Effect of murine strain on metabolic pathways of glucose production after brief or prolonged fasting. *Am. J. Physiol. Endocrinol. Metab.* **2005**, *289*, E53–E61. [CrossRef] [PubMed]
96. Gannon, K.S.; Smith, J.C.; Henderson, R.; Hendrick, P. A system for studying the microstructure of ingestive behavior in mice. *Physiol. Behav.* **1992**, *51*, 515–521. [CrossRef]
97. Ellacott, K.L.; Morton, G.J.; Woods, S.C.; Tso, P.; Schwartz, M.W. Assessment of Feeding Behavior in Laboratory Mice. *Cell Metab.* **2010**, *12*, 10–17. [CrossRef]
98. Perelis, M.; Ramsey, K.M.; Marcheva, B.; Bass, J. Circadian Transcription from Beta Cell Function to Diabetes Pathophysiology. *J. Biol. Rhythm.* **2016**, *31*, 323–336. [CrossRef]
99. Qian, J.; Yeh, B.; Rakshit, K.; Colwell, C.S.; Matveyenko, A.V. Circadian Disruption and Diet-Induced Obesity Synergize to Promote Development of β-Cell Failure and Diabetes in Male Rats. *Endocrinology* **2015**, *156*, 4426–4436. [CrossRef]
100. Johnston, J.D.; Ordovás, J.M.; Scheer, F.A.; Turek, F.W. Circadian Rhythms, Metabolism, and Chrononutrition in Rodents and Humans. *Adv. Nutr.* **2016**, *7*, 399–406. [CrossRef]
101. Luo, S.; Zhang, Y.; Ezrokhi, M.; Li, Y.; Tsai, T.-H.; Cincotta, A.H. Circadian peak dopaminergic activity response at the biological clock pacemaker (suprachiasmatic nucleus) area mediates the metabolic responsiveness to a high-fat diet. *J. Neuroendocr.* **2018**, *30*, e12563. [CrossRef]

102. Vadiveloo, M.; Scott, M.; Quatromoni, P.; Jacques, P.; Parekh, N. Trends in dietary fat and high-fat food intakes from 1991 to 2008 in the Framingham Heart Study participants. *Br. J. Nutr.* **2014**, *111*, 724–734. [CrossRef] [PubMed]
103. Kalupahana, N.S.; Voy, B.H.; Saxton, A.M.; Moustaid-Moussa, N. Energy-Restricted High-Fat Diets Only Partially Improve Markers of Systemic and Adipose Tissue Inflammation. *Obesity (Silver Spring)* **2011**, *19*, 245–254. [CrossRef] [PubMed]
104. Salinero, A.E.; Anderson, B.M.; Zuloaga, K.L. Sex differences in the metabolic effects of diet-induced obesity vary by age of onset. *Int. J. Obes.* **2018**, *42*, 1088–1091. [CrossRef] [PubMed]

2

Low Reported Adherence to the 2019 American Diabetes Association Nutrition Recommendations among Patients with Type 2 Diabetes Mellitus, Indicating the Need for Improved Nutrition Education and Diet Care

Savvas Katsaridis [1], Maria G. Grammatikopoulou [1,2], Konstantinos Gkiouras [3], Christos Tzimos [4], Stefanos T. Papageorgiou [5], Anastasia G. Markaki [6], Triada Exiara [7], Dimitrios G. Goulis [2,*,†] and Theodora Papamitsou [8,*,†]

1 Department of Nutritional Sciences & Dietetics, Faculty of Health Sciences, Alexander Campus, International Hellenic University, Sindos, GR-57400 Thessaloniki, Greece; savvaskatsaridis@gmail.com (S.K.); mariagram@auth.gr (M.G.G.)
2 Unit of Reproductive Endocrinology, 1st Department of Obstetrics and Gynecology, Medical School, Aristotle University of Thessaloniki, Papageorgiou General Hospital, GR-56429 Thessaloniki, Greece
3 Laboratory of Clinical Pharmacology, Faculty of Health Sciences, Medical School, Aristotle University of Thessaloniki, GR-54124 Thessaloniki, Greece; kostasgkiouras@hotmail.com
4 Northern Greece Statistics Directorate, Hellenic Statistical Authority, 218 Delfon Str, GR-54646 Thessaloniki, Greece; ctzimos@gmail.com
5 Faculty of Health Sciences, Medical School, Aristotle University of Thessaloniki, GR-54124 Thessaloniki, Greece; papagesn@auth.gr
6 Department of Nutrition and Dietetics, Faculty of Health Sciences, Hellenic Mediterranean University, PO Box 8556, Trypitos, GR-72300 Sitia, Greece; markakin@hotmail.com
7 Department of Internal Medicine, Sismanoglio General Hospital, 45 Sismanogliou Str, GR-69133 Komotini, Greece; texiara@otenet.gr
8 Laboratory of Histology and Embryology, Medical School, Aristotle University of Thessaloniki, GR-54124 Thessaloniki, Greece
* Correspondence: dgg@auth.gr (D.G.G.); thpapami@auth.gr (T.P.)
† These authors contributed equally to this work.

Abstract: Patient adherence to guidelines is important for improved outcomes and prognosis. Nevertheless, many patients with type 2 diabetes mellitus (T2DM) do not comply with the recommendations regarding medication, physical activity, diet or self-care. The present cross-sectional study aimed to assess the level of adherence to the dietary recommendations issued by the American Diabetes Association (ADA) among patients with T2DM in Komotini, Greece. A total of 162 adults with T2DM (64.7 ± 10.6 years old), of which 41.4% were men, were recruited from the Sismanoglio Hospital and participated in the study. The level of adherence to individual recommendations issued by the ADA was assessed using yes/no questions. The overall adherence rate to the guidelines was low (41.2%). According to the multivariable analysis, age and medication therapy were identified as contributors to the compliance rate. No differences were noted in the total compliance rate between patients of different religious denominations (Muslims/Christians). Patients on oral antidiabetic agents (OAA) were more adherent compared with those on insulin therapy. A mere 3.7% of the participants had received nutrition education by a registered dietitian, 9.9% were following an individualized diet plan to improve glycemia, and 3.1% had set specific energy goals to reduce body weight. These findings are indicative of the need for the delivery of improved nutrition education.

Keywords: diabetes guidelines; nutrition guidelines; dietary supplements; lifestyle medicine; carbohydrate counting; diabetes education; HbA_{1c}; medical nutrition therapy; glucose-lowering drugs; health equity

---

1. Introduction

Diabetes mellitus (DM) is a chronic condition affecting more than 451 million adults worldwide [1]. In Greece, type 2 diabetes mellitus (T2DM) has been estimated to affect 12% of the total adult population [2], demonstrating an increased prevalence as compared to older cross-sectional studies [3,4]. Depending on the type of the disease and the age of patients, treatment options include medication or insulin, self-management and lifestyle advice [5]. For patients with T2DM, adherence to non-insulin medication therapy is a challenging task, greatly dependent on the disease's duration, with newly diagnosed patients being the less adherent ones [6,7]. In addition, 4% of patients with T2DM are "primary" non-adherents (i.e., they have never filled their prescriptions) [8]. Regarding insulin, only 62–64% of patients with T2DM comply with the prescribed dose [7], leaving approximately 1/3 of them without therapy. Among insulin-naïve patients, the rate of non-adherence is high: 4.5% are "primary" and an additional 25.5% "secondary" non-adherents (i.e., they fill their prescriptions in an inconsistent way) [7,9,10].

With regard to self-management, assessment of blood glucose concentrations is performed on average on 0.2–2.2 days each week, whereas foot care is implemented for approximately 2.2–4.3 days/weekly [11].

Following the lifestyle recommendations is another issue of concern among patients with DM [12]. Anxiety, depression and stress are associated with reduced compliance to the lifestyle-recommendations [13]. Long-term compliance to exercise goals can vary greatly, ranging between 10 to 80%, mainly due to lack of motivation and the fact that exercise is not monitored [10,14]. Concerning diet, patients often report disliking the foods listed in their meal plans [10] and tend to comply with the dietary recommendations for approximately 2.3–4.6 days every week [11]. Longer disease duration and the attainment of nutrition education appear to positively affect the rate of adherence [15].

Poor compliance is associated with poorer disease prognosis, an increased risk for developing comorbidities and complications [16], and a higher mortality ratio [10,17]. Understanding the level of adherence to the treatment recommendations is important to evaluate the quality of provided care, implement changes in the delivery of care and related education, and identify those less likely to adhere and improve patient outcomes. With this in mind, the present cross-sectional study aimed to evaluate adherence to the American Diabetes Association (ADA) nutrition recommendations among patients with T2DM.

2. Materials and Methods

2.1. Sample Recruitment and Inclusion and Exclusion Criteria

A total of 171 patients with a diagnosis of DM were recruited from the "Sismanoglio" General Hospital in Komotini, Northern Greece, during the year 2019 (25 June to 16 December). All out-patients visiting the clinic at the time of the study, fulfilling the inclusion criteria, were recruited. Pre-existing nutrition education was not a pre-requisite for participation. Given that the number of recruited patients with type 1 DM was low ($n = 9$), they were excluded from the analysis. Thus, the final sample consisted of 162 patients with T2DM.

Inclusion criteria were as follows: (1) adult patients, (2) diagnosis of T2DM, (3) ability to understand and articulate effortlessly in the Greek language, (4) willingness to participate, and (5) provision of informed consent. Exclusion criteria involved (1) patients not capable of consenting, (2) those unable to understand and communicate in Greek and (3) underage patients. The characteristics of the sample are provided in Table 1.

Table 1. Patient characteristics (*n* and %, or mean ± SD) (*n* = 162).

Men/Women (*n*, %)	67 (41.4%)/95 (58.6%)
Age (years)	64.7 ± 10.6
Bodyweight (kg)	86.7 ± 18.0
Height (cm)	164 ± 8
BMI (kg/m^2)	32.4 ± 6.6
Weight status (normoweight/overweight/obese) (*n*, %)	13 (8%)/60 (37%)/89 (55%)
Educational level (primary/secondary/tertiary) (*n*, %)	122 (75.3%)/24 (14.8%)/16 (9.9%)
Religion (Christian/Muslim)	101 (62.3%)/61 (37.7%)
Diabetes diagnosis (years)	10.7 ± 7.3
HbA_{1c} (%)	7.1 ± 1.6
Therapy (insulin/pharmacotherapy/both)	22 (13.6%)/104 (64.4%)/36 (22.2%)
SBP (mm Hg)	129.1 ± 18.3
DBP (mm Hg)	80.3 ± 7.6
Triglycerides (mg/dL)	157.8 ± 98.5
HDL (mg/dL)	46.5 ± 11.9
LDL (mg/dL)	95.0 ± 31.4
TSH (mU/L)	2.2 ± 1.0

BMI, body mass index; DBP, diastolic blood pressure; HbA_{1c}, glycosylated hemoglobin; HDL, high-density lipoprotein; LDL, low-density lipoprotein; SBP, systolic blood pressure; SD, standard deviation; TSH, thyroid-stimulating hormone. Missing values: LDL (*n* = 41), HDL (*n* = 37), Triglycerides (*n* = 70), SBP (*n* = 24), DBP (*n* = 24), and TSH (*n* = 137).

The study's permission was granted by the "Sismanoglio" General Hospital Directorate (Approval ID: 457/20-June-2020), and all patients provided informed consent before participation. Data were handled according to the Helsinki Declaration for research on humans.

2.2. Adherence to the ADA Dietary Recommendations

According to the World Health Organization (WHO) [18,19], adherence for long-term treatment refers to "the extent to which a person's behavior—taking medication, following a diet, and/or executing lifestyle changes, corresponds with agreed recommendations from a health care provider". With this in mind, all ADA [20] nutrition recommendations issued in the same year of the present research (2019) were extracted by two researchers independently and included in a questionnaire with binary answers (yes/no). A total of 17 distinct recommendations were extracted from the guidelines [20] (Table 2). These were used to assess the degree of adherence to the guidelines. Two questions referring to insulin use were only addressed to those on insulin therapy (numbers 6 and 7—Table 2). No time restrictions were applied to participants regarding the completion of the questionnaire.

Table 2. Patient adherence to individual nutrition recommendations suggested by the American Diabetes Association (ADA) (n = 162) (n, % or median, interquartile range (IQR)).

	Individual Nutrition Recommendations:	Therapy		Sex		Religious Denomination		Age Group		Total (n = 162)
		On OAA Only (n = 104)	On Insulin $ (n = 58)	Men (n = 67)	Women (n = 95)	Christian (n = 101)	Muslim (n = 61)	<60 Years Old (n = 50)	≥60 Years Old (n = 112)	
1	Follow an individualized diet plan based on personal needs to improve glycemia	12 (11.5%)	4 (6.9%)	9 (13.4%)	7 (7.4%)	12 (11.9%)	4 (6.6%)	8 (16%)	8 (7.1%)	16 (9.9%)
2	Consumption of nutrient-dense foods in appropriate portion sizes in order to improve overall health	33 (56.9%)	55 (52.9%)	35 (52.2%)	53 (55.8%)	59 (58.4%)	29 (47.5%)	27 (54%)	61 (54.5%)	88 (54.3%)
3	Follow an intensive lifestyle intervention program including individualized goals and/or to individualized MNT (for people with prediabetes or overweight/obesity)	37 (35.6%) *	11 (19%)	22 (32.8%)	26 (27.4%)	36 (35.6%) *	12 (19.7%)	19 (38%)	29 (25.9%)	48 (29.6%)
4	Consumption of a specific energy target each day based on the individualized body weight goals and needs	4 (3.8%)	1 (1.7%)	3 (4.5%)	2 (2.1%)	5 (5%)	0 (0%)	3 (6%)	2 (1.8%)	5 (3.1%)
5	Consumption of adequate dietary fiber (preferably through food (vegetables, pulses (beans, peas and lentils), fruits, and whole intact grains)	96 (92.3%)	46 (79.3%)	62 (92.5%)	80 (84.2%)	91 (90.1%)	51 (83.6%)	43 (86%)	99 (88.4%)	142 (87.7%)
6	Able to count carbohydrate content of foods to calculate appropriate insulin dose	0 (0%) ∂	2 (3.4%)	2 (3%) *	0 (0%)	1 (1%)	1 (1.6%)	2 (4%) **	0 (0%)	2 (1.2%)
7	Use fixed daily insulin doses, consistent carbohydrate intake with respect to time and amount	0 (0%) ∂	6 (10.3%)	5 (7.5%)	1 (1.1%)	4 (4%)	2 (3.3%)	5 (10%)	1 (0.9%)	6 (3.7%)

Table 2. *Cont.*

	Individual Nutrition Recommendations:	Therapy		Sex		Religious Denomination		Age Group		Total (n = 162)
		On OAA Only (n = 104)	On Insulin [$] ($n$ = 58)	Men (n = 67)	Women (n = 95)	Christian (n = 101)	Muslim (n = 61)	<60 Years Old (n = 50)	≥60 Years Old (n = 112)	
8	Consumption of SSBs (including juice with sugar, energy drinks and soft-drinks) [#]	35 (33.7%)	22 (37.9%)	22 (32.8%)	35 (36.8%)	30 (29.7%)	27 (44.3%)	22 (44%)	35 (31.3%)	57 (35.2%)
9	In the case of hypoglycemic episodes:									
	a. Consumption of carbohydrate in the form of juice or sugar	101 (97.1%)	57 (98.3%)	63 (94%) *	95 (100%)	99 (98%)	59 (96.7%)	49 (89%)	109 (97.3%)	258 (97.5%)
	b. Consumption of carbohydrate food with high protein content (i.e., bread or cereals)	3 (2.9%)	1 (1.7%)	4 (6%) *	0 (0%)	2 (2%)	2 (3.3%)	5 (10%)	1 (0.9%)	4 (2.5%)
10	Consumption of one serving of fish (particularly fatty fish), at least twice/weekly	83 (79.8%)	44 (75.9%)	53 (79.1%)	74 (77.9%)	84 (83.2%)	43 (70.5%)	36 (72%)	91 (81.3%)	127 (78.4%)
11	Routine use of the following supplements for improving glycemia:									
	Vitamin D [‡]	3 (2.9%)	2 (3.4%)	0 (0%)	5 (5.3%)	4 (4%)	1 (1.6%)	1 (2%)	4 (3.6%)	5 (3.1%)
	Chromium [‡]	0 (0%)	0 (0%)	0 (0%)	0 (0%)	0 (0%)	0 (0%)	0 (0%)	0 (0%)	0 (0%)
	Curcumin [‡]	1 (1%)	0 (0%)	1 (1.5%)	0 (0%)	0 (0%)	1 (1.6%)	1 (2%)	4 (3.6%)	1 (0.6%)
	Cinnamon [‡]	9 (8.7%)	2 (3.4%)	3 (4.5%)	8 (8.4%)	9 (8.9%)	2 (3.3%)	6 (12%)	5 (4.5%)	11 (6.8%)
	Aloe vera [‡]	3 (2.9%)	0 (0%)	2 (3%)	1 (1.1%)	3 (3%)	0 (0%)	1 (2%)	2 (1.8%)	3 (1.9%)
	Any supplement [f]	6 (5.8%)	7 (12.1%)	6 (9%)	7 (7.4%)	12 (11.9%)	1 (1.6%)	4 (8%)	9 (8%)	13 (8%)
	No supplement	82 (78.8%)	47 (81%)	55 (82.1%)	74 (77.9%)	73 (72.3%)	56 (91.8%)	37 (74%) **	92 (82.1%)	129 (79.6%)

Table 2. *Cont.*

	Individual Nutrition Recommendations:	Therapy		Sex		Religious Denomination		Age Group		Total (n = 162)
		On OAA Only (n = 104)	On Insulin [$] ($n$ = 58)	Men (n = 67)	Women (n = 95)	Christian (n = 101)	Muslim (n = 61)	<60 Years Old (n = 50)	≥60 Years Old (n = 112)	
12	When alcohol is consumed, this is done in moderation (≤1 drink/day for women and ≤2 drinks/day for men)	4 (3.8%)	2 (3.4%)	6 (9%) **	0 (0%)	4 (4%)	2 (3.3%)	1 (2%)	5 (4.5%)	6 (3.7%)
13	Use of sugar substitutes (i.e., stevia, saccharin, acesulfame-K, aspartame, sucralose, etc.) †	18 (17.3%) *	20 (34.5%)	20 (29.9%)	18 (18.9%)	29 (28.7%) *	9 (14.8%)	12 (24%)	26 (23.2%)	38 (23.5%)
14	Maintenance of the pleasure of eating	96 (92.3%)	46 (79.3%)	62 (92.5%)	80 (84.2%)	91 (90.1%)	51 (83.6%)	45 (90%)	97 (86.6%)	142 (87.7%)
15	Controlling blood lipid levels through diet	22 (21.2%)	7 (12.1%)	17 (25.4%)	12 (12.6%)	21 (20.8%)	8 (13.1%)	14 (28%)	15 (13.4%)	29 (17.9%)
16	Controlling arterial blood pressure with diet	27 (26%)	8 (13.8%)	21 (31.3%) *	14 (14.7%)	26 (25.7%)	9 (14.8%)	20 (40%) ***	15 (13.4%)	35 (21.6%)
17	Received comprehensive nutrition education provided by a RDN, preferably one with DM knowledge and experience	4 (3.8%)	2 (3.4%)	4 (6%)	2 (2.1%)	6 (5.9%)	0 (0%)	3 (6%)	3 (2.7%)	6 (3.7%)
	Adherence to the recommendations (% of correct answers) ∝§	46.7 (40, 53.3) ***	38.2 (29.4, 41.2)	46.7 (40, 53.3) **	41.2 (35.3, 52.9)	46.7 (40, 53.3)	41.2 (35.3, 47.1)	46.9 (40, 53.3) **	41.2 (35.3, 50.2)	41.2 (35.3, 53.3)

ADA, American Diabetes Association; CVD, cardiovascular; DM, diabetes mellitus; IQR, interquartile range; MNT, medical nutrition therapy; OAA, oral antidiabetic agents; RDN, registered dietitian -nutritionist; SSBs, sugar-sweetened beverages. [$] Some were additionally receiving OAA; [#] should be avoided; [†] do not appear to reduce long-term CVD risk or body weight; [‡] not recommended; [f] not recommended, unless a deficiency is present; [∂] For those on OAA, these two questions were omitted from the adherence score; [∝] Based on 17 questions for those on insulin and 15 questions for those on OAA therapy only; * Significantly different compared to the opposite group (on insulin therapy/women/Muslim denomination/age ≥ 60 years old) as follows *** $p \leq 0.001$, ** $p \leq 0.01$, * $p \leq 0.05$; [§] Tested with the Mann–Whitney test.

The percentage (%) of adherence to the ADA's recommendations was calculated based on the sum of adherence (positive answers; "yes") according to the 17 questions for patients on insulin therapy and based on the sum adherence of 15 questions for patients on therapy with oral antidiabetic agents (OAA) only.

For the purpose of the study, an experienced registered nutritionist dietitian (RDN) (S.K.) was present at the outpatient clinic for DM every day, throughout the study's recruitment period. Participating patients were interviewed by the RDN on a one-on-one basis, and their reported adherence to the ADA recommendations was recorded on the questionnaire, on paper form, by the same RDN. No training was provided to the participants prior to participation.

For specific questions, participants were assisted with photographs of common food portion sizes and the micronutrient content of selected food groups, by the RDN. For instance, with regard to fiber, adequate intake was presented as daily portions of vegetables, fruit, or grains. Concerning sugar-sweetened beverages (SSBs), commercially available choices were presented to participants in order for them to report their intake. Alcohol portions were also presented in picture format, for participants to better understand and report their consumption. Commercially available sugar substitutes and dietary supplements were also presented, to achieve a more valid reporting.

2.3. *Anthropometric and Other Characteristics of the Participants*

The participants' body weight and height were measured during morning hours with a digital scale (SECA 813, SECA Group, Hamburg, Germany) and a wall-mounted stadiometer (SECA 216, SECA Group, Hamburg, Germany). Body mass index (BMI) was calculated for each patient by dividing body weight (kg) by the stature (m) squared. Weight status was identified according to the World Health Organization thresholds for BMI [21].

Data concerning disease duration, comorbidities, latest HbA_{1c} assessment, education level, and medication therapy for DM were recorded for each participant. Given that Komotini has the greatest Muslim population in Greece, the religious denomination of participants was also recorded.

2.4. *Statistical Analyses*

Normality in distribution was assessed both visually and with the Shapiro–Wilk test. Normally distributed variables are presented as mean ± standard deviation (SD) and non-normally distributed as median with the respective interquartile range (IQR). Descriptive statistics for qualitative data are presented as frequencies (n) with their respective percentages in parentheses. Chi-square tests and the Mann–Whitney test were utilized to examine differences among qualitative and quantitative variables, respectively.

A univariable linear regression analysis was conducted in order to assess the impact on percentage adherence to the ADA's recommendations total score (dependent variable) of the following study variables: age in years (continuous), sex (male vs. female), BMI in kg/m^2 (continuous), educational level (primary vs. secondary or tertiary), religious denomination (Christian vs. Muslim), diabetes duration in years (continuous), HbA_{1c} in % (continuous), and therapy type (insulin vs. OAA only). A multivariable linear regression analysis was conducted, which included those independent variables selected by the augmented backward selection procedure as previously described [22]. Normality assumption and homoscedasticity were examined on the residuals, and multicollinearity was assessed by calculating tolerance and variance inflation factor (VIF). All analyses were carried out on the Statistical Software for Social Studies (SPSS) v. 25.0 (IBM SPSS Statistics, Armonk, NY, USA) and the SAS University Edition (SAS Institute, Cary, NC, USA). The significance level was set at $\alpha = 0.05$.

3. Results

3.1. Adherence to the Dietary Recommendations

Total sample adherence to the ADA dietary recommendations [20] and adherence per participant group are presented in Table 2. The sample's median percentage of adherence to the ADA dietary recommendations was suboptimal, reaching 41.2% (35.3%, 53.3%).

A mere 3.7% of the sample had received nutrition education by an RDN. The majority of participants reported adhering to the fiber (87.7%) and fish intake (78.4%) recommendations; most reported being aware of how to combat hypoglycemia (97.5%) and of the fact that supplements cannot improve glycemic control (79.6%). Only 9.9% of the patients followed an individualized diet plan to improve glycemic control, and 3.1% had specific energy targets set to reduce their body weight. Among those on insulin therapy, only 1.2% were competent to count their meals' carbohydrate content, and 3.7% were receiving fixed insulin doses paired with a consistent carbohydrate intake. Recommendations regarding alcohol intake were only adhered to by 3.7% of the sample. The vast majority (87.7%) reported maintaining the pleasure of eating. Only 17.9% and 21.6% of the participants were able to control their blood lipid and blood pressure levels by diet alone, without pharmacotherapy.

Patients on OAA therapy only, exhibited increased adherence compared with those receiving insulin (medians: 46.7% vs. 38.2% respectively; $p \leq 0.001$). In parallel, men were more compliant compared with women (medians: 46.7% vs. 41.2%, respectively; $p \leq 0.01$) and younger patients compared with the older ones (medians: 46.9% vs. 41.2%, respectively; $p \leq 0.01$).

3.2. Assessment of the Impact of Study Variables on Percentage of ADA Adherence Score

In a univariable assessment (Table 3), patients on OAA were associated with an increased percentage of ADA adherence score (β = 9.56, 95% CI = 6.45 to 12.63). A positive association was also observed among participants having attained education on the secondary or tertiary level (β = 6.28, 95% CI = 2.61 to 9.95). On the other hand, female sex and age were associated with a decreased percentage of ADA adherence score (β = −4.30, 95% CI = −7.56 to −1.04, and β = −0.22, 95% CI = −0.37 to −0.04). DM-related variables including diabetes duration (years) and HbA_{1c} (%) demonstrated a negative association with percentage of ADA adherence score (β = −0.51, 95% CI = −0.72 to −0.30, and β = 1.48, 95% CI = −2.50 to −0.46). Religious beliefs and BMI were not associated with the ADA adherence score (p-values > 0.05).

Table 3. Univariable and multivariable linear regression assessment of the impact of study variables on the percentage of the total adherence score.

Independent Variable	Univariable		Multivariable †	
	β Coef (95% CI)	Significance	β Coef (95% CI)	*p*-Value
Age	−0.22 (−0.37 to−0.04)	0.006	−0.13 (−0.29 to 0.03)	0.115
Female	−4.30 (−7.56 to −1.04)	0.010	−2.26 (−5.15 to 0.63)	0.125
BMI (kg/m^2)	−0.10 (−0.35 to 0.15)	0.450	-	
Secondary/tertiary education	6.28 (2.61 to 9.95)	0.001	3.84 (−0.003 to 7.69)	0.050
Muslim denomination	−3.01 (−6.36 to 0.34)	0.077	−2.31 (−5.58 to 0.96)	0.165
Diabetes duration (years)	−0.51 (−0.72 to −0.30)	<0.001	−0.23 (−0.46 to −0.01)	0.042
HbA_{1c} (%)	−1.48 (−2.50 to −0.46)	0.005	-	
OAA therapy only	9.56 (6.48 to 12.63)	<0.001	8.36 (5.24 to 11.74)	<0.001

β Coef, linear regression coefficients; BMI, body mass index; CI, confidence intervals; HbA_{1c}, glycosylated hemoglobin; OAA, oral antidiabetic agents. † included variables selected by the augmented backward selection procedure [22] with adjusted R^2: 0.306.

In the multivariable model (Table 3), patients on OAA therapy demonstrated increased adherence to the guidelines (by 8.36%), whereas adherence was decreased by 0.23% with every year of increasing age.

4. Discussion

Patients with T2DM exhibited low compliance to the ADA dietary recommendations for DM. Among those on OAA therapy only, men and younger patients reported a better adherence rate compared with patients receiving insulin, women and older patients. Based on the univariable analysis, age, BMI, DM duration, HbA_{1c}, and Muslin denomination reduced compliance, whereas, having attained secondary or tertiary education and being on OAA therapy only, were associated with increased compliance. In the multivariable analysis, only OAA therapy and DM duration were associated with the rate of adherence to the recommendations.

In the present sample, only 3.7% of the participants had received nutrition education by an RDN. According to a systematic review and meta-analysis, the delivery of dietary education by RDNs consists of the most effective medium to improve patient outcomes [23]. Previous studies in Greece have revealed suboptimal nutrition knowledge among patients with DM [24–26], highlighting the need for an integrated approach to patient education. In parallel, randomized controlled trials (RCTs) have unanimously revealed improvements in glycemic control and disease prognosis following the implementation of nutrition education sessions [27,28]. In a study conducted in the USA [29] (Table 4), patients with T1DM and T2DM were educated on nutritional issues by an RDN and set individual goals based on the ADA/Morrison Health Care (MHC) recommendations. Post-intervention, 40% of participants attained the dietary goals excellently, 32.7% were adequately meeting their goals, and the remaining 27% adhered to the dietary goals fairly. A similar pattern was observed for exercise goals. After the intervention, an improvement was noted in the HbA_{1c} concentrations. In an RCT comparing adherence to the ADA dietary recommendations against a low-fat vegan diet, an improved overall adherence rate was noted in the latter compared with the former [30], indicating that many factors impeding adherence to the guidelines may exist. Interestingly, a mixed-methods study [31] failed to correlate DM knowledge to the rate of compliance with the guidelines (assessed by personal interviews). Several barriers were identified affecting the degree of compliance to the recommendations, including external stress, a conflict between advice and personal beliefs, lack of time and personal motivation, gaps in knowledge and living in an obesogenic environment [31]. Based on the latter observation, according to a recent meta-analysis [32], changing the dietary environment is more important for glycemic control compared with changing the dietary behavior; nevertheless, both are clinically effective for managing HbA_{1c} concentrations.

Apart from nutrition education, delivery of medical nutrition therapy (MNT) is important, as it involves the nutrition care process model, setting individual goals and guiding patients towards their attainment, close monitoring and evaluation. In the present sample, 9.9% of the patients were following an individualized diet plan to improve glycemia, whereas 3.1% had set specific energy targets and adhered to an MNT scheme aiming to reduce body weight. Individualized nutrition therapy carries more benefits for the patient than receiving dietary advice alone [33]. This is due to the low nutrition-related competencies and often inadequate education received by medical doctors in Greece and throughout the world [34,35] and the fact that RDNs are the most competent professionals for the delivery of MNT [36,37]. According to an econometric study [38], MNT is associated with a 9.5% reduction in the hospitalization of patients with DM, and a concurrent 23.5% decline in the use of physician services; thus, it should be considered as necessary instead of optimal, for all patients with DM [39].

Among participants in the present sample, complying with the alcohol recommendations proved to be a difficult task, as only 3.7% of them reported adhering to this goal. In contrast to the findings herein, in Northern California [40], most patients with DM complied with the ADA recommendations regarding alcohol intake. Alcohol intake is considered an indicator of poorer adherence to DM self-care behaviors [40]. In Greece, although alcohol use is not widespread, it holds a prominent position at celebrations and family meal tables. Thus, it might be difficult for patients with T2DM to control alcohol consumption in such habitual cases. Based on studies performed on humans and preclinical models, acute ethanol intake induces either a reduction, or a null effect on circulating glucose concentrations [41]. The first appears more likely to occur in fasted individuals, with only a small amount of evidence suggesting alcohol hypoglycemia in well-nourished patients [41–44]. Among patients with T2DM on different treatment regimes, it has been suggested that those on diet therapy do not experience hypoglycemia, whereas sulphonylurea-treated individuals might carry this risk [45].

Concerning the use of oral nutrient supplements (ONS) to improve glycemic control, most participants (79.6%) were aware that they are not efficient unless a deficiency is apparent, and subsequently, most patients herein abstained from their use. Nevertheless, 6.8% reported consuming cinnamon supplements, 1.9% received aloe vera ONS, 0.6% were reliant on curcumin to aid glycemic control, and 8% were consuming other supplements, with a special focus on poly-unsaturated fatty acids (PUFA). According to a recent scoping review [46], for many of the ONS postulated as efficient for DM care, a lack of scientific background is apparent. Thus, it is important to elaborate that these supplements often carry adverse effects and increase the cost of DM care, without offering any positive outcomes [47]. These issues can only be realized by educating patients on topics related to nutrition.

An individual's diet is greatly dependent on an interplay of religious, familial, psychological, financial, and personal factors [48]. According to the ADA [49,50], structured interventions destined for patients with DM should be offered for diverse populations and audiences, integrating both culture and religion. In particular, religion is an integral part of the culture, often directing food habits through Lent, fasting or beliefs related to certain foods [48]. Concerning the effect of the religious denomination on the rate of adherence to the dietary guidelines, no differences were observed in the total compliance score herein, apart from a greater proportion of patients with Christian denomination following specific energy targets for bodyweight reduction and reporting using sugar substitutes to a greater extend. Although having a Muslim denomination was associated with a decreased adherence score in the univariable analysis, this effect failed to remain significant when all other factors were considered. This fact indicates that in Komotini's multicultural community, healthcare equity does not allow for disparities based on religion, offering an individually adapted DM-care model.

Based on the multivariable model, each yearly increment in the age reduced total adherence score by −0.23%, whereas those on OAA therapy only had an increased dietary compliance score by 8.36%. These findings agree with previous research on patients with T2DM, suggesting that the use of insulin is associated with a decreased adherence to the therapy [51]. With regard to age, although a study in Rio de Janeiro revealed a decreased compliance rate among older patients [52], conflicting evidence exists in the literature concerning this issue. Concerning diet, studies have revealed an improved adherence rate with a more recent DM diagnosis (and subsequently, younger age) [53]; concerning medication, increasing age appears to ameliorate adherence [6,7,54,55].

The results also indicated a reduced adherence rate among women participants as compared to their male counterparts. Previous research on Greek patients with DM has also revealed a reduced nutritional knowledge and self-management practices among women with T2DM inhabiting the city of Agrinio, in Central Greece [24,26]. Apart from the fact that older women inhabiting mainland Greece are likely to have received less education in general, women are also responsible for preparing the meals for all the family. This increased preoccupation with food, including frequent tasting of the prepared dishes, is likely a factor reducing adherence to the dietary recommendations among women [25]. In parallel, according to Fitzgerald [56], gender differences are also apparent in diabetes attitudes. On the other hand, according to a study in Singapore [57], lower adherence was demonstrated in men with DM as compared to women. Therefore, the exact extent of the effect of gender on DM adherence remains unclear.

Table 4 summarizes available evidence assessing adherence to the dietary recommendations among patients with DM. In Canada [58], patients with T2DM exceeded daily sodium and saturated fatty acid (SFA) recommendations issued by the Canadian Diabetes Association (CDA). Cured meats, fast foods and snack foods were all major contributors to the intake of sodium and saturated fat [58]. In Pakistan [59], 36.5% of patients with DM complied with the ADA dietary recommendations. In further detail, greater adherence was noted among those feeling comfortable with their diet plan, and those aware of which diet was harmful to them. In Italy, a great proportion of patients with T2DM adhered to the recommendations for protein and added sugars, but the respective percentage of those meeting SFA and fiber goals was lower [60]. A similar pattern was noted in Thailand [61], with the majority of patients with T2DM failing to meet local SFA and fiber recommendations, issued based on the ADA respective guidelines. In Finland [62], a mere 28% of patients with T1DM with nephropathy restricted their SFA intake according to the recommended levels of less than 10% of the total energy intake based on the Finish Diabetes Association (FDA) guidelines. In parallel, 4% of the participants met the recommended fiber intake values, and 25% exceeded the suggested goal regarding sugar intake [62]. Nevertheless, more than 50% of the participants perceived themselves as adherers to the dietary recommendations either "most of the time", or "always" [62].

Concerning adolescents with T1DM [64], according to a study from Norway, apart from the intake of fat and fiber, which were over- and under-consumed, respectively, all intakes of remaining macronutrients were adequate according to the recommendations of the relevant International Society for Pediatric and Adolescent Diabetes (ISPAD). Improved dietary intakes were also noted among adolescents with better glycemic control.

The present study indicates that MNT and nutrition education are often neglected areas of DM care in Greece. Most hospitals fail to employ an adequate number of RDNs, and, thus, nutritional education and care are often offered in private practice to those patients who have the financial means to address relevant out-of-pocket expenses. On the other hand, multidisciplinary teams are required for the management of all conditions/diseases, and as far as DM is concerned, systematic reviews and meta-analyses have highlighted the importance of including RDNs in routine DM care for improved patient outcomes [65].

The limitations of this study include the assessment of adherence to the ADA guidelines instead of relevant recommendations from a Greek society/authority. Furthermore, the cross-sectional design does not allow for causal associations. In parallel, using a relatively small sample from one hospital only might not allow for extrapolation of the findings (external validity).

Table 4. Cross-sectional studies assessing adherence to the dietary guidelines among patients with diabetes.

First Author	Origin	Recruitment	Patient Characteristics			RR (%)	Guidelines Evaluated	Tools	Results
			DM Type	Age (Years)	N				
Ahmed [40]	US	Kaiser Permanente Northern California Diabetes Registry, and patients from the pharmacy, laboratory, outpatient clinics, ER and hospitalization	T1DM and T2DM	58.1 ± 13 *	77,722 (Alcohol drinkers: 38,564)	83	ADA	Survey by mail, computer-assisted telephone interview, HbA_{1c} and further DM-related tests	Among current drinkers, 92% of men (2 drinks/day) and 94% of women (1 drink/day) adhered to the guidelines. Alcohol consumption was inversely associated with HbA_{1c}.
Ahola [62]	FI	Patients of the Finnish Diabetic Nephropathy Study "FinnDiane"	T1DM	Men: 51 (40–60) † Women: 47 (37–54) †	817	63	FDA	FFQ, self-reported compliance with guidelines, 3-day food records concerning food intake, PA, Ins dose, and BG levels	Only 28% of participants restricted SFA to the recommendation. Almost 1/4 had higher than recommended sucrose intake. Fiber goals were met by 4% of participants.
Gillani [59]	PK	Patients from hospitals in Multan, Bahawalpur, and Rahim Yar Khan	T1DM and T2DM	48.8 ± 14.6 *	398	44.3	ADA	3-day recalls were used to assess dietary history and diet compliance	Diet compliance was 36.5%. Patients feeling comfortable with their diet plan and those aware of which diet was harmful to them were more compliant.
Krige [63]	ZA	Women were diagnosed during pregnancy from two hospitals	GDM/IGT	32.2 ± 5.3 *	239	–	SEMDSA	Interview administered picture-quantified FFQ and beliefs concerning food consumption	The average protein constituted 14.7% of TEI (goal 20%), with 93.5% of patients consuming protein below the cut-off point. The average carbohydrate intake was 53% (goal 40%), with 92.2% exceeding the goal. Mean fat intake was 33% of TEI (goal 40%), and 80.4% of patients were below the goal. Overall, patients demonstrated moderate adherence.
Nedra [29]	US	Hospital outpatients, a freestanding and an endocrinology clinic	T1DM and T2DM	56 ± 16.7 *	102	NR	ADA and MHC	Data from chart notes and phone calls for patients' self-rating of their DM knowledge, before and after nutrition education by an RDN	Approximately 40% of participants attained their goals excellently, 32.7% rated meeting their goals as good, and the remaining 27% considered their adherence as fair.

Table 4. *Cont.*

First Author	Origin	Recruitment	Patient Characteristics			RR (%)	Guidelines Evaluated	Tools	Results
			DM Type	Age (Years)	N				
Øverby [64]	NO	Norwegian Childhood Diabetes and Quality project	T1DM	11.3 ± 3.4 *	550	34	DNSG	4-day food records, FFQ, questionnaire on parental education, diabetes examinations	Apart from the intake of fat and fiber, which were higher and lower respectively than recommended, all intakes of macronutrients were adequate according to current recommendations.
Raj [58]	CA	Through advertising	T2DM	61.2 ± 10.4 *	80	80	CDA	PDAQ, 3-day food records, anthropometry and DM examinations	Reported mean daily intakes of Na and SFA exceeded the recommendations. Cured meats, fast foods and snack foods were all major contributors to intake of Na and SFA. SFA, Na intakes and total PDAQ scores did not correlate with HbA_{1c} concentration.
Thewjitcharoen [61]	YH	Outpatients of the DM clinics from the Theptarin and Ramathibodi hospitals	T2DM	57.4 (25–85) †	304	NR	Thailand guidelines based on the ADA	3- or 7-day food records, nutritional knowledge and a dietary self-care behavior questionnaire	Low adherence to the local guidelines was observed. The recommended intake of SFA was met by only 32.7% of free sugars by 11.8% and fiber by 1.6%.
Vitale [60]	IT	57 centers throughout Italy	T2DM	62.1 ± 6.5 *	2568	NR	DNSG and SID	EPIC FFQ, and specific software to convert dietary data to average daily amounts of foods	Adherence to the recommendations was high for the consumption of protein (77.8%) and added sugars (97.3%), while adherence for the intake of recommended quantities of SFA (17.9%) and fiber (6.9%) was lower.

ADA, American Diabetes Association; BG, blood glucose; CDA, Canadian Diabetes Association; DGA, Dietary Guidelines for Americans; DNSG, Diabetes and Nutrition Study Group; DM, diabetes mellitus; EPIC, European Prospective Investigation into Cancer and Nutrition; ER, emergency room; FDA, Finish Diabetes Association; FFQ, food frequency questionnaire; GDM, gestational diabetes mellitus; HbA_{1c}, glycosylated hemoglobin; HEI, Healthy Eating Index; IGT, impaired glucose tolerance; Ins, insulin; ISPAD, International Society for Pediatric and Adolescent Diabetes; MDG, Malaysian Dietary Guidelines; MHC, Morrison Health Care; Na, sodium; NCDQ, Norwegian Childhood Diabetes and Quality; NR, not reported; PA, physical activity; PDAQ, Perceived Dietary Adherence Questionnaire; RDN, registered nutritionist dietitian; RR, response rate; SD, standard deviation; SEMDSA, Society for Endocrinology Metabolism an Diabetes of South Africa; SID, Italian Diabetes Society; SFA, saturated fatty acids; T1DM, type 1 diabetes mellitus; T2DM, type 2 diabetes mellitus; TEI, total energy intake; USDA, United States Department of Agriculture. † Mean (range); * Mean ± SD.

5. Conclusions

According to the WHO, among patients with chronic disease, the rate of adherence to lifestyle recommendations is lower as compared to medication ones [19]. A salient explanation for this phenomenon might be that medication therapy does not require particular effort from the part of the patient, whereas on the other hand, lifestyle treatment is greatly dependent on the stage of motivational readiness [66,67]. The present cross-sectional study demonstrated a low reported adherence rate to the dietary recommendations for DM among patients with T2DM, indicating the need for improved nutrition education and diet care.

Author Contributions: Conceptualization, D.G.G. and M.G.G.; methodology, D.G.G. and M.G.G.; formal analysis, K.G. and C.T.; investigation, S.K. and T.E.; resources, T.P.; data curation, S.K.; writing—original draft preparation, M.G.G., D.G.G. and S.T.P.; writing—review and editing, D.G.G., M.G.G. and A.G.M.; supervision, T.P., M.G.G. and D.G.G.; project administration, T.P.; funding acquisition, T.P. All authors have read and agreed to the published version of the manuscript.

Acknowledgments: The authors appreciate the help and cooperation of all participating patients.

References

1. Cho, N.H.; Shaw, J.E.; Karuranga, S.; Huang, Y.; da Rocha Fernandes, J.D.; Ohlrogge, A.W.; Malanda, B. IDF Diabetes Atlas: Global estimates of diabetes prevalence for 2017 and projections for 2045. *Diabetes Res. Clin. Pract.* **2018**, *138*, 271–281. [CrossRef]
2. Tsirona, S.; Katsaros, F.; Alexandra, A.; Polyzos, S.; Arapoglou, G.; Koukoulis, G. Prevalence and determinants of type 2 diabetes mellitus in a Greek adult population. *Hormones* **2016**. [CrossRef]
3. Panagiotakos, D.B.; Pitsavos, C.; Chrysohoou, C.; Stefanadis, C. The epidemiology of Type 2 diabetes mellitus in Greek adults: The ATTICA study. *Diabet. Med.* **2005**, *22*, 1581–1588. [CrossRef] [PubMed]
4. Lionis, C.D.; Sasarolis, S.M.; Koutis, A.D.; Antonakis, N.A.; Benos, A.; Papavasiliou, S.; Fioretos, M. Measuring the prevalence of diabetes mellitus in a Greek primary health care district. *Fam. Pract.* **1996**, *13*, 18–21. [CrossRef] [PubMed]
5. Paschou, S.A.; Ljlijana, M.V.; Spartalis, E.; Anagnostis, P.; Alexandrou, A.; Goulis, D.G.; Lambrinoudaki, I. Therapeutic strategies for type 2 diabetes mellitus in women after menopause. *Maturitas* **2019**, *126*. [CrossRef] [PubMed]
6. Kirkman, M.S.; Rowan-Martin, M.T.; Levin, R.; Fonseca, V.A.; Schmittdiel, J.A.; Herman, W.H.; Aubert, R.E. Determinants of adherence to diabetes medications: Findings from a large pharmacy claims database. *Diabetes Care* **2015**, *38*, 604–609. [CrossRef] [PubMed]
7. Cramer, J.A. A systematic review of adherence with medications for diabetes. *Diabetes Care* **2004**, *27*, 1218–1224. [CrossRef] [PubMed]
8. Karter, A.J.; Parker, M.M.; Moffet, H.H.; Ahmed, A.T.; Schmittdiel, J.A.; Selby, J. New prescription medication gaps: A comprehensive measure of adherence to new prescriptions. *Health Serv. Res.* **2009**, *44*, 1640–1661. [CrossRef]
9. Karter, A.J.; Subramanian, U.; Saha, C.; Crosson, J.C.; Parker, M.M.; Swain, B.E.; Moffet, H.H.; Marrero, D.G. Barriers to insulin initiation: The translating research into action for diabetes insulin starts project. *Diabetes Care* **2010**, *33*, 733–735. [CrossRef]
10. García-Pérez, L.-E.; Alvarez, M.; Dilla, T.; Gil-Guillén, V.; Orozco-Beltrán, D. Adherence to therapies in patients with type 2 diabetes. *Diabetes Ther.* **2013**, *4*, 175–194. [CrossRef]
11. Mogre, V.; Johnson, N.A.; Tzelepis, F.; Shaw, J.E.; Paul, C. A systematic review of adherence to diabetes self-care behaviours: Evidence from low- and middle-income countries. *J. Adv. Nurs.* **2019**, *75*, 3374–3389. [CrossRef] [PubMed]
12. Aladhab, R.A.; Alabbood, M.H. Adherence of Patients with Diabetes to a Lifestyle Advice and Management Plan in Basra, Southern Iraq. *Int. J. Diabetes Metab.* **2019**, *25*, 1–6. [CrossRef]
13. Albuquerque, C.; Correia, C.; Ferreira, M.; Centro, B.; Tondela-Viseu, H.; Rei, A.; Duarte, D. Adherence to the therapeutic regime in person with type 2 diabetes. *Procedia Soc. Behav. Sci.* **2015**, *171*, 350–358. [CrossRef]
14. Praet, S.F.E.; van Loon, L.J.C. Exercise therapy in type 2 diabetes. *Acta Diabetol.* **2009**, *46*, 263–278. [CrossRef] [PubMed]

15. Mohammed, M.A.; Sharew, N.T. Adherence to dietary recommendation and associated factors among diabetic patients in Ethiopian teaching hospitals. *Pan Afr. Med. J.* **2019**, *33*. [CrossRef]
16. Katsiki, N.; Anagnostis, P.; Kotsa, K.; Goulis, D.G.; Mikhailidis, D.P. Obesity, Metabolic Syndrome and the Risk of Microvascular Complications in Patients with Diabetes mellitus. *Curr. Pharm. Des.* **2019**, *25*, 2051–2059. [CrossRef]
17. Bailey, C.J.; Kodack, M. Patient adherence to medication requirements for therapy of type 2 diabetes. *Int. J. Clin. Pract.* **2011**, *65*, 314–322. [CrossRef]
18. Osterberg, L.; Blaschke, T. Adherence to medication. *N. Engl. J. Med.* **2005**, *353*, 487–497. [CrossRef]
19. Sabaté, E. *Adherence to Long-Term Therapy: Evidence for Action*; World Health Organization: Geneva, Switzerland, 2003; ISBN 9241545992.
20. Evert, A.B.; Dennison, M.; Gardner, C.D.; Garvey, W.T.; Lau, K.H.K.; MacLeod, J.; Mitri, J.; Pereira, R.F.; Rawlings, K.; Robinson, S.; et al. Nutrition Therapy for Adults With Diabetes or Prediabetes: A Consensus Report. *Diabetes Care* **2019**, *42*, 731–754. [CrossRef]
21. World Health Organization. Obesity: Preventing and managing the global epidemic. Report of a WHO consultation. *World Health Organ. Tech. Rep. Ser.* **2000**, *894*, 1–253.
22. Dunkler, D.; Plischke, M.; Leffondré, K.; Heinze, G. Augmented Backward Elimination: A Pragmatic and Purposeful Way to Develop Statistical Models. *PLoS ONE* **2014**, *9*, e113677. [CrossRef] [PubMed]
23. Sun, Y.; You, W.; Almeida, F.; Estabrooks, P.; Davy, B. The Effectiveness and Cost of Lifestyle Interventions Including Nutrition Education for Diabetes Prevention: A Systematic Review and Meta-Analysis. *J. Acad. Nutr. Diet.* **2017**, *117*, 404–421.e36. [CrossRef] [PubMed]
24. Poulimeneas, D.; Grammatikopoulou, M.G.; Bougioukli, V.; Iosifidou, P.; Vasiloglou, M.F.; Gerama, M.A.; Mitsos, D.; Chrysanthakopoulou, I.; Tsigga, M.; Kazakos, K. Diabetes knowledge among Greek Type 2 Diabetes Mellitus patients. *Endocrinol. Nutr.* **2016**, *63*, 320–326. [CrossRef] [PubMed]
25. Digkliou, L.; Kazakos, K.; Kotsa, K.; Goulis, D.G. Disease-specific knowledge and lifestyle behavior in patients with diabetes mellitus. *Obes. Med.* **2016**, *1*, 29–32. [CrossRef]
26. Grammatikopoulou, M.G.; Iosifidou, P.; Maraki, M.I.; Baltzis, D.; Mitsos, D.; Tsigga, M. Nutritional surveillance and diabetes knowledge among patients with type 2 diabetes. *Obes. Med.* **2017**, *5*, 44–49. [CrossRef]
27. Vasconcelos, C.; Almeida, A.; Cabral, M.; Ramos, E.; Mendes, R. The Impact of a Community-Based Food Education Program on Nutrition-Related Knowledge in Middle-Aged and Older Patients with Type 2 Diabetes: Results of a Pilot Randomized Controlled Trial. *Int. J. Environ. Res. Public Health* **2019**, *16*, 2403. [CrossRef]
28. Thuita, A.W.; Kiage, B.N.; Onyango, A.N.; Makokha, A.O. Effect of a nutrition education programme on the metabolic syndrome in type 2 diabetes mellitus patients at a level 5 Hospital in Kenya: "A randomized controlled trial". *BMC Nutr.* **2020**, *6*, 30. [CrossRef]
29. Christensen, N.K.; Steiner, J.; Whalen, J.; Pfister, R. Contribution of Medical Nutrition Therapy and Diabetes Self-Management Education to Diabetes Control as Assessed by Hemoglobin A1c. *Diabetes Spectr.* **2000**, *13*, 72.
30. Barnard, N.D.; Gloede, L.; Cohen, J.; Jenkins, D.J.A.; Turner-McGrievy, G.; Green, A.A.; Ferdowsian, H. A Low-Fat Vegan Diet Elicits Greater Macronutrient Changes, but Is Comparable in Adherence and Acceptability, Compared with a More Conventional Diabetes Diet among Individuals with Type 2 Diabetes. *J. Am. Diet. Assoc.* **2009**, *109*, 263–272. [CrossRef]
31. Han, C.Y.; Chan, C.G.B.; Lim, S.L.; Zheng, X.; Woon, Z.W.; Chan, Y.T.; Bhaskaran, K.; Tan, K.F.; Mangaikarasu, K.; Chong, M.F.-F. Diabetes-related nutrition knowledge and dietary adherence in patients with Type 2 diabetes mellitus: A mixed-methods exploratory study. *Proc. Singapore Healthc.* **2020**, *29*, 81–90. [CrossRef]
32. Cradock, K.A.; Gearóid, G.G.; Gearóid´olaighin, G.; Finucane, F.M.; Mckay, R.; Quinlan, L.R.; Ginis, K.A.M.; Gainforth, H.L. Diet Behavior Change Techniques in Type 2 Diabetes: A Systematic Review and Meta-analysis. *Diabetes Care* **2017**, *40*, 1800–1810. [CrossRef] [PubMed]
33. Møller, G.; Andersen, H.K.; Snorgaard, O. A systematic review and meta-analysis of nutrition therapy compared with dietary advice in patients with type 2 diabetes. *Am. J. Clin. Nutr.* **2017**, *106*, 1394–1400. [CrossRef] [PubMed]

34. Crowley, J.; Ball, L.; Hiddink, G.J. Nutrition in medical education: A systematic review. *Lancet Planet. Health* **2019**, *3*, e379–e389. [CrossRef]
35. Grammatikopoulou, M.G.; Katsouda, A.; Lekka, K.; Tsantekidis, K.; Bouras, E.; Kasapidou, E.; Poulia, K.-A.; Chourdakis, M. Is continuing medical education sufficient? Assessing the clinical nutrition knowledge of medical doctors. *Nutrition* **2018**. [CrossRef]
36. Raynor, H.A.; Davidson, P.G.; Burns, H.; Nadelson, M.D.H.; Mesznik, S.; Uhley, V.; Moloney, L. Medical Nutrition Therapy and Weight Loss Questions for the Evidence Analysis Library Prevention of Type 2 Diabetes Project: Systematic Reviews. *J. Acad. Nutr. Diet.* **2017**, *117*, 1578–1611. [CrossRef] [PubMed]
37. Early, K.B.; Stanley, K. Position Paper Position of the Academy of Nutrition and Dietetics: The Role of Medical Nutrition Therapy and Registered Dietitian Nutritionists in the Prevention and Treatment of Prediabetes and Type 2 Diabetes. *J. Acad. Nutr. Diet.* **2018**, *118*. [CrossRef]
38. Sheils, J.F.; Rubin, R.; Stapleton, D.C. The estimated costs and savings of medical nutrition therapy: The Medicare population. *J. Am. Diet. Assoc.* **1999**, *99*, 428–435. [CrossRef]
39. Pastors, J.G.; Warshaw, H.; Daly, A.; Franz, M.; Kulkarni, K. The evidence for the effectiveness of medical nutrition therapy in diabetes management. *Diabetes Care* **2002**, *25*, 608–613. [CrossRef]
40. Ahmed, A.T.; Karter, A.J.; Warton, E.M.; Doan, J.U.; Weisner, C.M. The relationship between alcohol consumption and glycemic control among patients with diabetes: The Kaiser Permanente Northern California diabetes registry. *J. Gen. Intern. Med.* **2008**. [CrossRef]
41. Steiner, J.L.; Crowell, K.T.; Lang, C.H. Impact of Alcohol on Glycemic Control and Insulin Action. *Biomolecules* **2015**, *5*, 2223. [CrossRef]
42. Searle, G.L.; Shames, D.; Cavalieri, R.R.; Bagdade, J.D.; Porte, D. Evaluation of ethanol hypoglycemia in man: Turnover studies with C-6 14C glucose. *Metabolism* **1974**, *23*, 1023–1035. [CrossRef]
43. Field, J.B.; Williams, H.E.; Mortimore, G.E. Studies on the mechanism of ethanol-induced hypoglycemia. *J. Clin. Investig.* **1963**, *42*, 497–506. [CrossRef] [PubMed]
44. Lang, C.H.; Derdak, Z.; Wands, J.R. Strain-dependent differences for suppression of insulin-stimulated glucose uptake in skeletal and cardiac muscle by ethanol. *Alcohol. Clin. Exp. Res.* **2014**, *38*, 897–910. [CrossRef] [PubMed]
45. Pietraszek, A.; Gregersen, S.; Hermansen, K. Alcohol and type 2 diabetes. A review. *Nutr. Metab. Cardiovasc. Dis.* **2010**, *20*, 366–375. [CrossRef]
46. Hannon, B.A.; Fairfield, W.D.; Adams, B.; Kyle, T.; Crow, M.; Thomas, D.M. Use and abuse of dietary supplements in persons with diabetes. *Nutr. Diabetes* **2020**, *10*, 14. [CrossRef]
47. Campbell, A.P. Diabetes and Dietary Supplements. *Clin. Diabetes* **2010**, *28*, 35–39. [CrossRef]
48. Tripp-Reimer, T.; Choi, E.; Kelley, L.S.; Enslein, J.C. Cultural Barriers to Care: Inverting the Problem. *Diabetes Spectr.* **2001**, *14*, 13–22. [CrossRef]
49. Zeh, P.; Sandhu, H.K.; Cannaby, A.M.; Sturt, J.A. The impact of culturally competent diabetes care interventions for improving diabetes-related outcomes in ethnic minority groups: A systematic review. *Diabet. Med.* **2012**, *29*, 1237–1252. [CrossRef]
50. American Diabetes Association (ADA). 1. Promoting Health and Reducing Disparities in Populations. *Diabetes Care* **2017**, *40*, S6–S10. [CrossRef]
51. Mendes, R.; Martins, S.; Fernandes, L. Adherence to Medication, Physical Activity and Diet in Older Adults With Diabetes: Its Association With Cognition, Anxiety and Depression. *J. Clin. Med. Res.* **2019**, *11*, 583–592. [CrossRef]
52. Marinho, F.S.; Moram, C.B.M.; Rodrigues, P.C.; Leite, N.C.; Salles, G.F.; Cardoso, C.R.L. Treatment Adherence and Its Associated Factors in Patients with Type 2 Diabetes: Results from the Rio de Janeiro Type 2 Diabetes Cohort Study. *J. Diabetes Res.* **2018**, *2018*, 1–8. [CrossRef] [PubMed]
53. Alhariri, A.; Daud, F.; Almaiman, A.; Ayesh, S.; Saghir, M. Diabetes Management Factors associated with adherence to diet and exercise among type 2 diabetes patients in Hodeidah city, Yemen. *Diabetes Manag.* **2017**, *7*, 264–271.
54. Patel, S.; Abreu, M.; Tumyan, A.; Adams-Huet, B.; Li, X.; Lingvay, I. Effect of medication adherence on clinical outcomes in type 2 diabetes: Analysis of the SIMPLE study. *BMJ Open Diabetes Res. Care* **2019**, *7*, e000761. [CrossRef] [PubMed]

55. Jannoo, Z.; Mamode Khan, N. Medication Adherence and Diabetes Self-Care Activities Among Patients With Type 2 Diabetes Mellitus. *Value Health Reg. Issues* **2019**, *18*, 30–35. [CrossRef]
56. Fitzgerald, J.T.; Anderson, R.M.; Davis, W.K. Gender differences in diabetes attitudes and adherence. *Diabetes Educ.* **1995**, *21*, 523–529. [CrossRef] [PubMed]
57. Lin, L.-K.; Sun, Y.; Heng, B.H.; Chew, D.E.K.; Chong, P.-N. Medication adherence and glycemic control among newly diagnosed diabetes patients. *BMJ Open Diabetes Res. Care* **2017**, *5*, e000429. [CrossRef]
58. Raj, G.D.; Hashemi, Z.; Soria Contreras, D.C.; Babwik, S.; Maxwell, D.; Bell, R.C.; Chan, C.B. Adherence to Diabetes Dietary Guidelines Assessed Using a Validated Questionnaire Predicts Glucose Control in Adults With Type 2 Diabetes. *Can. J. Diabetes* **2018**, *42*, 78–87. [CrossRef]
59. Gillani, A.H.; Ahmed, A.B.; Bashir, S.; Ibrahim, M.I.M.; Fang, Y. Associated Factors with Diet and Exercise Compliance and Smoking Habits in Diabetic Patients of Punjab, Pakistan. *Rev. Med. Univ.* **2019**, *20*. [CrossRef]
60. Vitale, M.; Masulli, M.; Calabrese, I.; Rivellese, A.A.; Bonora, E.; Signorini, S.; Perriello, G.; Squatrito, S.; Buzzetti, R.; Sartore, G.; et al. Impact of a mediterranean dietary pattern and its components on cardiovascular risk factors, glucose control, and body weight in people with type 2 diabetes: A real-life study. *Nutrients* **2018**, *10*, 1067. [CrossRef]
61. Thewjitcharoen, Y.; Chotwanvirat, P.; Jantawan, A.; Siwasaranond, N.; Saetung, S.; Nimitphong, H.; Himathongkam, T.; Reutrakul, S. Evaluation of dietary intakes and nutritional knowledge in Thai patients with type 2 diabetes mellitus. *J. Diabetes Res.* **2018**, *2018*. [CrossRef]
62. Ahola, A.J.; Mikkilä, V.; Mäkimattila, S.; Forsblom, C.; Freese, R.; Groop, P.H. Energy and nutrient intakes and adherence to dietary guidelines among Finnish adults with type 1 diabetes. *Ann. Med.* **2012**, *44*, 73–81. [CrossRef] [PubMed]
63. Krige, S.M.; Booley, S.; Levitt, N.S.; Chivese, T.; Murphy, K.; Harbron, J. Dietary Intake and Beliefs of Pregnant Women with Gestational Diabetes in Cape Town, South Africa. *Nutrients* **2018**, *10*, 1183. [CrossRef] [PubMed]
64. Øverby, N.C.; Margeirsdottir, H.D.; Brunborg, C.; Andersen, L.F.; Dahl-Jørgensen, K. The influence of dietary intake and meal pattern on blood glucose control in children and adolescents using intensive insulin treatment. *Diabetologia* **2007**. [CrossRef] [PubMed]
65. García-Molina, L.; Lewis-Mikhael, A.-M.; Riquelme-Gallego, B.; Cano-Ibáñez, N.; Oliveras-López, M.-J.; Bueno-Cavanillas, A. Improving type 2 diabetes mellitus glycaemic control through lifestyle modification implementing diet intervention: A systematic review and meta-analysis. *Eur. J. Nutr.* **2020**, *59*, 1313–1328. [CrossRef] [PubMed]
66. Bulc, M.; Švab, I.; Godycki-Cwirko, M. Factors that affect readiness to change lifestyle: A 22-country survey from primary care. *Eur. J. Gen. Pract.* **2015**, *21*, 33–38. [CrossRef] [PubMed]
67. Livia, B.; Elisa, R.; Claudia, R.; Roberto, P.; Cristina, A.; Emilia, S.T.; Chiara, P.; Alberto, T.; Angelo, R.; Pierpaolo, D.F.; et al. Stage of Change and Motivation to a Healthier Lifestyle before and after an Intensive Lifestyle Intervention. *J. Obes.* **2016**, *2016*, 6421265. [CrossRef]

3

Early-Life Nutritional Programming of Type 2 Diabetes: Experimental and Quasi-Experimental Evidence

Alexander M. Vaiserman

D.F. Chebotarev Institute of Gerontology, Kiev 04114, NAMS, Ukraine; vaiserman@geront.kiev.ua

Abstract: Consistent evidence from both experimental and human studies suggest that inadequate nutrition in early life can contribute to risk of developing metabolic disorders including type 2 diabetes (T2D) in adult life. In human populations, most findings supporting a causative relationship between early-life malnutrition and subsequent risk of T2D were obtained from quasi-experimental studies ('natural experiments'). Prenatal and/or early postnatal exposures to famine were demonstrated to be associated with higher risk of T2D in many cohorts around the world. Recent studies have highlighted the importance of epigenetic regulation of gene expression as a possible major contributor to the link between the early-life famine exposure and T2D in adulthood. Findings from these studies suggest that prenatal exposure to the famine may result in induction of persistent epigenetic changes that have adaptive significance in postnatal development but can predispose to metabolic disorders including T2D at the late stages of life. In this review, quasi-experimental data on the developmental programming of T2D are summarized and recent research findings on changes in DNA methylation that mediate these effects are discussed.

Keywords: type 2 diabetes; famine; natural experiment; quasi-experimental design; epigenetics

---

1. Introduction

Type 2 diabetes (T2D) is one of most common chronic diseases, constituting a serious social and economic problem in modern societies, both developed and developing. It is caused by insulin resistance resulting from decreased activity and enhanced obesity levels that occur with increasing age. T2D is considered to be adult-onset disease, since it typically occurred in middle-age and old adults. Generally, T2D occurs after the age of 40, although it is now increasingly diagnosed in younger patients [1]. Over the last decades, a rapid increase in the prevalence of obesity arising from high caloric diet intake and sedentary lifestyle is driving a global pandemic of T2D. Currently, 415 million people (about 9% of whole adult population) across the world have T2D. During the next decade, the number of T2D patients is expected to rise to around 642 million persons [2]. Obviously, genetics plays a crucial role in driving this disease; however, the dramatic increase in T2D incidence across the globe cannot be explained by genetic factors alone but must involve environmental factors as well [3]. There is increasing experimental and epidemiological evidence that the risk of development of T2D can be influenced not only by actual adult-life environmental conditions (primarily, lifestyle ones) but also by conditions in early life [3]. Convincing evidence that risk of T2D cannot be completely attributable to genetic predisposition and/or adult-life environmental factors was obtained, e.g., in a study on Pima Indian nuclear families in which at least one sibling was born before and other after the mother was diagnosed with T2D [4]. In this research, those siblings conceived after the mother has been diagnosed with T2D were 3.7 times more likely to have T2D compared to siblings born before their mother developed diabetes, even though they lived in similar conditions the rest of their life.

In the present review, we have summarized and discussed findings on this topic from epidemiological studies conducted with quasi-experimental design ('natural experiments').

2. Conceptual Framework for Developmental Nutritional Programming of Type 2 Diabetes (T2D)

According to the developmental programming of health and disease (DOHaD) hypothesis, which has been confirmed by many research findings over the past decades, the physiology and structure of the developing organism may be adapted in response to unfavourable environmental conditions, thereby predisposing it to many pathological conditions in adult life [5]. In particular, poor nutritional environments in early life can induce structural and functional changes in key organs responsible for nutrient regulation, including brain, liver, adipose tissue, muscle and pancreas [6]. Presently, this view is commonly referred to as the 'predictive adaptive response (PAR)' concept [7]. Exposure to adverse environmental factors such as inadequate or unbalanced nutrient supply during in utero development may 'program' for the long term appetite regulation, feeding behaviour, as well as adipose tissue and pancreatic beta cell dysfunction in the developing foetus [3]. As a result of these processes, the foetus may be adapted to adverse nutritional conditions by reducing ability to produce insulin and by occurrence of insulin resistance. According to the 'thrifty phenotype' hypothesis [8], such metabolic adaptation may provide short-term survival benefit in a poor postnatal environment via enhanced capacity to store fat in conditions of irregular availability of food resources, but may predispose the child to T2D development in conditions of food abundance in postnatal life. More specifically, in malnourished conditions when the foetus exhibits poor growth in utero (commonly referred to as intrauterine growth restriction, IUGR), the foetal adaptation to undernutrition is realized by a variety of mechanisms responsible for the energy and glucose metabolism, such as enhanced peripheral insulin sensitivity for glucose utilization, increased hepatic glucose production, lowered insulin sensitivity for protein synthesis in muscle, and impaired pancreatic development [9]. All these mechanisms provide obvious survival benefit for the IUGR foetuses by promoting both energy uptake and utilization, reducing the demand for amino acids and anabolic hormone production, and elevating glucose production to maintain glucose supply to vital organs, primarily the heart and brain. These adaptations lead to asymmetrical growth restriction of the foetus. The muscle and subcutaneous tissues exhibit the most pronounced growth restriction, while the least pronounced growth restriction is peculiar to the growing brain. Collectively, such adaptations allow IUGR foetal tissues to maintain the energy-dependent basal metabolic functions at the expense of body growth in conditions of reduced nutrient supply. If these adaptive modifications persist, or are more readily inducible later in life, they have the potential to promote energy absorption beyond metabolic capability when energy supplies increase, thereby causing insulin resistance, obesity and T2D in adulthood [9]. Among the factors affecting the risk of metabolic dysfunctions, including T2D, in adulthood, the prenatal and early postnatal malnutrition (both under- and overnutrition) is currently believed to be most important [10,11]. It should be noted that in this review only one aspect of malnutrition i.e., undernutrition but not overnutrition will be discussed.

The majority of early population studies used birth weight as a proxy for foetal conditions. From the data obtained, it has been initially concluded that low birth weight is a risk factor for T2D and that birth weight is inversely related to the disease risk [12]. In addition to T2D, low birth weight is a predictor of other T2D-associated conditions and complications later in life, including the impaired body composition and fat distribution [13], fasting lipid profile, blood pressure and insulin resistance [14], life-long activation of the hypothalamic-pituitary-adrenal axis [15], as well as coronary heart disease in adulthood [16]. Several more recent studies, however, found that a relationship between birth weight and risk of T2D is not linear but rather U-shaped, and high birth weight (>4000 g) is associated with an increased risk of T2D to the same extent as low birth weight (<2500 g) [17].

An association between low birth weight and risk of T2D in later life is most thoroughly studied to date. This association is apparently mediated by catch-up growth early in life which is an important risk factor for later T2D. The catch-up growth leads to a disproportionately enhanced rate of fat gain in comparison with lean tissue gain [18]. Such preferential catch-up fat is partly driven by mechanisms of energy conservation operating through suppression of thermogenesis and resulting in the development of thrifty 'catch-up fat' phenotype generally characterized by insulin and leptin resistance. Abnormalities in the growth hormone/insulin-like growth factor-1 (GH/IGF-1) axis, known to play a central role in promoting human growth and development, have been repeatedly reported in children born small for gestational age (SGA) [19]. Such long-lasting abnormalities of IGF-1 in SGA children with catch-up growth are believed to be critically implicated in the association with metabolic disorders, including T2D, later in life.

Precise molecular mechanisms responsible for the nutritional developmental programming of T2D are not yet thoroughly characterized. In many recent studies, compelling evidence was provided that changes in epigenetic regulation of gene expression (heritable alterations in gene function without changes in the nucleotide sequence) is the most plausible mechanism for the link between unfavourable conditions in early development and adverse health outcomes in later life [20]. The main epigenetic mechanisms are DNA methylation and post-translational modifications of histone tails, as well as regulation by non-coding RNAs (microRNAs and long non-coding RNAs) [21]. Evidence for the key role of DNA methylation and other epigenetic mechanisms in mediating the risk of T2D and obesity has been repeatedly documented over the past years [22]. Initial evidence for the role of epigenetic regulation in obesity and T2D has been mainly provided by studies in animal models. These studies reported changes in epigenetic marks in key metabolic tissues following feeding with high-fat diet and by human investigation that demonstrated epigenetic alterations in T2D and obesity candidate genes in obese and/or diabetic persons. More recently, rapid technological advances and price reduction in epigenetic methodologies led to a rapid expansion of epigenome-wide association studies (EWAS) in human epidemiological examinations [22]. These studies clearly demonstrated epigenetic differences between diabetic and healthy control individuals, as well as epigenetic alterations associated with lifestyle interventions.

Within the DOHaD concept, an important point is that throughout embryonic and foetal development, intense epigenetic remodelling takes place that is necessary for the establishment of transcriptional programs responsible for cellular proliferation and differentiation. During these sensitive developmental periods, the epigenome is especially plastic and most sensitive to environmental disturbances [23]. Numerous research findings suggest that early-life adverse events (i.e., insufficient nutrition in utero) might be epigenetically 'imprinted' and 'remembered' decades later, thereby permanently influencing the metabolic phenotype [24]. There is convincing evidence that epigenetic alterations, including those triggered by early-life events and persisting through adulthood, is an important etiological factor in the development of T2D. Changes in DNA methylation and associated changes in patterns of expression of genes implicated in various aspects of glucose metabolism such as β-cell dysfunction, glucose intolerance and insulin resistance, have been shown to be critically involved in the pathogenesis of T2D [25]. The specific DNA methylation markers have been repeatedly identified in peripheral blood and pancreatic islets of the T2D patients (for review, see [26]).

A schematic representation of hypothetical regulatory pathways responsible for developmental nutritional programming of T2D is presented in Figure 1.

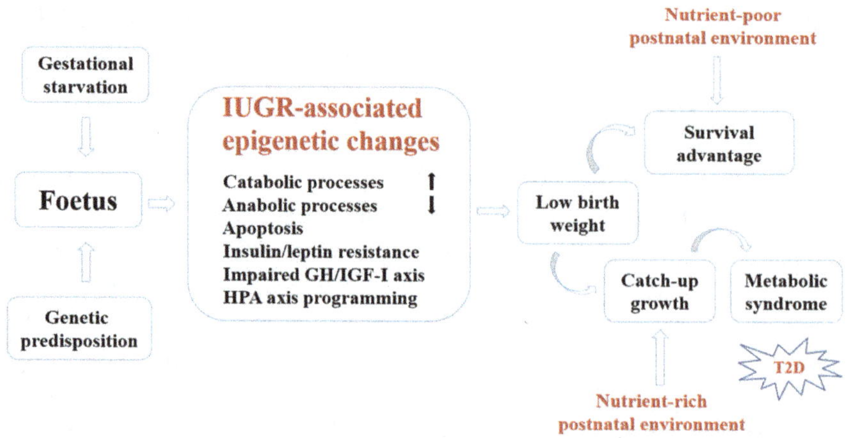

Figure 1. Schematic representation of hypothetical regulatory pathways responsible for developmental programming of type 2 diabetes (T2D) through prenatal undernutrition followed by catch-up growth in a nutrient-rich postnatal environment.

3. Evidence from Animal Models

The bulk of evidence linking intrauterine and/or early postnatal nutrient environment and predisposition to beta-cell failure and T2D in adulthood comes from animal models (for review, see [27–29]). Most of these studies have used rodent models of 50% maternal dietary restriction (DR) during pregnancy to examine the postnatal beta-cell mass development in pups exposed to either normal or restricted post-natal nutritional conditions. Rodents exposed to intrauterine DR and subsequent normal or restricted post-natal nutrition exhibited diminished beta-cell mass both at birth (30%–50% vs. control) and throughout the early postnatal development (50%–70% vs. control) [30–33]. In adulthood, these animals were unable to adaptively enhance beta-cell mass in response to rising metabolic demand and consequent insulin resistance. As a result, they developed diabetic phenotypes characterized by beta-cell failure due to insufficient expansion of beta-cell mass, impaired insulin secretion, glucose intolerance and fasting hyperglycaemia [34,35]. For example, in a study using cross-fostering methodology to isolate effects of selective pre- and postnatal 50% DR [36,37], prenatal DR resulted in a ~50% reduction in beta-cell mass whereas postnatal DR led to decreased body weight, but both beta-cell mass and beta-cell fractional area were increased compared with control animals. These findings indicate that prenatal DR largely determines endocrine cell development while postnatal DR primarily impacts development of the exocrine pancreas [37].

Currently, molecular mechanisms responsible for impaired formation of beta-cell mass in response to early-life DR have come under intensive investigation. Among them, mechanisms of epigenetic regulation of gene activity seem to play a dominant role [38–40]. Inadequate nutritional environment during intrauterine development suppressed transcription of key genes regulating beta-cell development in rats [39]. Feeding pregnant females with a low-protein diet led to hypomethylation of genes encoding glucocorticoid receptor and peroxisome proliferator-activated receptor gamma in the offspring livers. In a rat model, maternal DR also resulted in a significant reduction in the levels of expression of genes encoding key transcription factors regulating embryonic beta-cell development such as the pancreatic and duodenal homeobox 1 (PDX-1) [41,42]. Such changes on the epigenetic level were accompanied by reduced postnatal beta-cell formation and incapability to expand beta-cell mass in response to metabolic stress. Moreover, maternal DR diminished the postnatal expression of *Pdx-1* gene in pancreatic exocrine ducts which is suspected to harbor a putative pool of pancreatic beta-cell progenitor population in adult rodents [39]. Other factors potentially contributing to these effects are hormones that operate during foetal life, such as insulin, insulin-like growth factors, glucocorticoids, as well as some specific molecules such as taurine [43].

In several studies, maternal protein restriction has been shown to program an insulin-resistant phenotype in rodents, especially in consequence of catch-up growth following intrauterine growth restriction. Such mode of malnutrition resulted in expression of early markers of insulin resistance and metabolic disease risk, including alterations in adipocyte cell size and expression levels of several insulin-signalling proteins through post-transcriptional mechanisms [44]. Catch-up growth following maternal protein restriction also favoured the development of obesity in adult male rat offspring [45]. In a mice model, a protein restriction during foetal life followed by catch-up growth led to obesity in adult male mice [46]. These changes were associated with increased relative fat mass, hypercholesterolemia, hyperglycaemia and hyperleptinemia, and also with altered expression profile of several gene-encoding enzymes involved in lipid metabolism.

4. Quasi-Experimental Design in Studying the Developmental Origin of T2D

The experimental research of developmental programming in human populations is not applicable, either for ethical reasons and because the long-term follow-up is required to observe life-long outcomes of early-life experiences. In this regard, an important point is that observational studies in appropriate populations may be realized. The consistent evidence linking the early-life conditions with adult health status has been accumulated from studies conducted with a quasi-experimental design ('natural experiments'), defined as "naturally occurring circumstances in which subsets of the population have different levels of exposure to a supposed causal factor, in a situation resembling an actual experiment where human subjects would be randomly allocated to groups" [47]. Both natural and man-made disasters such as famine obviously provide a lot of advantages to their use in quasi-experimental studies. In the sections below, empirical findings from such a line of research across countries are reviewed.

4.1. Dutch Famine of 1944–1945

The long-term health consequences of the Dutch famine ('Hunger Winter') are the most comprehensively studied up to now. This famine, caused by the Nazi food embargo, affected the western Netherlands from November 1944 to May 1945. Many features of the Dutch famine can be used in a quasi-experimental design. It was a severe famine, distinctly defined in time and place and occurred in a society with a well-developed structure of administrative control. Therefore, exposure to this famine may be accurately defined by region and date of birth in relation to distribution of the food rations and the level of calories consumed. Such circumstances of the Hunger Winter famine provide the opportunity to thoroughly examine the link between inadequate maternal nutrition during particular trimesters of pregnancy and the offspring's adult health status. While a normal daily ration is 2000 kcal and 2500 kcal for women and men, respectively, the average daily rations during the famine were less than 700 kcal [48]. The population that suffered from severe food shortage throughout the famine was generally well fed before and after this period. These features of the Dutch famine provide the researchers with a near-ideal quasi-experimental research design to examine how maternal malnutrition throughout the critical early-life time windows can affect the life-course offspring health status. The prenatal exposure to the Dutch famine has been repeatedly shown to be related to the impaired metabolic phenotypes such as elevated levels of plasma lipids and body mass index (BMI), as well as enhanced risks of obesity and cardiovascular disease (CVD) later in life (for reviews, see refs. [48–50]). Most of these associations have been critically dependent on the timing of exposure. In the majority of the studies, early gestation was found to be the most vulnerable period [48–51]. Childhood and puberty are other sensitive periods with high potential to trigger programming effects. The link between exposure to the Dutch famine between age 0 and 21 years and T2D in adulthood was clearly evident, e.g., from the study by van Abeelen et al. [52]. This relationship was found to be dose-dependent: in those women who self-reported moderate famine exposure during their childhood and young adulthood, the age-adjusted hazard ratio for T2D was 1.36, and in those who reported severe famine exposure, the hazard ratio was 1.64 compared to unexposed women. The exposure to severe malnutrition during the Dutch famine at ages 11−14 was found to be considerably associated with enhanced probability of developing T2D and/or peripheral arterial diseases at ages 60—76 in women, but not in men [53].

In the Dutch famine study, compelling evidence has been obtained that exposure to famine during prenatal development may result in persistent epigenetic changes. Although no relationship between the prenatal exposure to the Dutch famine and overall global DNA methylation in adulthood was observed [54], levels of methylation of particular genes were clearly associated with prenatal famine exposure. The methylation levels of the imprinted gene encoding an insulin-like growth factor 2 (IGF2), known to play a crucial role in human growth and development, have been estimated by Heijmans et al. [51]. This gene was selected for analysis because its methylation marks are stable up to adult age, making *IGF2* gene a good candidate for such a study. In this research, those subjects exposed to the Dutch famine during their early gestation period had much lower *IGF2* methylation levels compared to control unexposed individuals six decades after the hunger exposure. Subsequently, this observation has been extended by examination of a set of 15 additional candidate loci responsible for development of metabolic and cardiovascular phenotypes [55]. Levels of methylation of six of these loci (*GNASAS, IL10, LEP, ABCA1, INSIGF* and *MEG3*) have been found to be associated with prenatal exposure to famine.

4.2. Famines in 20th-Century Austria

Findings from the Dutch Hunger Winter Study on the developmental origin of T2D were also confirmed in populations of other countries such as Austria, which has been subjected to three massive famine episodes during the 20th century. These famines occurred in 1918–19 during the collapse of the Austro-Hungarian Empire; in 1938, following the economic crisis, harvest failure, and food embargo from Nazi Germany; and in 1946–1947 in the period following the Second World War. Based on the data set including 325,000 Austrian diabetic patients, Thurner et al. [56] observed an excess risk of T2D in those persons who were born during or immediately after the periods of these famine episodes. For instance, up to 40% higher chances of having T2D in those individuals who were born in 1919–1921 compared to those who were born in 1918 or 1922, have been revealed in different Austrian regions. Noteworthy, the excess risk of T2D was practically absent in those Austrian provinces that were less affected by hunger. Furthermore, T2D rates have been correlated with the economic wealth of particular regions. The authors concluded that the revealed peaks of T2D in subjects born during and after the periods of severe starvation obviously demonstrate importance of environmental determinants in the period from conception to early childhood, in addition to genetic predisposition and shared life-course factors. These determinants clearly include nutritional triggers, although contribution of other triggering factors such as the famine-related stress and infectious factors, including rodent-borne viral infections, cannot be excluded [57]. The data obtained from this research, however, collectively favoured the hunger hypothesis as the leading explanation for the effects observed [56,58].

4.3. Ukrainian Famine of 1932–1933

The association between prenatal exposure to the famine and adult risk of T2D has been recently examined in large birth cohorts (total n = 43,150) born before, during and after the Great Ukrainian Famine of 1932–1933 ('Holodomor') [59]. This famine was caused by the Soviet Union government's forced agriculture collectivization throughout the early 1930s and led to the deaths from starvation of several million people with a ten-fold increase of mortality rate in April—July 1933 compared to the pre- and post-famine times. The cohorts born during the famine can be well defined with respect to the timing of the famine exposure in relation to the stage of pregnancy and the severity of the famine around the birth date. The odds ratios (ORs) for developing T2D were 1.47 in those individuals born in the first half of 1934 in regions affected by extreme famine, 1.26 in those born in regions with severe famine, and there was no increase (OR = 1.0) in those born in regions with no famine, compared to the births in other examined time periods. The associations observed between T2D and famine exposure around the time of birth have been found to be similar in men and women. The data obtained showed a dose-response relationship between the famine severity during the prenatal development and the risk of T2D later in life, and assumed that early gestational stage is a critical time window for modulating the prenatal environment to affect the adult T2D risk.

4.4. Leningrad Siege of 1941–1944

The Nazi Siege of the Russian city of Leningrad (the modern-day St. Petersburg) in 1941–1944 resulted in extreme hunger and death of about a million city residents. The siege-induced starvation caused an average fall in birth weight of 500–600 g [60]. Follow-up of 549 subjects born in Leningrad before or during the siege, however, demonstrated no effect of intrauterine undernutrition during the siege on dyslipidaemia, glucose intolerance, hypertension and the risk of CVD in adulthood [61,62]. Starvation-exposed individuals demonstrated only evidence for endothelial dysfunction and for a stronger influence of obesity on blood pressure. These results seem to contradict the thrifty phenotype concept since in utero undernutrition was not related to glucose intolerance in adult persons, although prenatal malnutrition influenced their blood pressure and differ from those obtained in the Dutch Hunger Winter study. One possible explanation for such a contradiction suggested by some authors in discussing these data is that the Leningrad siege research was complicated by the fact that malnutrition extended into the postnatal period. Thus, the conflict between prenatal and postnatal environments did not occur [63]. Indeed, in the Netherlands, the food supplies become fully adequate after the war ended, while those babies who were born throughout the Leningrad siege remained malnourished during all their childhood, since this famine lasted for years rather than months and nutrition was poor in subsequent years as well. The association between starvation during the Leningrad siege in early life and the risk of T2D development in adulthood was, however, observed in several more recent studies. Both the increasing incidence and decreasing age of onset of T2D without obesity have been found in women exposed to starvation throughout the Siege of Leningrad during their childhood [64]. This cohort was characterized by higher incidence of conditions associated with metabolic dysregulation such as severe arterial hypertension, and also atherosclerosis of coronary, brain and carotid arteries [65]. Similar health problems were also demonstrated in cohorts exposed to starvation during the Leningrad Siege in their childhood and puberty. Women who were 6−8 years old and men who were 9−15 years old throughout the peak of the famine demonstrated higher systolic blood pressure in their adulthood as compared with unexposed individuals who were born during the same period. Moreover, men exposed to hunger at age 6−8 and 9−15 were characterized by increased mortality from ischaemic heart disease and cerebrovascular disease, respectively [66].

4.5. Chinese Famine of 1959–1961

The long-term health consequences of the Chinese Famine of 1959–1961 ('Great Leap Forward Famine') are extensively studied now. This massive famine occurred in China in the late 1950s following the disastrous social agricultural reform commonly referred to as 'Great Leap Forward.' Over the years of the famine, 25 to 30 million more deaths and 30 to 35 million fewer births were registered in China than would have been expected under normal conditions [67]. In recent years, the Great Leap Forward Famine is the most actively studied famine episode across the globe. It should be noted, however, that one methodological limitation of the Chinese Famine study is that famine exposure data are not available by month; therefore, the periods of the famine exposure cannot be as precisely defined as in the Dutch famine study or in the Ukrainian study.

In most of the studies of long-term impacts of the Chinese Famine, the evidence was obtained that T2D as well as associated metabolic abnormalities were more common among adult Chinese residents born during the famine than among control individuals born after the famine (for a systematic review, see [68]). More specifically, in areas which were severely affected by famine, those subjects who were exposed to famine prenatally had a 3.9-fold enhanced risk of hyperglycaemia in comparison with non-exposed individuals; this difference was not seen in less severely affected regions. Remarkably, the hyperglycaemia risk was 7.6-fold higher in those prenatally exposed subjects who followed an affluent/Western dietary pattern and 6.2-fold higher in those who had a higher economic status in later life compared to non-exposed controls [69]. In a more recent study by Wang et al. [70], both prenatal and childhood exposures to famine were shown to result in higher risk of being diagnosed with T2D in adulthood (1.5-times and 1.8-times, respectively), compared with non-exposed subjects. Individuals residing in Chinese regions with high economic status had a greater T2D risk (OR = 1.46). Interestingly, the timing of association between the famine exposure in early life and adult T2D was gender-specific: an elevated risk of T2D development was evident in the foetal-exposed men (OR = 1.64) and childhood-exposed women (OR = 2.81). These findings were further confirmed in subsequent research by the same authors, where a significant association between the famine severity in the areas of exposure and the risk of T2D was found [71]. Those subjects who were exposed to severe famine during the foetal and childhood periods had substantially higher odds estimates (1.90 and 1.44, respectively). A significant interaction between the level of famine severity in the areas of exposure throughout the prenatal and childhood periods and the risk of T2D in adulthood has been observed. In another Chinese population, 1.44-fold higher risk of T2D development in the middle-childhood-exposed group, and 1.5-fold higher risks of hyperglycaemia in both the middle- and late-childhood-exposed groups were demonstrated compared to the unexposed group [72]. Remarkably, those individuals who experienced more severe famine in childhood had a 38% higher risk of T2D development than those exposed to less severe famine. The revealed association was, however, sex-specific and has been found in women, but not in men. Similar associations have been observed for the hyperglycaemia risk as well.

In a recent study conducted in Suihua, China, the evidence was obtained that programming effects can be manifested not only in those prenatally exposed to famine population (F1 generation), but also in the F2 progeny [73]. In this research, prenatal exposure to the Chinese Famine has been linked to a 1.75-fold enhanced risk of T2D and 1.93-fold enhanced risk of hyperglycaemia in F1 adult offspring in comparison with unexposed individuals. Furthermore, F2 offspring of exposed ancestors had a 2.02-fold elevated risk of adult hyperglycaemia compared to the offspring of non-exposed ancestors. These findings suggest that famine-induced effects can be transmitted via the germ line across generations and translated into increased T2D susceptibility in the descendants of the famine-exposed individuals.

4.6. Nigerian Famine of 1967–1970

The Nigerian Famine (commonly referred to as 'Biafran Famine') occurred during the Nigerian Civil War from 1967–1970. Of the one to three million Nigerians that died during this civil war, only a relatively small fraction (about 10%) had lost their lives from military action as such; the majority died from war-associated starvation [74]. The risks of glucose intolerance, hypertension and being overweight 40 years after prenatal exposure to the Biafran Famine have been assessed in the Hult et al. study [75]. The studied cohorts (total n = 1339) included those adults born before (1965—1967), during (1968—1970), or after (1971—1973) the years of famine. The exposure to famine during both foetal and infant periods has been found to be associated with significantly increased systolic and diastolic blood pressure, higher levels of p-glucose and waist circumference, as well as with substantially elevated risks of systolic hypertension (OR = 2.87), impaired glucose regulation (OR = 1.65) and overweight (OR = 1.41) in adulthood compared with persons who were born after the famine. As in the case of the Chinese Famine study, the lack of birth weight data and the resulting impossibility to separate effects of prenatal and infant famine exposure is the main methodological weakness of Biafran Famine research.

4.7. Holocaust (1939—1945)

The Holocaust was a genocide in which Nazi Germany and its collaborators killed about six million Jews. It was obviously associated with severe starvation and stress in affected populations. The long-term health outcomes of exposure to the Holocaust in the period from preconception to early infancy were determined in recent studies conducted in Israel. The pilot study involved 70 European

Jews born in countries under Nazi rule during the period 1940−1945 (exposed group) and 230 age- and sex-matched Israeli-born individuals (non-exposed group) who self-reported the presence of chronic diseases [76]. The exposed individuals have been shown to be at a higher risk of adult metabolic disturbances, including enhanced BMI, as well as 1.46-fold increased risk of hypertension, 1.58-fold increased risk for dyslipidaemia, and 1.89-fold increased risk of T2D compared to the Holocaust-unexposed group. The associations observed were further confirmed on larger groups of participants (exposed group, n = 653; non-exposed group, n = 433) [77]. The higher risks of hypertension (OR = 1.52), T2D (OR = 1.60), metabolic syndrome (OR = 2.14) and vascular disease (OR = 1.99) were found in exposed individuals.

In general, findings from quasi-experimental studies suggest that exposure to famine in early life may result in serious metabolic disturbances in later life including high risk of development of T2D and associated conditions. The main findings from these studies are summarized in Table 1.

Table 1. Summary of main findings from research on long-term metabolic health consequences of early-life undernutrition exposure

Country	Cause of Starvation	Period	Adult consequence	Ref.
Netherlands ('Dutch Hunger Winter')	Nazi food embargo	1944–1945	Impaired glucose regulation Atherogenic lipid profiles Obesity, CVD T2D Lower *IGF2* methylation Changed methylation of *ABCA1, GNASAS, IL10, LEP, INSIGF* and *MEG3* genes	[78] [79–81] [49,81] [49] [51] [55]
Austria	Empire's collapse Nazi food embargo Post-war period	1918–1919 1938 1946–1947	High risk of T2D	[56]
Ukraine ('Holodomor')	Agriculture collectivization	1932–1933	High risk of T2D	[59]
Russia	Leningrad Siege	1941–1944	Endothelial dysfunction, stronger influence of obesity on blood pressure Increasing incidence of T2D Atherosclerosis, arterial hypertension	[61,62] [64] [65,66]
China ('Great Leap Forward Famine')	Disastrous social agricultural reform	1959–1961	Hyperglycemia High risk of T2D	[69,73] [70–73]
Nigeria ('Biafran Famine')	Civil war	1967–1970	Increased blood pressure, higher levels of p-glucose, increased waist circumference, overweight, high risks of impaired glucose regulation and systolic hypertension	[75]
Europe ('Holocaust')	Nazi genocide	1939–1945	Enhanced BMI, hypertension, dyslipidemia, high risk of T2D and CVD	[76,77]
Spain	Seasonal malnutrition	1935−1954	High systolic blood pressure	[82]
United Kingdom	Seasonal malnutrition	1920–1930	Obesity	[83]
Canada	Seasonal malnutrition	1943–1995	Obesity	[84]
United Kingdom	Seasonal malnutrition	1924–1943	Dyslipidaemia, insulin resistance and CVD	[85]
USA	Seasonal malnutrition	1968–1995	High risk of T2D	[86]
Netherlands	Seasonal malnutrition	1920–1948	High risk of T2D	[87]
Ukraine	Seasonal malnutrition	1930–1938	High risk of T2D	[88]

5. Seasonality of Birth

Season of birth also can be used in quasi-experimental design to examine associations between early-life exposures, including nutritional ones, and later-life health outcomes. In this regard, month of birth presents a good instrument which may help to examine later-life outcomes of early-life exposures independently of life-course factors. This is true since decades ago there were strong seasonal variations in nutrition, especially in developing countries. Availability of cereals, vegetables, fruits and animal proteins varied significantly according to the season. Such differences in the supply of high-quality food might potentially affect the foetal and neonatal development depending on the month of gestation [89]. Other potentially confounding factors for early-life disease programming, including temperature [90], infections [91], sunlight/photoperiod and, correspondingly, production of melatonin and vitamin D [92], as well as maternal lifestyle factors such as physical activity [93] and alcohol intake [94], also tend to vary seasonally.

Seasonal conditions around the period of birth were demonstrated to significantly determine birth weight: lower birth weights were observed in the winter-born newborns and higher birth weights in summer-born newborns in the high- and low-latitude areas, while the summer birth was associated with relatively lower birth weight in the mid-latitude areas [95]. Seasonality of birth has been demonstrated for many aspects of metabolic syndrome, including high systolic blood pressure [82], obesity [83,84] and also dyslipidaemia, insulin resistance and CVD [85]. The seasonal pattern of birth for childhood autoimmune (type 1) diabetic patients was reported repeatedly (see, e.g., [96]), while the seasonality of birth for T2D adult persons was observed only in a few studies. Seasonal patterns of birth were reported, e.g., in small-sample studies conducted in 155 adolescent African-Americans [86] and in 282 T2D patients in the Netherlands [87].

By now, the most obvious evidence for the seasonality of birth in T2D patients is provided in research conducted in a Ukrainian population [88]. In this study, those persons who were born in April—May had increased risk ofT2D development. In the climatic conditions characteristic of the Ukraine, these subjects ordinarily experienced their foetal life in the nutritionally marginal period from late autumn to early spring and passed the first neonatal months during the relatively plentiful season. In contrast, a decreased risk of T2D was observed in those born in November–December. In these individuals, prenatal development in a nutritionally abundant season would have been followed by early infancy in the season of relative scarcity (winter—spring). The first scenario is apparently more high-risk for developing T2D than the second one. These results are highly consistent with the thrifty phenotype hypothesis [8]. Interestingly, the seasonal pattern of birth was found to be very similar in type 1 and type 2 diabetic patients, suggesting shared early-life etiological causation for both disorders [97]. In more recent research by Jensen et al. [98], no evidence for seasonality of birth in Danish patients with T2D was found. The authors assumed that difference in effects obtained in Denmark and the Ukraine may be explained by standards of living or by differences in latitude between the countries. Indeed, as the seasonal variations in both weather and nutrition were much more pronounced in the Ukraine than in Denmark throughout the study periods, and since the Ukraine belonged to low-income countries for much of that time, its residents experienced more pronounced seasonal extremes than those experienced by people in a more prosperous country like Denmark.

In discussing the mechanistic basis for seasonal programming of adult-life diseases, one possible explanation is that seasonal factors operating around the time of birth may trigger persistent epigenetic changes that have adaptive significance in postnatal development but can predispose to chronic disorders, including the metabolic ones, at the late stages of life. The evidence for the link between season of birth and long-term changes in DNA methylation has been recently obtained in the epigenome-wide association study (EWAS) by Lockett et al. [99], where methylation at 92 CpG dinucleotides was significantly associated with season of birth. The networks related to the cell cycle, development and apoptosis have been found to be enriched among these differentially methylated CpG sites. Interestingly, the season-associated methylation patterns have been mainly absent in newborns, suggesting they arise postnatally. Although these findings were not confirmed in a more recent study by Dugué et al. [100], they, however, suggest that changes in DNA methylation might mechanistically underlie the season-of-birth effects on the risk of later-life disease.

6. Conclusions and Future Perspectives

A trend to a dramatic enhancing incidence of type 2 diabetes (T2D) has become a serious problem across the globe over the past years. Metabolic syndrome and associated risk factors including dyslipidaemia, high blood pressure, impaired glucose metabolism and T2D, are among the main causes of death in both developed and developing countries. It is widely believed that risk of T2D is mostly dependent on genetic and lifestyle factors. However, while genetic factors undoubtedly contribute to an individual susceptibility to development of obesity and T2D, the identified genetic variants can explain only part of the variation [22,101]. Recent research has demonstrated that exposure to unfavourable environmental stimuli early in life is another important determinant of the risk of T2D and associated conditions during adulthood. Findings from several of these studies suggest that epigenetic regulation can be largely contributed to development of these pathological states. Since epigenetic marks may persist long term, epigenetic modifications triggered by environmental cues throughout early sensitive stages may lead to lasting effects on the metabolic functioning, thereby affecting the risk of metabolic disorders, including T2D, later in life [102]. Prenatal and early postnatal nutrition is likely the most important factor affecting the adult risk of T2D. For instance, in studying the long-term health consequences of prenatal exposure to the Dutch famine, a link between poor nutritional intake in utero and impaired glucose regulation, atherogenic lipid profiles and obesity later in life, all known to be risk factors for development of T2D, has been demonstrated [99–102]. Therefore, it is not surprising that cohorts exposed to starvation in early life are at higher risk of T2D development. In a very recent meta-analysis of 11 published articles, a strong association between exposure to famine in early life and increased risk of T2D in adulthood has been observed (the pooled relative risk (RR) = 1.38, 95% CI 1.17−1.63) [103]. RRs for T2D development were 1.36 (95% CI 1.12−1.65) for cohorts exposed prenatally or during the early postnatal period and 1.40 (95% CI 0.98−1.99) for those cohorts who were exposed in their childhood compared to the unexposed cohorts.

In offspring born to mothers experiencing famine during pregnancy, differential methylation of genes, including those associated with pathogenesis of T2D, has been observed [51,55], indicating the importance of epigenetic processes in mediating early-life starvation exposure to the risk of later-life disease. Data from reviewed studies suggest that a focus on very early periods of gestation, and perhaps even on the periconceptional period, should constitute the next frontier for prevention of T2D over the human life course [104]. Some studies have indicated that epigenetic effects contributing to development of T2D could be transmitted across several generations. In research conducted in the Överkalix, an isolated community in northern Sweden, the possibility of transgenerational effects on T2D mortality was observed. The transgenerational consequences of the ancestors' nutrition throughout their slow growth period (SGP, aged 9 to 12 years), the period of higher susceptibility of organism to environmental influences, were investigated in cohorts born in this region in 1890, 1905 and 1920 [105,106]. In case of limited food availability in the father's SGP, then the descendant cardiovascular mortality was low, while the overeating of paternal grandfathers led to a four-fold increase in diabetes mortality in the offspring [105,106]. Such transgenerational effects were shown to be gender-specific: the paternal grandmother's nutrient supply affected granddaughters' mortality risk, while the paternal grandfather's nutrient supply was shown to be associated with the mortality risk in grandsons [106]. Since epigenetic alterations unlike genetic mutations are potentially reversible [107], pharmacological modification of epigenetic marks contributing to T2D development can provide a novel approach to prevention and treatment of T2D and associated disorders.

Acknowledgments: The author would like to thank Oksana Zabuga for the technical assistance in preparing this manuscript.

References

1. Wilmot, E.; Idris, I. Early onset type 2 diabetes: Risk factors, clinical impact and management. *Ther. Adv. Chronic. Dis.* **2014**, *5*, 234–244. [CrossRef] [PubMed]
2. Jaacks, L.M.; Siegel, K.R.; Gujral, U.P.; Narayan, K.M. Type 2 diabetes: A 21st century epidemic. *Best Pract. Res. Clin. Endocrinol. Metab.* **2016**, *30*, 331–343. [CrossRef] [PubMed]
3. Nielsen, J.H.; Haase, T.N.; Jaksch, C.; Nalla, A.; Søstrup, B.; Nalla, A.A.; Larsen, L.; Rasmussen, M.; Dalgaard, L.T.; Gaarn, L.W. Impact of fetal and neonatal environment on beta cell function and development of diabetes. *Acta Obstet. Gynecol. Scand.* **2014**, *93*, 1109–1122. [CrossRef] [PubMed]

4. Dabelea, D.; Hanson, R.L.; Lindsay, R.S.; Pettitt, D.J.; Imperatore, G.; Gabir, M.M.; Roumain, J.; Bennett, P.H.; Knowler, W.C. Intrauterine exposure to diabetes conveys risks for type 2 diabetes and obesity: A study of discordant sibships. *Diabetes* **2000**, *49*, 2208–2211. [CrossRef] [PubMed]
5. Eriksson, J.G. Developmental Origins of Health and Disease—From a small body size at birth to epigenetics. *Ann. Med.* **2016**, *48*, 456–467. [CrossRef] [PubMed]
6. Kim, J.B. Dynamic cross talk between metabolic organs in obesity and metabolic diseases. *Exp. Mol. Med.* **2016**, *48*, e214. [CrossRef] [PubMed]
7. Nettle, D.; Bateson, M. Adaptive developmental plasticity: What is it, how can we recognize it and when can it evolve? *Proc. Biol. Sci.* **2015**, *282*, 20151005. [CrossRef] [PubMed]
8. Hales, C.N.; Barker, D.J. Type 2 (non-insulin-dependent) diabetes mellitus: The thrifty phenotype hypothesis. 1992. *Int. J. Epidemiol.* **2013**, *42*, 1215–1222. [CrossRef] [PubMed]
9. Thorn, S.R.; Rozance, P.J.; Brown, L.D.; Hay, W.W., Jr. The intrauterine growth restriction phenotype: Fetal adaptations and potential implications for later life insulin resistance and diabetes. *Semin. Reprod. Med.* **2011**, *29*, 225–236. [CrossRef] [PubMed]
10. Carolan-Olah, M.; Duarte-Gardea, M.; Lechuga, J. A critical review: Early life nutrition and prenatal programming for adult disease. *J. Clin. Nurs.* **2015**, *24*, 3716–3729. [CrossRef] [PubMed]
11. Tarry-Adkins, J.L.; Ozanne, S.E. Nutrition in early life and age-associated diseases. *Ageing Res. Rev.* **2016**. [CrossRef] [PubMed]
12. Whincup, P.H.; Kaye, S.J.; Owen, C.G.; Huxley, R.; Cook, D.G.; Anazawa, S.; Barrett-Connor, E.; Bhargava, S.K.; Birgisdottir, B.E.; Carlsson, S.; et al. Birth weight and risk of type 2 diabetes: A systematic review. *J. Am. Med. Assoc.* **2008**, *300*, 2886–2897. [PubMed]
13. Kensara, O.A.; Wootton, S.A.; Phillips, D.I.; Patel, M.; Jackson, A.A.; Elia, M.; Hertfordshire Study Group. Fetal programming of body composition: Relation between birth weight and body composition measured with dual-energy X-ray absorptiometry and anthropometric methods in older Englishmen. *Am. J. Clin. Nutr.* **2005**, *82*, 980–987. [PubMed]
14. Morrison, K.M.; Ramsingh, L.; Gunn, E.; Streiner, D.; van Lieshout, R.; Boyle, M.; Gerstein, H.; Schmidt, L.; Saigal, S. Cardiometabolic health in adults born premature with extremely low birth weight. *Pediatrics* **2016**, *138*. [CrossRef] [PubMed]
15. Stirrat, L.I.; Reynolds, R.M. The effect of fetal growth and nutrient stresses on steroid pathways. *J. Steroid. Biochem. Mol. Biol.* **2016**, *160*, 214–220. [CrossRef] [PubMed]
16. Frankel, S.; Elwood, P.; Sweetnam, P.; Yarnell, J.; Smith, G.D. Birthweight, body-mass index in middle age and incident coronary heart disease. *Lancet* **1996**, *348*, 1478–1480. [CrossRef]
17. Harder, T.; Rodekamp, E.; Schellong, K.; Dudenhausen, J.W.; Plagemann, A. Birth weight and subsequent risk of type 2 diabetes: A meta-analysis. *Am. J. Epidemiol.* **2007**, *165*, 849–857. [CrossRef] [PubMed]
18. Dulloo, A.G. Thrifty energy metabolism in catch-up growth trajectories to insulin and leptin resistance. *Best Pract. Res. Clin. Endocrinol. Metab.* **2008**, *22*, 155–171. [CrossRef] [PubMed]
19. Cho, W.K.; Suh, B.K. Catch-up growth and catch-up fat in children born small for gestational age. *Korean J. Pediatr.* **2016**, *59*, 1–7. [CrossRef] [PubMed]
20. Ong, T.P.; Ozanne, S.E. Developmental programming of type 2 diabetes: Early nutrition and epigenetic mechanisms. *Curr. Opin. Clin. Nutr. Metab. Care* **2015**, *18*, 354–360. [CrossRef] [PubMed]
21. Paluch, B.E.; Naqash, A.R.; Brumberger, Z.; Nemeth, M.J.; Griffiths, E.A. Epigenetics: A primer for clinicians. *Blood Rev.* **2016**, *30*, 285–295. [CrossRef] [PubMed]
22. Van Dijk, S.J.; Tellam, R.L.; Morrison, J.L.; Muhlhausler, B.S.; Molloy, P.L. Recent developments on the role of epigenetics in obesity and metabolic disease. *Clin. Epigenet.* **2015**, *7*, 66. [CrossRef] [PubMed]
23. Vaiserman, A. Epidemiologic evidence for association between adverse environmental exposures in early life and epigenetic variation: A potential link to disease susceptibility? *Clin. Epigenet.* **2015**, *7*, 9. [CrossRef] [PubMed]
24. Geraghty, A.A.; Lindsay, K.L.; Alberdi, G.; McAuliffe, F.M.; Gibney, E.R. Nutrition during pregnancy impacts offspring's epigenetic status—Evidence from human and animal studies. *Nutr. Metab. Insights* **2016**, *8*, 41–47. [CrossRef] [PubMed]
25. Alam, F.; Islam, M.A.; Gan, S.H.; Mohamed, M.; Sasongko, T.H. DNA methylation: An epigenetic insight into Type 2 diabetes mellitus. *Curr. Pharm. Des.* **2016**, *22*, 4398–4419. [CrossRef] [PubMed]

26. Kwak, S.H.; Park, K.S. Recent progress in genetic and epigenetic research on type 2 diabetes. *Exp. Mol. Med.* **2016**, *48*, e220. [CrossRef] [PubMed]
27. Green, A.S.; Rozance, P.J.; Limesand, S.W. Consequences of a compromised intrauterine environment on islet function. *J. Endocrinol.* **2010**, *205*, 211–224. [CrossRef] [PubMed]
28. Portha, B.; Chavey, A.; Movassat, J. Early-life origins of type 2 diabetes: Fetal programming of the beta-cell mass. *Exp. Diabetes Res.* **2011**. [CrossRef] [PubMed]
29. Pinney, S.E. Intrauterine growth retardation–A developmental model of type 2 diabetes. *Drug Discov Today Dis. Models.* **2013**, *10*, e71–e77. [CrossRef] [PubMed]
30. Dumortier, O.; Blondeau, B.; Duvillie, B.; Reusens, B.; Breant, B.; Remacle, C. Different mechanisms operating during different critical time-windows reduce rat fetal beta cell mass due to a maternal low-protein or low-energy diet. *Diabetologia* **2007**, *50*, 2495–2503. [CrossRef] [PubMed]
31. Garofano, A.; Czernichow, P.; Breant, B. In utero undernutrition impairs rat beta-cell development. *Diabetologia* **1997**, *40*, 1231–1234. [CrossRef] [PubMed]
32. Garofano, A.; Czernichow, P.; Breant, B. Beta-cell mass and proliferation following late fetal and early postnatal malnutrition in the rat. *Diabetologia* **1998**, *41*, 1114–1120. [CrossRef] [PubMed]
33. Petrik, J.; Reusens, B.; Arany, E.; Remacle, C.; Coelho, C.; Hoet, J.J.; Hill, D.J. A low protein diet alters the balance of islet cell replication and apoptosis in the fetal and neonatal rat and is associated with a reduced pancreatic expression of insulin-like growth factor-II. *Endocrinology* **1999**, *140*, 4861–4873. [CrossRef] [PubMed]
34. Garofano, A.; Czernichow, P.; Breant, B. Effect of ageing on beta-cell mass and function in rats malnourished during the perinatal period. *Diabetologia* **1999**, *42*, 711–718. [CrossRef] [PubMed]
35. Blondeau, B.; Garofano, A.; Czernichow, P.; Breant, B. Age-dependent inability of the endocrine pancreas to adapt to pregnancy: A long-term consequence of perinatal malnutrition in the rat. *Endocrinology* **1999**, *140*, 4208–4213. [CrossRef] [PubMed]
36. Thamotharan, M.; Shin, B.C.; Suddirikku, D.T.; Thamotharan, S.; Garg, M.; Devaskar, S.U. GLUT4 expression and subcellular localization in the intrauterine growth-restricted adult rat female offspring. *Am. J. Physiol. Endocrinol. Metab.* **2005**, *288*, E935–E947. [CrossRef] [PubMed]
37. Matveyenko, A.V.; Singh, I.; Shin, B.C.; Georgia, S.; Devaskar, S.U. Differential effects of prenatal and postnatal nutritional environment on ss-cell mass development and turnover in male and female rats. *Endocrinology* **2010**, *151*, 5647–5656. [CrossRef] [PubMed]
38. Ong, T.P.; Ozanne, S.E. Developmental programming of type 2 diabetes: Early nutrition and epigenetic mechanisms. *Curr. Opin. Clin. Nutr. Metab Care* **2015**, *18*, 354–360. [CrossRef] [PubMed]
39. Simmons, R.A. Developmental origins of diabetes: The role of epigenetic mechanisms. *Curr Opin. Endocrinol. Diabetes Obes.* **2007**, *14*, 13–16. [CrossRef] [PubMed]
40. Simmons, R.A. Developmental origins of adult disease. *Pediatr. Clin. N. Am.* **2009**, *56*, 449–466. [CrossRef] [PubMed]
41. Blondeau, B.; Avril, I.; Duchene, B.; Breant, B. Endocrine pancreas development is altered in foetuses from rats previously showing intra-uterine growth retardation in response to malnutrition. *Diabetologia* **2002**, *45*, 394–401. [CrossRef] [PubMed]
42. Park, J.H.; Stoffers, D.A.; Nicholls, R.D.; Simmons, R.A. Development of type 2 diabetes following intrauterine growth retardation in rats is associated with progressive epigenetic silencing of Pdx1. *J. Clin. Investig.* **2008**, *118*, 2316–2324. [CrossRef] [PubMed]
43. Reusens, B.; Theys, N.; Dumortier, O.; Goosse, K.; Remacle, C. Maternal malnutrition programs the endocrine pancreas in progeny. *Am. J. Clin. Nutr.* **2011**, *94*, 1824S–1829S. [CrossRef] [PubMed]
44. Berends, L.M.; Fernandez-Twinn, D.S.; Martin-Gronert, M.S.; Cripps, R.L.; Ozanne, S.E. Catch-up growth following intra-uterine growth-restriction programmes an insulin-resistant phenotype in adipose tissue. *Int. J. Obes. (Lond.)* **2013**, *37*, 1051–1057. [CrossRef] [PubMed]
45. Bieswal, F.; Ahn, M.T.; Reusens, B.; Holvoet, P.; Raes, M.; Rees, W.D.; Remacle, C. The importance of catch-up growth after early malnutrition for the programming of obesity in male rat. *Obesity (Silver Spring)* **2006**, *14*, 1330–1343. [CrossRef] [PubMed]
46. Bol, V.V.; Delattre, A.I.; Reusens, B.; Raes, M.; Remacle, C. Forced catch-up growth after fetal protein restriction alters the adipose tissue gene expression program leading to obesity in adult mice. *Am. J. Physiol. Regul. Integr. Comp. Physiol.* **2009**, *297*, R291–R299. [CrossRef] [PubMed]

47. Last, J.M. *A Dictionary of Epidemiology*, 3rd ed.; Oxford University Press: New York, NY, USA, 1995.
48. Heijmans, B.T.; Tobi, E.W.; Lumey, L.H.; Slagboom, P.E. The epigenome: Archive of the prenatal environment. *Epigenetics* **2009**, *4*, 526–531. [CrossRef] [PubMed]
49. Lumey, L.H.; Stein, A.D.; Susser, E. Prenatal famine and adult health. *Annu. Rev. Public Health* **2011**, *32*, 237–262. [CrossRef] [PubMed]
50. Roseboom, T.J.; Painter, R.C.; van Abeelen, A.F.; Veenendaal, M.V.; de Rooij, S.R. Hungry in the womb: What are the consequences? Lessons from the Dutch famine. *Maturitas* **2011**, *70*, 141–145. [CrossRef] [PubMed]
51. Heijmans, B.T.; Tobi, E.W.; Stein, A.D.; Putter, H.; Blauw, G.J.; Susser, E.S.; Slagboom, P.E.; Lumey, L.H. Persistent epigenetic differences associated with prenatal exposure to famine in humans. *Proc. Natl Acad. Sci. USA* **2008**, *105*, 17046–17049. [CrossRef] [PubMed]
52. Van Abeelen, A.F.; Elias, S.G.; Bossuyt, P.M.; Grobbee, D.E.; van der Schouw, Y.T.; Roseboom, T.J.; Uiterwaal, C.S. Famine exposure in the young and the risk of type 2 diabetes in adulthood. *Diabetes* **2012**, *61*, 2255–2260. [CrossRef] [PubMed]
53. Portrait, F.; Teeuwiszen, E.; Deeg, D. Early life undernutrition and chronic diseases at older ages: The effects of the Dutch famine on cardiovascular diseases and diabetes. *Soc. Sci. Med.* **2011**, *73*, 711–718. [CrossRef] [PubMed]
54. Lumey, L.H.; Terry, M.B.; Delgado-Cruzata, L.; Liao, Y.; Wang, Q.; Susser, E.; McKeague, I.; Santella, R.M. Adult global DNA methylation in relation to pre-natal nutrition. *Int. J. Epidemiol.* **2012**, *41*, 116–123. [CrossRef] [PubMed]
55. Tobi, E.W.; Lumey, L.H.; Talens, R.P.; Kremer, D.; Putter, H.; Stein, A.D.; Slagboom, P.E.; Heijmans, B.T. DNA methylation differences after exposure to prenatal famine are common and timing- and sex-specific. *Hum. Mol. Genet.* **2009**, *18*, 4046–4053. [CrossRef] [PubMed]
56. Thurner, S.; Klimek, P.; Szell, M.; Duftschmid, G.; Endel, G.; Kautzky-Willer, A.; Kasper, D.C. Quantification of excess risk for diabetes for those born in times of hunger, in an entire population of a nation, across a century. *Proc. Natl. Acad. Sci. USA* **2013**, *110*, 4703–4707. [CrossRef] [PubMed]
57. Klitz, W.; Niklasson, B. Viral underpinning to the Austrian record of type 2 diabetes? *Proc. Natl. Acad. Sci. USA* **2013**, *110*, E2750. [CrossRef] [PubMed]
58. Thurner, S.; Klimek, P.; Szell, M.; Duftschmid, G.; Endel, G.; Kautzky-Willer, A.; Kasper, D.C. Reply to Klitz and Niklasson: Can viral infections explain the cross-sectional Austrian diabetes data? *Proc. Natl. Acad. Sci. USA* **2013**, *110*, E2751. [CrossRef]
59. Lumey, L.H.; Khalangot, M.D.; Vaiserman, A.M. Association between type 2 diabetes and prenatal exposure to the Ukraine famine of 1932–33: A retrospective cohort study. *Lancet Diabetes Endocrinol.* **2015**, *3*, 787–794. [CrossRef]
60. Sparén, P.; Vågerö, D.; Shestov, D.B.; Plavinskaja, S.; Parfenova, N.; Hoptiar, V.; Paturot, D.; Galanti, M.R. Long term mortality after severe starvation during the siege of Leningrad: Prospective cohort study. *Br. Med. J.* **2004**, *328*, 11. [CrossRef] [PubMed]
61. Stanner, S.A.; Bulmer, K.; Andrès, C.; Lantseva, O.E.; Borodina, V.; Poteen, V.V.; Yudkin, J.S. Does malnutrition in utero determine diabetes and coronary heart disease in adulthood? Results from the Leningrad siege study: A cross sectional study. *Br. Med. J.* **1997**, *315*, 1342–1348. [CrossRef] [PubMed]
62. Stanner, S.A.; Yudkin, J.S. Fetal programming and the Leningrad Siege study. *Twin Res.* **2001**, *4*, 287–292. [CrossRef] [PubMed]
63. Bateson, P. Fetal experience and good adult design. *Int. J. Epidemiol.* **2001**, *30*, 928–934. [CrossRef] [PubMed]
64. Khoroshinina, L.P.; Zhavoronkova, N.V. Starving in childhood and diabetes mellitus in elderly age. *Adv. Gerontol.* **2008**, *21*, 684–687.
65. Khoroshinina, L.P. Peculiarities of somatic diseases in people of middle and old age survived Leningrad siege at childhood. *Adv. Gerontol.* **2004**, *14*, 55–65. (In Russian)
66. Koupil, I.; Shestov, D.B.; Sparén, P.; Plavinskaja, S.; Parfenova, N.; Vågerö, D. Blood pressure, hypertension and mortality from circulatory disease in men and women who survived the siege of Leningrad. *Eur. J. Epidemiol.* **2007**, *22*, 223–234. [CrossRef] [PubMed]
67. Jowett, A.J. The demographic responses to famine: The case of China 1958-61. *GeoJournal* **1991**, *23*, 135–146. [CrossRef] [PubMed]
68. Li, C.; Lumey, L.H. Exposure to the Chinese famine of 1959–61 in early life and current health conditions: A systematic review and meta-analysis. *Lancet* **2016**, *388*, S63. [CrossRef]

69. Li, Y.; He, Y.; Qi, L.; Jaddoe, V.W.; Feskens, E.J.; Yang, X.; Ma, G.; Hu, F.B. Exposure to the Chinese famine in early life and the risk of hyperglycemia and type 2 diabetes in adulthood. *Diabetes* **2010**, *59*, 2400–2406. [CrossRef] [PubMed]
70. Wang, N.; Wang, X.; Han, B.; Li, Q.; Chen, Y.; Zhu, C.; Chen, Y.; Xia, F.; Cang, Z.; Zhu, C.; et al. Is exposure to famine in childhood and economic development in adulthood associated with diabetes? *J. Clin. Endocrinol. Metab.* **2015**, *100*, 4514–4523. [CrossRef] [PubMed]
71. Wang, N.; Cheng, J.; Han, B.; Li, Q.; Chen, Y.; Xia, F.; Jiang, B.; Jensen, M.D.; Lu, Y. Exposure to severe famine in the prenatal or postnatal period and the development of diabetes in adulthood: An observational study. *Diabetologia* **2017**, *60*, 262–269. [CrossRef] [PubMed]
72. Wang, J.; Li, Y.; Han, X.; Liu, B.; Hu, H.; Wang, F.; Li, X.; Yang, K.; Yuan, J.; Yao, P.; et al. Exposure to the Chinese Famine in childhood increases type 2 diabetes risk in adults. *J. Nutr.* **2016**, *146*, 2289–2295. [CrossRef] [PubMed]
73. Li, J.; Liu, S.; Li, S.; Feng, R.; Na, L.; Chu, X.; Wu, X.; Niu, Y.; Sun, Z.; Han, T.; et al. Prenatal exposure to famine and the development of hyperglycemia and type 2 diabetes in adulthood across consecutive generations: A population-based cohort study of families in Suihua, China. *Am. J. Clin. Nutr.* **2016**, *105*, 221–227. [CrossRef] [PubMed]
74. Miller, J.P. Medical relief in the Nigerian civil war. *Lancet* **1970**, *760*, 1330–1334. [CrossRef]
75. Hult, M.; Tornhammar, P.; Ueda, P.; Chima, C.; Bonamy, A.K.; Ozumba, B.; Norman, M. Hypertension, diabetes and overweight: Looming legacies of the Biafran famine. *PLoS ONE* **2010**, *5*, e13582. [CrossRef] [PubMed]
76. Bercovich, E.; Keinan-Boker, L.; Shasha, S.M. Long-term health effects in adults born during the Holocaust. *Isr. Med. Assoc. J.* **2014**, *16*, 203–207. [PubMed]
77. Keinan-Boker, L.; Shasha-Lavsky, H.; Eilat-Zanani, S.; Edri-Shur, A.; Shasha, S.M. Chronic health conditions in Jewish Holocaust survivors born during World War II. *Isr. Med. Assoc. J.* **2015**, *17*, 206–212. [PubMed]
78. Watson, P.E.; McDonald, B.W. Seasonal variation of nutrient intake in pregnancy: Effects on infant measures and possible influence on diseases related to season of birth. *Eur. J. Clin. Nutr.* **2007**, *61*, 1271–1280. [CrossRef] [PubMed]
79. Flouris, A.D.; Spiropoulos, Y.; Sakellariou, G.J.; Koutedakis, Y. Effect of seasonal programming on fetal development and longevity: Links with environmental temperature. *Am. J. Hum. Biol.* **2009**, *21*, 214–216. [CrossRef] [PubMed]
80. Finch, C.E.; Crimmins, E.M. Inflammatory exposure and historical changes in human life-spans. *Science* **2004**, *305*, 1736–1739. [CrossRef] [PubMed]
81. Lowell, W.E.; Davis, G.E., Jr. The light of life: Evidence that the sun modulates human lifespan. *Med. Hypotheses.* **2008**, *70*, 501–507. [CrossRef] [PubMed]
82. Smith, A.D.; Crippa, A.; Woodcock, J.; Brage, S. Physical activity and incident type 2 diabetes mellitus: A systematic review and dose-response meta-analysis of prospective cohort studies. *Diabetologia* **2016**, *59*, 2527–2545. [CrossRef] [PubMed]
83. Vaiserman, A.M. Early-life exposure to substance abuse and risk of type 2 diabetes in adulthood. *Curr. Diabetes Rep.* **2015**, *15*, 48. [CrossRef] [PubMed]
84. Chodick, G.; Flash, S.; Deoitch, Y.; Shalev, V. Seasonality in birth weight: Review of global patterns and potential causes. *Hum. Biol.* **2009**, *81*, 463–477. [CrossRef] [PubMed]
85. Banegas, J.R.; Rodríguez-Artalejo, F.; de la Cruz, J.J.; Graciani, A.; Villar, F.; del Rey-Calero, J. Adult men born in spring have lower blood pressure. *J. Hypertens.* **2000**, *18*, 1763–1766. [CrossRef] [PubMed]
86. Phillips, D.I.; Young, J.B. Birth weight: Climate at birth and the risk of obesity in adult life. *Int. J. Obes. Relat. Metab. Disord.* **2000**, *24*, 281–287. [CrossRef] [PubMed]
87. Wattie, N.; Ardern, C.I.; Baker, J. Season of birth and prevalence of overweight and obesity in Canada. *Early Hum. Dev.* **2008**, *84*, 539–547. [CrossRef] [PubMed]
88. Lawlor, D.A.; Davey-Smith, G.; Mitchell, R.; Ebrahim, S. Temperature at birth, coronary heart disease, and insulin resistance: Cross sectional analyses of the British women's heart and health study. *Heart* **2004**, *90*, 381–388. [CrossRef] [PubMed]
89. Laron, Z.; Lewy, H.; Wilderman, I.; Casu, A.; Willis, J.; Redondo, M.J.; Libman, I.; White, N.; Craig, M. Seasonality of month of birth of children and adolescents with type 1 diabetes mellitus in homogenous and heterogeneous populations. *Isr. Med. Assoc. J.* **2005**, *7*, 381–384. [PubMed]

90. Grover, V.; Lipton, R.B.; Sclove, S.L. Seasonality of month of birth among African American children with diabetes mellitus in the City of Chicago. *J. Pediatr. Endocrinol. Metab.* **2004**, *17*, 289–296. [CrossRef] [PubMed]
91. Jongbloet, P.H.; van Soestbergen, M.; van der Veen, E.A. Month-of-birth distribution of diabetics and ovopathy: A new aetiological view. *Diabetes Res.* **1988**, *9*, 51–58. [PubMed]
92. Vaiserman, A.M.; Khalangot, M.D.; Carstensen, B.; Tronko, M.D.; Kravchenko, V.I.; Voitenko, V.P.; Mechova, L.V.; Koshel, N.M.; Grigoriev, P.E. Seasonality of birth in adult type 2 diabetic patients in three Ukrainian regions. *Diabetologia* **2009**, *52*, 2665–2667. [CrossRef] [PubMed]
93. Vaiserman, A.M.; Khalangot, M.D. Similar seasonality of birth in type 1 and type 2 diabetes patients: A sign for common etiology? *Med. Hypotheses* **2008**, *71*, 604–605. [CrossRef] [PubMed]
94. Jensen, C.B.; Zimmermann, E.; Gamborg, M.; Heitmann, B.L.; Baker, J.L.; Vaag, A.; Sørensen, T.I. No evidence of seasonality of birth in adult type 2 diabetes in Denmark. *Diabetologia* **2015**, *58*, 2045–2050.
95. Lockett, G.A.; Soto-Ramírez, N.; Ray, M.A.; Everson, T.M.; Xu, C.J.; Patil, V.K.; Terry, W.; Kaushal, A.; Rezwan, F.I.; Ewart, S.L.; et al. Association of season of birth with DNA methylation and allergic disease. *Allergy* **2016**, *71*, 1314–1324. [CrossRef] [PubMed]
96. Dugué, P.A.; Geurts, Y.M.; Milne, R.L.; Lockett, G.A.; Zhang, H.; Karmaus, W.; Holloway, J.W. Is there an association between season of birth and blood DNA methylation in adulthood? *Allergy* **2016**, *71*, 1501–1504. [CrossRef] [PubMed]
97. Desiderio, A.; Spinelli, R.; Ciccarelli, M.; Nigro, C.; Miele, C.; Beguinot, F.; Raciti, G.A. Epigenetics: Spotlight on type 2 diabetes and obesity. *J. Endocrinol. Investig.* **2016**, *39*, 1095–1103. [CrossRef] [PubMed]
98. Sterns, J.D.; Smith, C.B.; Steele, J.R.; Stevenson, K.L.; Gallicano, G.I. Epigenetics and type II diabetes mellitus: Underlying mechanisms of prenatal predisposition. *Front. Cell Dev. Biol.* **2014**, *2*, 15. [CrossRef] [PubMed]
99. Ravelli, A.C.; van der Meulen, J.H.; Michels, R.P.; Osmond, C.; Barker, D.J.; Hales, C.N.; Bleker, O.P. Glucose tolerance in adults after prenatal exposure to famine. *Lancet* **1998**, *351*, 173–177. [CrossRef]
100. Lussana, F.; Painter, R.C.; Ocke, M.C.; Buller, H.R.; Bossuyt, P.M.; Roseboom, T.J. Prenatal exposure to the Dutch famine is associated with a preference for fatty foods and a more atherogenic lipid profile. *Am. J. Clin. Nutr.* **2008**, *88*, 1648–1652. [CrossRef] [PubMed]
101. Lumey, L.H.; Stein, A.D.; Kahn, H.S.; Romijn, J.A. Lipid profiles in middle-aged men and women after famine exposure during gestation: The dutch hunger winter families study. *Am. J. Clin. Nutr.* **2009**, *89*, 1737–1743. [CrossRef] [PubMed]
102. Roseboom, T.; de Rooij, S.; Painter, R. The Dutch famine and its long-term consequences for adult health. *Early Hum. Dev.* **2006**, *82*, 485–491. [CrossRef] [PubMed]
103. Liu, L.; Wang, W.; Sun, J.; Pang, Z. Association of famine exposure during early life with the risk of type 2 diabetes in adulthood: A meta-analysis. *Eur. J. Nutr.* **2016**. [CrossRef] [PubMed]
104. Gillman, M.W. Prenatal famine and developmental origins of type 2 diabetes. *Lancet Diabetes Endocrinol.* **2015**, *3*, 751–752. [CrossRef]
105. Kaati, G.; Bygren, L.O.; Edvinsson, S. Cardiovascular and diabetes mortality determined by nutrition during parents' and grandparents' slow growth period. *Eur. J. Hum. Genet.* **2002**, *10*, 682–688. [CrossRef] [PubMed]
106. Pembrey, M.E. Male-line transgenerational responses in humans. *Hum. Fertil. (Camb.)* **2010**, *13*, 268–271. [CrossRef] [PubMed]
107. Vaiserman, A.M.; Pasyukova, E.G. Epigenetic drugs: A novel anti-aging strategy? *Front. Genet.* **2012**, *3*, 224. [CrossRef] [PubMed]

4

Vitamin D Status, Calcium Intake and Risk of Developing Type 2 Diabetes: An Unresolved Issue

Araceli Muñoz-Garach [1,2,*], Beatriz García-Fontana [3,4] and Manuel Muñoz-Torres [3,4,5,6,*]

1 Department of Endocrinology and Nutrition, Virgen de la Victoria University Hospital, Institute of Biomedical Research in Malaga (IBIMA), 29010 Malaga, Spain
2 Instituto de Salud Carlos III, 28029 Madrid, Spain
3 Instituto de Investigación Biosanitaria (Ibs.GRANADA), 18106 Granada, Spain; bgfontana@fibao.es
4 Centro de Investigación Biomédica en Red sobre Fragilidad y Envejecimiento Saludable (CIBERFES), Instituto de Salud Carlos III, 28029 Madrid, Spain
5 Unidad de Gestión Clínica Endocrinología y Nutrición, Hospital Universitario San Cecilio de Granada, Avenida de la Innovacion, 18016 Granada, Spain
6 Department of Medicine, University of Granada, 18016 Granada, Spain
* Correspondence: aracelimugar@gmail.com (A.M.-G.); mmt@mamuto.es (M.M.-T.)

Abstract: The relationship between vitamin D status, calcium intake and the risk of developing type 2 diabetes (T2D) is a topic of growing interest. One of the most interesting non-skeletal functions of vitamin D is its potential role in glucose homeostasis. This possible association is related to the secretion of insulin by pancreatic beta cells, insulin resistance in different tissues and its influence on systemic inflammation. However, despite multiple observational studies and several meta-analyses that have shown a positive association between circulating 25-hydroxyvitamin D concentrations and the risk of T2D, no randomized clinical trials supplementing with different doses of vitamin D have confirmed this hypothesis definitively. An important question is the identification of what 25-hydroxyvitamin D levels are necessary to influence glycemic homeostasis and the risk of developing T2D. These values of vitamin D can be significantly higher than vitamin D levels required for bone health, but the currently available data do not allow us to answer this question adequately. Furthermore, a large number of observational studies show that dairy consumption is linked to a lower risk of T2D, but the components responsible for this relationship are not well established. Therefore, the importance of calcium intake in the risk of developing T2D has not yet been established. Although there is a biological plausibility linking the status of vitamin D and calcium intake with the risk of T2D, well-designed randomized clinical trials are necessary to answer this important question.

Keywords: calcium intake; dairy products; vitamin D; type 2 diabetes

---

1. Introduction

The incidence of type 2 diabetes (T2D) has increased substantially in recent years related, in part, to higher obesity rates. If current trends continue, more than 642 million people will have diabetes by 2040 [1]. The management and early treatment of T2D are essential to prevent further complications involving loss of quality of life and premature death. It is unclear whether vitamin D deficiency might be contributing to an increased T2D risk [2].

A vast body of evidence associates vitamin D deficiency and T2D [3]. This relationship could be mediated by the direct and indirect effects of vitamin D on glucose homeostasis such as insulin secretion, insulin sensitivity, and systemic inflammation. However, the extent of this relationship and its clinical relevance are not well established.

There is no doubt that vitamin D homeostasis is of vital importance for skeletal health, being especially important for bone mineralization. Moreover, recent studies have demonstrated that low vitamin D concentrations are related to other pathologic conditions that were not previously considered, such as insulin resistance, T2D, metabolic syndrome and cardiovascular diseases. All these diseases could potentially be developed as a result of vitamin D deficiency [4–6].

Moreover, the evidence linking milk and, in particular, calcium intake, insulin secretion and sensitivity has been related to glucose homeostasis in both prediabetes and T2D [7–9]. However, the main clinical studies conducted to confirm this hypothesis have yielded inconsistent results.

The aim of the present review is to summarize the recent evidence linking vitamin D and calcium intake with the development of T2D. We also analyzed different intervention studies with vitamin D supplements to determine their influence on glucose metabolism.

2. Methods

We performed a comprehensive literature search on PubMed to identify peer-reviewed articles on vitamin D levels, vitamin D supplementation and T2D prevention published until December 2018. Search strategies included the following search terms: vitamin D intake, vitamin D supplementation, 25-hydroxyvitamin D, calcium intake, dairy products, type 2 diabetes, impaired glucose tolerance, insulin resistance, insulin sensitivity, β-cell function and obesity.

We included a selection of papers that showed original research articles in humans mainly published in English language; and also in vitro studies, observational studies (prospective and retrospective) and randomized controlled trials. Finally, we reviewed meta-analyses published compiling all studies information. Priority was given to larger studies (according to number of patients included) and the most recent and strongest available evidence.

3. Vitamin D and Type 2 Diabetes (T2D)

3.1. *Vitamin D Physiology and Glucose Homeostasis*

The term vitamin D includes vitamin D2 or ergocalciferol and vitamin D3 or cholecalciferol. The main metabolites of vitamin D, which differ in their hydroxylation patterns, are 25-hydroxyvitamin D or calcidiol (25(OH)D) and 1,25-dihydroxyvitamin D3 or calcitriol (1,25-$(OH)_2D_3$). In humans, the main sources of vitamin D come from the skin through the cutaneous synthesis of vitamin D3 and, to a lesser extent, from the intake of foods rich in vitamins D2 and D3 or supplements. Circulating vitamin D is bound to vitamin D binding protein (DBP), which transports it to the liver, there vitamin D25-hydroxylase converts it to 25(OH)D. This form of vitamin D is primarily converted to the most biologically active form, 1,25-$(OH)_2D$ in the kidneys. This transformation is done by the enzyme 25-hydroxyvitamin D-1alpha-hydroxylase (CYP27B1). The presence of CYP27B1 in multiple tissues, which also express the vitamin D receptor, suggests that vitamin D could play an important function beyond bone metabolism.

Both in vitro and in vivo studies have reported that vitamin D may play an important role in the maintenance of pancreatic beta cell function [10]. This effect could have different explanations. It could be induced by the activation of the vitamin D receptor (VDR) located in pancreatic beta cells. It was suggested by the study results that showed how mice without VDR have impaired insulin secretion [11] and the addition of calcitriol to the culture medium stimulated pancreatic islets and resulted in an increased insulin secretion [12].

Moreover, vitamin D could also influence insulin secretion by regulating calcium channel opening and closure. Calcitriol participates as a chemical messenger interacting with different receptors regulating calcium flux in beta cells. They are located on the phospholipid layers of plasma membranes. For this reason, calcium is essential for appropriate insulin secretion by pancreatic beta cells; and, therefore, insufficient vitamin D may alter normal insulin secretion through alterations in calcium flux in beta cells [13,14]. In relation to this, the regulation of the protein calbindin, a calcium-binding protein, by vitamin D may be another mechanism influencing insulin secretion. In addition, preclinical studies show that vitamin D can reduce the hyperactivity of the renin angiotensin system and, thus, improve the functioning of beta cells (Leung PS. Nutrients 2016 [15]).

An adequate vitamin D level can also improve insulin resistance pathways associated with diabetes. It is caused mainly by alterations in calcium flux and concentration through the cell membranes of insulin-responsive tissues [16]. The regulation of extracellular and intracellular calcium concentrations may promote dephosphorylation of glucose transporter-4 (GLUT-4) driving a reduced insulin-stimulated glucose transport [14,17]. The 1,25-$(OH)_2D$ stimulates the expression of insulin receptors and, therefore, stimulates insulin sensitivity. In addition, calcitriol could also improve insulin sensitivity activating the peroxisome proliferator-activated delta receptor (PPAR-d), a transcription factor that regulates fatty acids metabolism in adipose tissue and the skeletal muscle. Another interesting study indicates that insulin resistance may also be reduced by the specific effects of calcitriol on hepatic lipid synthesis and glucose output, and on skeletal muscle (Leung PS. Nutrients 2016 [15]).

Calcitriol has a central role in a wide variety of metabolic pathways by binding to the VDR, and the measurement of its substrate 25(OH)D is an important marker for health risks. This receptor is expressed in an assortment of cells, such as in the pancreatic beta cells of Langerhans, but also in liver, adipose tissue, and muscle cells [18,19]. The VDR and the 1α-hydroxylase, the enzyme catalyzing calcidiol to calcitriol conversion, are expressed in primary preadipocytes and recently differentiated adipocytes [18]. Therefore, in vitro studies suggest that calcitriol regulates the growth of human adipose tissue and its remodeling. Moreover, fat tissue is a storage site for vitamin D [19]. In contrast, a higher body mass index (BMI) is associated to lower vitamin D concentrations. Vitamin D, a fat-soluble hormone, is sequestered in the adipose tissue and, consequently, only small quantities are available for circulation [20]. On the other hand, since the concentrations of 25(OH)D in serum and adipose tissue are closely related, obesity can reduce serum 25(OH)D through volumetric dilution and the distribution of 25(OH)D in larger fat volumes [21].

Vitamin D could also shorten the effects of chronic inflammation, and it is well established that it plays a key role in the pathogenesis of T2D. Therefore, 1,25$(OH)_2D$ can protect against cytokine-induced apoptosis of beta cells directly regulating the activity and expression of cytokines, with an improvement in insulin sensitivity [22]. Moreover, vitamin D demonstrated the possibility of deactivating inflammatory cytokines associated with insulin resistance and promoting calbindin expression which involves protection from apoptosis [23]. Finally, vitamin D also reduces the accumulation of advanced glycation products in experimental studies [24]. These products are related with the development of T2D complications and have been involved with insulin resistance. Vitamin D functions related with glucose homeostasis are summarized in Figure 1.

3.2. Vitamin D Status and Its Relationship with T2D in Cross-Sectional and Longitudinal Studies

Serum 25(OH)D concentrations have been noticed to be inversely associated with glucose homeostasis, insulin resistance, and beta cell function, and forecast lower risks of both metabolic syndrome and T2D [25–27]. Numerous clinical studies have associated vitamin D inadequacy with the development of insulin resistance in different populations, not only in adults [5,28,29] but also in children [30,31].

Consistently, higher baseline 25(OH)D levels have been found to predict better beta cell function and lower glucose levels in subjects at risk for T2D in longitudinal studies [32]. Overall, data from observational studies strongly support an association between low vitamin D status and incidence of T2D [33–35].

We discuss in this review the largest prospective articles and some meta-analyses. In 2013, Afzal et al. published the results of a prospective cohort study that included 9841 participants who were followed-up for 29 years. They found an odds ratio for the development of T2D of 1.5 (95% CI 1.33–1.70) between the lowest and the highest quartile of 25(OH)D [34]. More recently, Park et al. measured 25(OH)D levels in a cohort of 903 adults without diabetes or prediabetes, these authors found an inverse dose-response association between 25(OH)D concentration and risk of diabetes. They proposed a target 25(OH)D of 50 ng/mL; higher than the levels previously suggested in other studies, in the attempt to influence and reduce the incidence rate of diabetes [36]. These data are consistent with the levels published recently by Avila-Rubio et al. in postmenopausal women, the authors link values of 25(OH)D > 45 ng/dL in these women with better glycemic indexes measured by homeostasis model assessment (HOMA) [37].

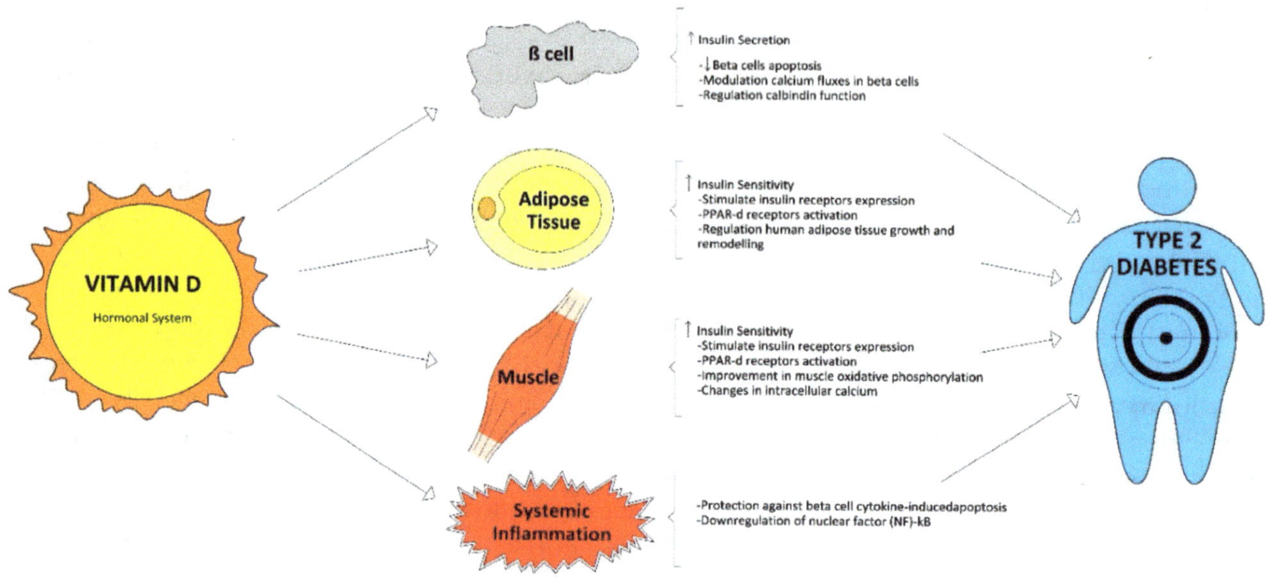

Figure 1. Vitamin D functions related with glucose homeostasis.

The multicenter EPIC-InterAct study measured plasma 25(OH)D metabolites: non-epimeric 25(OH)D_3, 3-epi-25(OH)D_3 and 25(OH)D_2. They identified that plasma non-epimeric 25(OH)D_3 (the major component of total 25(OH)D) was inversely associated with T2D, whereas 3-epi-25(OH)D_3 was positively associated with the incidence of T2D, and 25(OH)D_2 was not associated with T2D [38].

Another large cohort was The Melbourne cohort, which included a sample of middle-aged Australians, the authors showed how vitamin D status was inversely associated with the risk of T2D and, apparently, this association cannot be explained by reverse causality [39]. If the association was due to reverse causality, then a much stronger association would be expected to be observed in the first few years of follow-up.

The meta-analysis conducted by Song et al. included 21 observational studies with 76,220 subjects in total; the authors found a 38% lesser risk of developing T2D in the highest baseline reference category of 25(OH)D compared to the lowest one (95% CI 0.54–0.70) [35].

Despite the consistency of these results, all these were observational studies and estimation of causality cannot be completely excluded because of residual confounding agents.

3.3. Vitamin D Supplementation and Risk of T2D: Randomized Trials and Meta-Analysis

In the last decade, more than ten well-designed, randomized trials evaluated the effect of vitamin D3 supplementation on glucose homeostasis in subjects at risk for T2D and showed inconsistent results. We have selected a set of studies that analyzed outcomes related to the objectives of this review. Table 1 summarizes the main results of these studies.

In Table 1 we describe the main findings of the largest trials. Sollid et al. [40] conducted a randomized clinical trial with approximately 500 prediabetes subjects comparing vitamin D versus placebo for the prevention of T2D. They supplemented with 20,000 IU cholecalciferol weekly and after one year, no significant differences were reported between those receiving vitamin D and those taking placebo in any of the glycemic or inflammatory markers and blood pressure, regardless of baseline serum 25(OH)D concentrations.

Two years later, Forouhi et al. [41] compared, in another large randomized trial including 340 prediabetes or at risk of developing T2D subjects, the effect of supplementation with cholecalciferol or ergocalciferol (both 100,000 IU/month) versus placebo, for four months. Prediabetes was estimated by the Cambridge Risk Score [42]. Despite vitamin D supplementation, neither ergocalciferol or cholecalciferol, resulted in increased $25(OH)D_2$ and $25(OH)D_3$ concentrations. No differences in HbA1c concentration were found between groups. It is important to point out that only half of the subjects had concentrations of 25(OH)D < 50 nmol/L. This data could influence the results.

Their results are in accordance with previous findings by Davidson et al. [43]. They supplemented a cohort of Latino and African Americans subjects with prediabetes and hypovitaminosis D at baseline for one year. They used a cholecalciferol dose sufficient to raise serum 25(OH)D levels into the upper-normal range versus placebo. They did not find any effect on insulin secretion or sensitivity, nor the proportion of subjects who developed T2D or whose oral glucose tolerance test became normal [43].

However, it is possible to find some positive effect on glycemic markers in some studies. In this line, Gagnon et al. [44] reported when they performed a post hoc analysis only including subjects with prediabetes, an improvement in insulin sensitivity indices was observed. Previously, they gave a supplement of calcium carbonate 1200 mg and cholecalciferol 2000–6000 UI daily to subjects with glucose intolerance or recently diagnosed diabetes, but they found no effect on insulin sensitivity or secretion, and beta cell function. So, despite most clinical randomized trials failing to show a favorable effect of vitamin D supplementation on glycemic control, insulin sensitivity indices, and incident T2D [40,41,43–49] in subjects at risk for diabetes, there is some interesting evidence supporting a beneficial effect of vitamin D on beta cell function. In fact, Mitri et al. [50] reported in 2011 a significant improvement in insulin secretion in 92 prediabetic subjects who were overweight or obese and at risk for T2D. They were supplemented with cholecalciferol 2000 IU daily and calcium carbonate versus placebo for four months. An important restriction of the above described studies is that they were not designed specifically to assess glycemic homeostasis and the results found correspond to post hoc analyses.

Although not being designed for this purpose, we would like to point out the results of the Vitamin D and Omega-3 Trial (VITAL), a large-scale trial that evaluated high-dose vitamin D supplementation. This study was designed to evaluate the effect of supplementation with vitamin D on incidence of invasive cancer or cardiovascular events versus placebo. Overall, no differences were found between groups. However, in Black Americans a potential beneficial effect was found in cancer mortality [51].

A recent meta-analysis conducted by Rafiq et al. showed an inverse relationship; higher vitamin D concentrations were associated with lower BMI in T2D patients and non-diabetic subjects at risk for T2D. But this association was more pronounced in T2D patients. Moreover, the correlation was directly associated to the BMI quartiles, so the highest BMI quartile had the greatest correlations in both populations, both T2D and non-diabetic [52].

Tang et al. [53] published a meta-analysis and did not find an effect of vitamin D supplementation on the incidence of T2D. However, the authors suggested a possible dose-response effect of vitamin D supplementation to improve glucose and insulin metabolism among non-diabetic adults. They postulated a possible benefit of taking vitamin D supplements in higher doses for the primary prevention of T2D.

In summary, studies were very heterogeneous in terms of design, duration, and type of supplement administered and participants characteristics. It is noteworthy that adherence to the treatment would have played a major role in arguing these results.

Table 1. Clinical trials investigating the association between vitamin D supplementation and risk of type 2 diabetes (T2D).

Study, Year	Country	Population Characteristics (Mean age/age range (years))	Type of Treatment	*N*	Duration (months)	Main Outcomes
LeBlanc et al. D2d Research Group [54] 2018	US	Prediabetes (59)	4000 IU D3/day vs. placebo	2423	36	Not yet published
Forouhi et al. [41] 2016	UK	Prediabetes IFG or IGT or positive diabetes risk score (53)	100,000 IU D2/month or 100,000 IU D3/month vs. placebo	340	4	No effect on HbA1c Improve pulse wave velocity (arterial stiffness)
Wagner et al. [48] 2016	Sweden	Prediabetes or diet-controlled T2D (67.3)	30,000 IU D3/week vs. placebo	44	2	No difference in insulin secretion/sensitivity, beta cell function and glucose tolerance
Tuomainen et al. [47] 2015	Finland	Prediabetes (65.7)	40 µg/day D3 or 80 µg/day D3 vs. placebo	68	5	No difference in glucose homeostasis indicators
Gagnon et al. [44] 2014	Australia	25(OH)D $\leq$ 22ng/ml at risk of T2D (54)	1200 mg calcium carbonate and 2000–6000 IU D3 day to target vs. placebo	95	6	No difference in insulin secretion/sensitivity and beta cell function. A post-hoc analysis (only prediabetes patients) showed a significant beneficial effect on insulin sensitivity
Sollid et al. [40] 2014	Norway	Prediabetes IFG or IGT (62.1)	20,000 IU D3/week vs. placebo	511	12	No difference in insulin secretion/sensitivity or glucose metabolism, blood pressure or lipid status
Oosterwerff et al. [45] 2014	Netherlands	Overweight, vitamin D deficient subjects with prediabetes (20–65)	Calcium carbonate 500 mg (all) and 1200 IU D3/day vs. placebo	130	4	No difference in insulin sensitivity or in beta cell function. A post hoc analysis (without diabetes patients at baseline), showed a significant increase in the insulinogenic index when 25(OH)D $\geq$ 60 nmol/L
Salehpour et al. [46] 2013	Iran	Healthy, overweight/obese women (38)	25 µg D3/daily vs. placebo	77	4	No effect in glycemic indices (glucose, insulin, HbA1c and HOMA-IR)
Belenchia et al. [55] 2013	US	Obese adolescents (14.1)	4000 IU D3/day vs. placebo	35	6	Significant effect in fasting insulin, HOMA-IR and leptin-to-adiponectin ratio
Davidson et al. [43] 2013	US	Prediabetes and hypovitaminosis D (52)	D3 to target serum 25OHD level of 65–90 ng/mL vs. placebo	109	12	No difference on insulin secretion/sensitivity or the development of diabetes or returning to normal glucose tolerance
Mitri et al. [50] 2011	US	Prediabetes. At risk for T2D (57)	2000 IU D3/daily vs. calcium carbonate 800 mg/day	92	4	Significant effect in beta cell function and improvement in insulin secretion
von Hurst et al. [49] 2010	New Zealand	Insulin resistance, At risk for T2D 25(OH)D < 20 ng/mL (23–68)	4000 IU D3/day vs. placebo	81	6.5	No difference in FPG, HOMA2%B; C-peptide Significant effect on HOMA IR and insulin
Jorde et al. [56] 2010	Norway	Overweight/Obese; At risk for T2D (21–70)	500 mg calcium/day plus D3, 40,000 IU/week or D3 20,000 IU/week	438	48	No difference in HbA1c, FPG, 2hs PG and HOMA-IR

BMI, body mass index; FPG, fasting plasma glucose; 2hs PG, 2 h plasma glucose; HbA1c, glycated hemoglobin; HOMA-IR, homeostatic model assessment of insulin resistance; IFG, impaired fasting glucose; IGT, impaired glucose tolerance; NAFLD, nonalcoholic fatty liver disease; T2D, type 2 diabetes.

Recently, the design of a new randomized clinical trial has been published and its results can be a determinant in clarifying many of the uncertainties that exist today. The D2d is a large randomized clinical trial (including participants from 22 sites across the U.S.) hypothesizing that supplementation with vitamin D_3 daily lowers risk of diabetes in adults with prediabetes [54]. This trial meets people with a large spectrum of diabetes risk, more convenient for testing the underlying hypothesis. D2d trial results are expected to answer two important questions: whether vitamin D supplementation is useful to prevent T2D and how the 2010 expanded American Diabetes Association (ADA) criteria for prediabetes would impact the natural history of this state previous to diabetes.

3.4. New Thresholds for the Relationship between Vitamin D and T2D

An important question that has arisen is what 25(OH)D levels are necessary to influence glycemic homeostasis and the risk of developing T2D. Three recent studies have addressed this issue. Von Horst et al. found that optimal 25OHD concentrations for reducing IR were around 50 ng/dL in a randomized controlled study with 81 Asian women [49]. Avila Rubio et al. [37], in a study conducted in women with postmenopausal osteoporosis, suggested that the established goal of reaching a level of 25(OH)D > 30 ng/mL was insufficient to improve glucose metabolism in these population. The data from this study indicates that 25(OH)D > 45 ng/mL are necessary to achieve this goal. These data are consistent with a cohort study of 903 adults of 12 years of duration in non-diabetic population where reaching values of 25(OH)D > 50 ng/mL contributed to reach the maximum benefits to reduce the risk of incident diabetes [36]. Therefore, it is important to establish what 25(OH)D values are necessary to achieve and, even more importantly, maintain all the potential benefits of vitamin D. The currently available studies do not allow us to answer this question with certainty.

4. Calcium Intake and T2D

4.1. Mechanistic Studies

To introduce and understand the underlying mechanisms that associates dairy products, and specifically dairy components to T2D prevention, mechanistic studies are essential. Further to the structural role it plays in the skeleton, calcium is an essential electrolyte necessary for many critical biological functions. Calcium may play a key role in a wide range of functions related to glucose homeostasis. Calcium regulates insulin-mediated intracellular processes in specific tissues that respond to insulin, participates in the secretory function of pancreatic beta cells and the phosphorylation of insulin receptors. Calcium also down-regulates specific regulatory genes encoding pro-inflammatory cytokines involved in insulin resistance [16,57,58].

Insulin secretion is a calcium-dependent process [59]. Calcium is vital for insulin-mediated intracellular processes in those tissues responding to insulin, such as muscle and fat [16,58]. There is a narrow range of intracellular calcium concentration needed for optimal insulin-mediated functions. When there are changes in intracellular calcium concentrations in insulin-responsive tissues there is a contribution to peripheral insulin resistance [17,60] through a dysregulated insulin signal transduction cascade that leads to a lower glucose transporter activity.

An appropriate range of intracellular calcium concentration is also required for some insulin-mediated activities in tissues such as liver, adipose and skeletal muscle [57]. It is important to maintain relatively low intracellular calcium concentrations in these target tissues to have a beneficial effect on the insulin signal transduction cascade [60] and peripheral insulin sensitivity. In addition, low intracellular calcium attenuates cytokine-induced inflammation, augments vascular relaxation and inhibits platelet aggregation. It is important to keep in mind that calcium intake should be considered in the context of dairy intake and dairy products, which provide other important nutrients besides calcium.

4.2. *Dairy Intake and T2D Risk*

Increased dairy consumption is linked to a lower risk of T2D, but the components responsible for this relation are not well established. The participation of specific dairy products needs to be further studied. Calcium, vitamin D, dairy fat, partially hydrogenated oils and specifically *trans*-palmitoleic acid (a natural *trans* fatty acid found in dairy) are key dairy components. They have been proposed to influence some metabolic pathways implicated in T2D prevention.

We have previously reported how vitamin D has a direct effect on insulin secretion by binding to VDR in pancreatic beta cells and an indirect effect via the regulation of extracellular calcium [13,57,61]. Moreover, vitamin D effects include suppression of inappropriately prolonged inflammation by modulating secretion of proinflammatory cytokines.

The role of dietary intake of *trans*-palmitoleic acid has been related to an improvement in metabolic regulation, hepatic and peripheral insulin resistance, and suppression of hepatic de novo lipogenesis and lower levels of fasting insulin, C-reactive protein, triglycerides and blood pressure [62,63]. In the Cardiovascular Health Study (CHS), a prospective cohort analysis about dietary intake of *trans*-palmitoleic acid, a significantly and considerably 62% risk reduction of incident T2D has been shown [62]. Moreover, the Multi-Ethnic Study of Atherosclerosis (MESA), a prospective cohort study, showed that dietary intake of *trans*-palmitoleic acid was associated with a 48% lower risk of incident T2D [63].

When we analyzed the fat content of dairy, the evidence finds relatively consistent results regarding a beneficial role of fatty dairy products in T2D prevention. But, to date, the differences between low, regular or high fat dairy are less known. Kratz et al. described in a systematic review including observational studies [64], that the majority of studies analyzed inversely associated high-fat dairy products with obesity, T2D and cardiometabolic disease, either significantly or insignificantly. However, the meta-analysis of cohort studies conducted by Alhazmi et al. showed that saturated fat ingestion was not associated with a risk of T2D [65].

Furthermore, the evidence regarding the role of specific types of dairy products (milk, yogurt, and cheese) is even more limited. Milk has generally been posted as part of total dairy consumption, and scarce evidence exists on milk particularly. It seems that milk consumption may be associated with a T2D risk reduction, with not well-established differences between regular-fat or whole fat milk and T2D [66–68]. The association between cheese consumption and a reduced risk of T2D still needs to be strongly supported because some findings are not statistically significant [68–71]. Finally, limited evidence suggested a protective role of fermented dairy products in general (including yogurt, cheese, buttermilk, and fermented milk), against T2D [69,71].

4.3. *Observational Studies*

More than twenty observational studies regarding calcium intake and T2D prevention were found. Different populations have investigated the association between calcium intake and T2D. The largest are four cohort studies. They were done in the United States (n = 83,779 [72], (n = 41,186) [73]), and the other two in Asian populations: China (n = 64,191) [74], and Japan (n = 59,796) [75]. They demonstrated an inverse association between dietary or total calcium intake and T2D risk among women but not in men, in the United States and in China. In the Japanese study, they found an inverse association in subjects with higher vitamin D intake.

In Korea, a smaller cohort study conducted in rural areas (n = 8313) also showed an inverse association between total and vegetable calcium intake and T2D risk among women, as previously reported [76]. Conversely, a relatively short study (n = 5200) in Australia did not find an association between dietary calcium and T2D [77]. Additionally, other studies provided mixed results when investigating the association between dairy products and the potential risk of T2D.

More recently, the Korean Genome study, a prospective cohort community-based trial followed for 10 years, explained the longitudinal associations between dietary calcium intake and the incidence of T2D [9]. The authors also associated dietary calcium intake and serum calcium levels at the baseline survey. They found that higher dietary calcium intake was associated with a lower risk of developing T2D. These results are important for public health and have implications for predicting and preventing T2D development. These findings can provide guidelines for calcium dietary and calcium supplementation.

At the same time, a Spanish study including more than 500 postmenopausal women without diabetes showed a decrease in fasting plasma glucose and glycated hemoglobin after the intervention. This supplementation consisted of a higher dose of vitamin D3 as part of an enriched milk, providing a daily intake of 600 IU of vitamin D3 and 900 mg of calcium [78].

Another population-based study using a prospective survey of 5582 adults, the Australian Diabetes Obesity and Lifestyle Study (AusDiab), showed a significant inverse association between the highest tertial of dairy intake and risk of diabetes in men after a following-up period of five years. They obtained these results after adjustment for confounding variables such as age, sex, energy intake, and other potential confounders (adjusted OR 0.53, 95% CI 0.29–0.96 [79]. This inverse association was non-significant in women (adjusted OR 0.71, 95% CI 0.48–1.05). When the authors analyzed different dairy products (low-fat milk, full-fat milk, yogurt, cheese), they only found significant inverse association with diabetes for low-fat milk (adjusted OR 0.65, 95% CI 0.44–0.94).

The Danish population-based lifestyle intervention study done by Struijk et al. called the Inter 99 Study, explained the association between specific types of dairy products and T2D incidence. They did not find a significant association between total dairy intake and T2D incidence (OR 0.95, 95% CI 0.86–1.06) and when they analyzed specific dairy products and T2D no association was reported. Particularly, cheese and other fermented dairy (including yogurt, and buttermilk) appeared to have a beneficial effect on glucose regulation markers, with an inverse association with fasting plasma glucose and glycated hemoglobin [69].

At the same time, the results of the Whitehall II prospective cohort study of working staff of Civil Service departments, were reported. They followed 4186 subjects for ten year and found that total dairy consumption was not significantly associated with T2D (hazard ratio (HR) 1.30, 95% CI 0.95–1.77). They analyzed all possible dairy (high-fat and low-fat dairy, total milk, yogurt, cheese and fermented products) and were not associated with T2D risk. But, nevertheless, fermented dairy products were significantly associated with an inverse risk of overall mortality [68].

In the French population, the Data from the Epidemiological Study on Insulin Resistance Syndrome (DESIR) study analyzed 3435 participants prospectively for nine years. This cohort study showed that global consumption of dairy products, but not cheese, was inversely associated with new impaired fasting glycemia diagnosis and T2D (adjusted OR 0.85, 95% CI 0.76–0.94). When analyzing cheese consumption, they did not find an association with T2D (adjusted OR 0.93, 95% CI 0.82–1.06). Curiously, they reported an inverse relationship between cheese and incident metabolic syndrome (adjusted OR 0.82, 95% CI 0.71–0.95) [70].

Moreover, data from the Nurses' Health Study II, including 37,038 women followed-up for seven years, evaluated the possible influence of dairy consumption during adolescence with the development of T2D later in adulthood. They adjusted for risk factors present in adolescence. Those women with the highest quintile intake of dairy during adolescence (two servings per day) had a 38% lower risk of T2D. They also adjusted for risk factors appearing in adulthood and still demonstrated a significant inverse association between adolescent dairy intake and T2D (RR 0.73, 95% CI 0.54–0.97). There was a 43% T2D risk reduction in women with high-dairy intakes for a long time (from adolescence to adulthood), highlighting the importance of persistence in dairy consumption. They also found a 25% risk reduction for the highest current dairy consumption (two servings per 1000 kcal), and a 26% and 28% risk reduction with low- and high-fat dairy consumption, respectively [80]. In contrast, the EPIC Study, including 16,835 participants in a nested case-cohort analysis including eight European countries, found no association between total dairy consumption and T2D (HR 1.01, 95% CI 0.83–1.34) [71]. There were an inverse association between the consumption of cheese and fermented dairy products (cheese, yogurt, and thick fermented milk) with T2D (HR 0.88, 95% CI 0.76–1.02 and HR 0.88, 95% CI 0.78–0.99, respectively).

Recently the PURE study was published [81]. It analyzes the association of dairy intake with cardiovascular disease and mortality in 21 countries from five continents. In this study, the dietary intake of dairy products of 136,384 individuals were recorded using country-specific validated food frequency questionnaires. During a follow-up period of 9.1 years, the incidence of cardiovascular events and mortality was evaluated. The authors concluded that higher consumption of dairy products is associated with lower risks of mortality and cardiovascular disease.

To date, there are no well-designed randomized controlled trials (RCTs) that have specifically studied the relationship between dairy products and the risk of incident T2D. However, there is a randomized crossover trial with 12 months follow up that need to be considered. It evaluated the consumption of low-fat dairy (four servings per day) and was associated with better insulin resistance, without negative effects on body weight and lipid profile [82].

4.4. Systematic Reviews and Meta-Analyses

Three meta-analyses of prospective cohort studies on dairy products and T2D are worth noting. In a meta-analysis conducted by Tong et al. the highest dairy consumption, compared to the lowest category, significantly reduced the risk of T2D by 14% [67]. They found a significant inverse association for low-fat dairy and yogurt with T2D. This association was not found for high-fat dairy and whole (regular-fat) milk. They described, in a dose-response analysis, how each additional daily serving of total dairy showed a decrease of 6% in T2D risk. Especially per each additional serving of low-fat dairy intake there was a 10% T2D risk reduction.

Elwood et al. have previously demonstrated in their meta-analysis including four prospective cohort studies on diabetes, that milk or dairy consumption played a protective role against T2D. Per each additional daily serving there was a 4%–9% risk reduction in diabetes incidence [66]. Pittas et al. found in their meta-analysis including mostly similar cohort studies that the highest versus lowest dairy intake (3–5 vs. 1.5 servings per day) was associated with a lower risk of incident T2D [57].

So, we can consider that, to date, there is some strong, consistent, and accumulating evidence about the influence of dairy intake on a reduced the risk of T2D [7].

However, it is important to notice possible confounding factors such as fat content in some dairy products, which can influence the protective effects of calcium [74,83]. Moreover, calcium intake may also depend on other products non-dairy foods (for example tofu, fish, rice, vegetables, and pulses). It is evident that the main source of dietary calcium differs between populations and different cultures.

5. Nutritional Recommendations for T2D Prevention

An important body of evidence has shown that dairy products can reduce the risk of T2D significantly and probably in a dose-response way.

The value of having an adequate intake of dairy products should be reinforced especially among those with prediabetes, obesity and metabolic syndrome.

In addition, cultural differences, nutritional habits, economic status and gender are related to the consumption of milk and dairy products. Unfortunately, a large percentage of the adult population, particularly older adults, do not to meet the international recommendations for optimal calcium intake and need to be encouraged to increase daily calcium intake.

Dairy products are largely under-consumed by all age groups and across populations. More than 80% Americans do not meet the minimum dairy requirements of the Dietary Guidelines for Americans (DGA) [84]. The same problems have been identified in other cultures, such as the Chinese population. Their milk intake is still quite low [85].

The amount of calcium needed daily varies by age. The recommendations given by the National Institutes of Health (NIH) proposed a daily intake of 1000 mg for men between 25 and 65 years [86]. This is the same recommendation for women between 25 and 50 years, with an exception for pregnant or lactating women or postmenopausal women not receiving estrogen replacement therapy. They should take 1500 mg/day [86]. For all subjects, men and women over 65 years, the NIH proposes a daily calcium intake of 1500 mg [86]. On the other hand, recently updated the US Institute of Medicine (IOM) recommendation of 1000 mg/day of calcium intake for all adults aged 19–50 years and for men until age 70 years. They recommend 1200 mg/day for women 51 years or older and both men and women aged >70 years [87]. They proposed in their guidelines that calcium-rich foods, especially milk and other dairy products, are the best source of calcium intake because they have showed a higher absorption efficiency. Alternatively, calcium supplementation may help reaching optimal intake for those subjects who cannot take adequate calcium through diet alone.

Although 25(OH)D blood concentration is the most commonly used biomarker to determine vitamin D status, there is no global consensus on what the 25(OH)D thresholds are for vitamin D deficiency or insufficiency. The main guidelines issued by the IOM and the Endocrine Society differ on their classification of vitamin D status. The differences can be explained because of the various populations recognized by the guidelines and the way evidence was described. The IOM guidelines focus on the general healthy population and emphasize on interventional studies. The IOM did not find appropriate evidence linking vitamin D and beneficial effects for non-skeletal outcomes, such as diabetes. Therefore, the IOM argued that a level of 25(OH)D >20 ng/mL is adequate and enough for skeletal outcomes, whereas only low evidence data ratify a higher level. Moreover, the IOM proposed that a level >50 ng/mL should be followed to avoid potential adverse events. In contrast, the Endocrine Society clinical practice guidelines focus on people at high risk for vitamin D deficiency and emphasize more on observational (epidemiological) studies. The latter guidelines determined that 25(OH)D concentrations >30 ng/mL are desirable for optimal skeletal outcomes without suggesting any upper limit to be concern for safety. However, the Endocrine Society guidelines have been criticized for the way they characterized several subgroups as a high-risk population and their wide recommendations for screening for vitamin D deficiency [88]. There is agreement between both guidelines about the requirement to reconsider current recommendations in the future when ongoing randomized trials become available. Thus, two important questions are raised. First, the existence of different thresholds for different beneficial effects. Second, the harmonization of techniques to determine circulating 25(OH)D concentrations to achieve comparable results [89].

6. Unsolved Questions

In this review, a large body of evidence has been discussed about the intake of calcium and vitamin D and its association with the incidence of T2D, although the results are inconsistent. To date, several observational studies and randomized trials have been performed including very heterogeneous subject populations. They differ in design and duration, and in which range of vitamin D types and calcium products and various dosing regimens used. Therefore, it seems necessary to clarify what vitamin D levels are needed to obtain a real benefit, if any, on glycemic status, and this concentration is probably higher than recommendations currently focused on obtaining a benefit on bone metabolism. Supplementation with vitamin D at doses around 4000 IU/day may be an option to increase 25(OH)D levels close to 50 ng/mL and improve homeostasis rates of glucose and insulin among non-diabetic subjects. Therefore, no consensus regarding whether the general population needs further supplementation of vitamin D to improve health outcomes has been found.

Furthermore, more research is needed to better understand the role of calcium intake from milk and specific types of dairy products (regular fat, skimmed, fermented, non-fermented) on the incidence of T2D and indices of glucose metabolism.

Establishing if specific populations such as those with prediabetes, the overweight or obese, could obtain significant benefits with nutritional recommendations regarding the intake of calcium and vitamin D has become a matter of special interest.

7. Conclusions and Perspectives

We conclude that the current literature is inadequate for drawing firm conclusions about the association between calcium intake and incident T2D, although it appears that a higher consumption of dairy products may be beneficial for glucose metabolism. Moreover, an adequate level of vitamin D may also have a helpful effect on T2D prevention, and a potential dose-response effect is suggested.

Nevertheless, specific studies with a close control of calcium intakes and higher vitamin D supplementation are needed to better understand their effects on glucose and insulin homeostasis.

Author Contributions: A.M.-G.: carried out the bibliographic search and wrote the manuscript. B.G.-F.: reviewed the manuscript. M.M.-T.: designed and revised the manuscript. All authors approved the manuscript.

Acknowledgments: This work was supported in part by grants from Instituto de Salud Carlos III (PI15/01207). This study has been co-funded by FEDER funds. A.M.G. is the recipient of a postdoctoral grant (Juan Rodes JR 17/00023) from the Spanish Ministry of Economy and Competitiveness. We acknowledge Nutraceutical Translations for English language editing of this review. All sources of funding of the study should be disclosed. We acknowledge Nutraceutical Translations for English language editing of this manuscript.

References

1. International Diabetes Federation. *IDF Diabetes Atlas*, 8th ed.; International Diabetes Federation: Brussels, Belgium, 2017; ISBN 978-2-930229-81-2.
2. Pittas, A.G.; Nelson, J.; Mitri, J.; Hillmann, W.; Garganta, C.; Nathan, D.M.; Hu, F.B.; Dawson-Hughes, B.; Diabetes Prevention Program Research Group. Plasma 25-hydroxyvitamin D and progression to diabetes in patients at risk for diabetes: An ancillary analysis in the Diabetes Prevention Program. *Diabetes Care* **2012**, *35*, 565–573. [CrossRef] [PubMed]
3. Maddaloni, E.; Cavallari, I.; Napoli, N.; Conte, C. Vitamin D and Diabetes Mellitus. *Front. Horm. Res.* **2018**, *50*, 161–176. [PubMed]
4. Ford, E.S.; Ajani, U.A.; McGuire, L.C.; Liu, S. Concentrations of serum vitamin D and the metabolic syndrome among U.S. adults. *Diabetes Care* **2005**, *28*, 1228–1230. [CrossRef]
5. Chiu, K.C.; Chu, A.; Go, V.L.W.; Saad, M.F. Hypovitaminosis D is associated with insulin resistance and β cell dysfunction. *Am. J. Clin. Nutr.* **2004**, *79*, 820–825. [CrossRef] [PubMed]
6. Lips, P.; Eekhoff, M.; van Schoor, N.; Oosterwerff, M.; de Jongh, R.; Krul-Poel, Y.; Simsek, S. Vitamin D and type 2 diabetes. *J. Steroid Biochem. Mol. Biol.* **2017**, *173*, 280–285. [CrossRef]
7. Kalergis, M.; Leung Yinko, S.S.L.; Nedelcu, R. Dairy products and prevention of type 2 diabetes: Implications for research and practice. *Front. Endocrinol.* **2013**, *4*, 90. [CrossRef] [PubMed]
8. Talaei, M.; Pan, A.; Yuan, J.M.; Koh, W.P. Dairy intake and risk of type 2 diabetes. *Clin. Nutr.* **2018**, *37*, 712–718. [CrossRef]
9. Kim, K.N.; Oh, S.Y.; Hong, Y.C. Associations of serum calcium levels and dietary calcium intake with incident type 2 diabetes over 10 years: The Korean Genome and Epidemiology Study (KoGES). *Diabetol. Metab. Syndr.* **2018**, *10*, 50. [CrossRef]
10. Cade, C.; Norman, A.W. Rapid normalization/stimulation by 1,25- dihydroxyvitamin d3 of insulin secretion and glucose tolerance in the vitamin d-deficient rat. *Endocrinology* **1987**, *120*, 1490–1497. [CrossRef]
11. Zeitz, U.; Weber, K.; Soegiarto, D.W.; Wolf, E.; Balling, R.; Erben, R.G. Impaired insulin secretory capacity in mice lacking a functional vitamin D receptor. *FASEB J.* **2003**, *17*, 509–511. [CrossRef]
12. Bouillon, R.; Carmeliet, G.; Verlinden, L.; Van Etten, E.; Verstuyf, A.; Luderer, H.F.; Lieben, L.; Mathieu, C.; Demay, M. Vitamin D and human health: Lessons from vitamin D receptor null mice. *Endocr. Rev.* **2008**, *29*, 726–776. [CrossRef] [PubMed]
13. Bland, R.; Markovic, D.; Hills, C.E.; Hughes, S.V.; Chan, S.L.F.; Squires, P.E.; Hewison, M. Expression of 25-hydroxyvitamin D3-1alpha-hydroxylase in pancreatic islets. *J. Steroid Biochem. Mol. Biol.* **2004**, *89–90*, 121–125. [CrossRef] [PubMed]
14. Reusch, J.E.; Begum, N.; Sussman, K.E.; Draznin, B. Regulation of GLUT-4 phosphorylation by intracellular calcium in adipocytes. *Endocrinology* **1991**, *129*, 3269–3273. [CrossRef] [PubMed]

15. Leung, P.S. The Potential Protective Action of Vitamin D in Hepatic Insulin Resistance and Pancreatic Islet Dysfunction in Type 2 Diabetes Mellitus. *Nutrients* **2016**, *8*, 147. [CrossRef] [PubMed]
16. Wright, D.C.; Hucker, K.A.; Holloszy, J.O.; Han, D.H. Ca^{2+} and AMPK both mediate stimulation of glucose transport by muscle contractions. *Diabetes* **2004**, *53*, 330–335. [CrossRef]
17. Draznin, B. Cytosolic calcium and insulin resistance. *Am. J. Kidney Dis.* **1993**, *21*, 32–38. [CrossRef]
18. Nimitphong, H.; Holick, M.F.; Fried, S.K.; Lee, M.-J. 25-hydroxyvitamin D(3) and 1,25-dihydroxyvitamin D(3) promote the differentiation of human subcutaneous preadipocytes. *PLoS ONE* **2012**, *7*, e52171. [CrossRef]
19. Blum, M.; Dolnikowski, G.; Seyoum, E.; Harris, S.S.; Booth, S.L.; Peterson, J.; Saltzman, E.; Dawson-Hughes, B. Vitamin D(3) in fat tissue. *Endocrine* **2008**, *33*, 90–94. [CrossRef]
20. Wamberg, L.; Christiansen, T.; Paulsen, S.K.; Fisker, S.; Rask, P.; Rejnmark, L.; Richelsen, B.; Pedersen, S.B. Expression of vitamin D-metabolizing enzymes in human adipose tissue—The effect of obesity and diet-induced weight loss. *Int. J. Obes.* **2013**, *37*, 651–657. [CrossRef]
21. Hyppönen, E.; Boucher, B.J. Adiposity, vitamin D requirements, and clinical implications for obesity-related metabolic abnormalities. *Nutr. Rev.* **2018**, *76*, 678–692. [CrossRef]
22. Chun, R.F.; Liu, P.T.; Modlin, R.L.; Adams, J.S.; Hewison, M. Impact of vitamin D on immune function: lessons learned from genome-wide analysis. *Front. Physiol.* **2014**, *5*, 151. [CrossRef] [PubMed]
23. Christakos, S.; Liu, Y. Biological actions and mechanism of action of calbindin in the process of apoptosis. *J. Steroid Biochem. Mol. Biol.* **2004**, *89–90*, 401–404. [CrossRef] [PubMed]
24. Salum, E.; Kals, J.; Kampus, P.; Salum, T.; Zilmer, K.; Aunapuu, M.; Arend, A.; Eha, J.; Zilmer, M. Vitamin D reduces deposition of advanced glycation end-products in the aortic wall and systemic oxidative stress in diabetic rats. *Diabetes Res. Clin. Pract.* **2013**, *100*, 243–249. [CrossRef] [PubMed]
25. Forouhi, N.G.; Luan, J.; Cooper, A.; Boucher, B.J.; Wareham, N.J. Baseline serum 25-hydroxy vitamin d is predictive of future glycemic status and insulin resistance: The Medical Research Council Ely Prospective Study 1990-2000. *Diabetes* **2008**, *57*, 2619–2625. [CrossRef] [PubMed]
26. Kayaniyil, S.; Vieth, R.; Retnakaran, R.; Knight, J.A.; Qi, Y.; Gerstein, H.C.; Perkins, B.A.; Harris, S.B.; Zinman, B.; Hanley, A.J. Association of vitamin D with insulin resistance and beta-cell dysfunction in subjects at risk for type 2 diabetes. *Diabetes Care* **2010**, *33*, 1379–1381. [CrossRef] [PubMed]
27. Maki, K.C.; Fulgoni, V.L., 3rd; Keast, D.R.; Rains, T.M.; Park, K.M.; Rubin, M.R. Vitamin D intake and status are associated with lower prevalence of metabolic syndrome in U.S. adults: National Health and Nutrition Examination Surveys 2003–2006. *Metab. Syndr. Relat. Disord.* **2012**, *10*, 363–372. [CrossRef]
28. Gannage-Yared, M.-H.; Chedid, R.; Khalife, S.; Azzi, E.; Zoghbi, F.; Halaby, G. Vitamin D in relation to metabolic risk factors, insulin sensitivity and adiponectin in a young Middle-Eastern population. *Eur. J. Endocrinol.* **2009**, *160*, 965–971. [CrossRef]
29. Scragg, R.; Holdaway, I.; Singh, V.; Metcalf, P.; Baker, J.; Dryson, E. Serum 25-hydroxyvitamin D3 levels decreased in impaired glucose tolerance and diabetes mellitus. *Diabetes Res. Clin. Pract.* **1995**, *27*, 181–188. [CrossRef]
30. Olson, M.L.; Maalouf, N.M.; Oden, J.D.; White, P.C.; Hutchison, M.R. Vitamin D deficiency in obese children and its relationship to glucose homeostasis. *J. Clin. Endocrinol. Metab.* **2012**, *97*, 279–285. [CrossRef]
31. Parikh, S.; Guo, D.-H.; Pollock, N.K.; Petty, K.; Bhagatwala, J.; Gutin, B.; Houk, C.; Zhu, H.; Dong, Y. Circulating 25-hydroxyvitamin D concentrations are correlated with cardiometabolic risk among American black and white adolescents living in a year-round sunny climate. *Diabetes Care* **2012**, *35*, 1133–1138. [CrossRef]
32. Kayaniyil, S.; Retnakaran, R.; Harris, S.B.; Vieth, R.; Knight, J.A.; Gerstein, H.C.; Perkins, B.A.; Zinman, B.; Hanley, A.J. Prospective associations of vitamin D with beta-cell function and glycemia: The PROspective Metabolism and ISlet cell Evaluation (PROMISE) cohort study. *Diabetes* **2011**, *60*, 2947–2953. [CrossRef] [PubMed]
33. Forouhi, N.G.; Ye, Z.; Rickard, A.P.; Khaw, K.T.; Luben, R.; Langenberg, C.; Wareham, N.J. Circulating 25-hydroxyvitamin D concentration and the risk of type 2 diabetes: Results from the European Prospective Investigation into Cancer (EPIC)-Norfolk cohort and updated meta-analysis of prospective studies. *Diabetologia* **2012**, *55*, 2173–2182. [CrossRef] [PubMed]

34. Afzal, S.; Bojesen, S.E.; Nordestgaard, B.G. Low 25-hydroxyvitamin D and risk of type 2 diabetes: A prospective cohort study and metaanalysis. *Clin. Chem.* **2013**, *59*, 381–391. [CrossRef]
35. Song, Y.; Wang, L.; Pittas, A.G.; Del Gobbo, L.C.; Zhang, C.; Manson, J.E.; Hu, F.B. Blood 25-hydroxy vitamin D levels and incident type 2 diabetes: A meta-analysis of prospective studies. *Diabetes Care* **2013**, *36*, 1422–1428. [CrossRef]
36. Park, S.K.; Garland, C.F.; Gorham, E.D.; BuDoff, L.; Barrett-Connor, E. Plasma 25-hydroxyvitamin D concentration and risk of type 2 diabetes and pre-diabetes: 12-year cohort study. *PLoS ONE* **2018**, *13*, e0193070. [CrossRef]
37. Avila-Rubio, V.; Garcia-Fontana, B.; Novo-Rodriguez, C.; Cantero-Hinojosa, J.; Reyes-Garcia, R.; Munoz-Torres, M. Higher Levels of Serum 25-Hydroxyvitamin D Are Related to Improved Glucose Homeostasis in Women with Postmenopausal Osteoporosis. *J. Women's Health* **2018**, *27*, 1007–1015. [CrossRef] [PubMed]
38. Zheng, J.-S.; Imamura, F.; Sharp, S.J.; van der Schouw, Y.T.; Sluijs, I.; Gundersen, T.E.; Ardanaz, E.; Boeing, H.; Bonet, C.; Gómez, J.H.; et al. Association of plasma vitamin D metabolites with incident type 2 diabetes: EPIC-InterAct case-cohort study. *J. Clin. Endocrinol. Metab.* **2019**, *104*, 1293–1303. [CrossRef]
39. Heath, A.K.; Williamson, E.J.; Hodge, A.M.; Ebeling, P.R.; Eyles, D.W.; Kvaskoff, D.; O'Dea, K.; Giles, G.G.; English, D.R. Vitamin D status and the risk of type 2 diabetes: The Melbourne Collaborative Cohort Study. *Diabetes Res. Clin. Pract.* **2018**, *149*, 179–187. [CrossRef] [PubMed]
40. Sollid, S.T.; Hutchinson, M.Y.S.; Fuskevag, O.M.; Figenschau, Y.; Joakimsen, R.M.; Schirmer, H.; Njolstad, I.; Svartberg, J.; Kamycheva, E.; Jorde, R. No effect of high-dose vitamin D supplementation on glycemic status or cardiovascular risk factors in subjects with prediabetes. *Diabetes Care* **2014**, *37*, 2123–2131. [CrossRef]
41. Forouhi, N.G.; Menon, R.K.; Sharp, S.J.; Mannan, N.; Timms, P.M.; Martineau, A.R.; Rickard, A.P.; Boucher, B.J.; Chowdhury, T.A.; Griffiths, C.J.; et al. Effects of vitamin D2 or D3 supplementation on glycaemic control and cardiometabolic risk among people at risk of type 2 diabetes: Results of a randomized double-blind placebo-controlled trial. *Diabetes Obes. Metab.* **2016**, *18*, 392–400. [CrossRef]
42. Griffin, S.J.; Little, P.S.; Hales, C.N.; Kinmonth, A.L.; Wareham, N.J. Diabetes risk score: Towards earlier detection of type 2 diabetes in general practice. *Diabetes. Metab. Res. Rev.* **2000**, *16*, 164–171. [CrossRef]
43. Davidson, M.B.; Duran, P.; Lee, M.L.; Friedman, T.C. High-dose vitamin D supplementation in people with prediabetes and hypovitaminosis D. *Diabetes Care* **2013**, *36*, 260–266. [CrossRef] [PubMed]
44. Gagnon, C.; Daly, R.M.; Carpentier, A.; Lu, Z.X.; Shore-Lorenti, C.; Sikaris, K.; Jean, S.; Ebeling, P.R. Effects of combined calcium and vitamin D supplementation on insulin secretion, insulin sensitivity and beta-cell function in multi-ethnic vitamin D-deficient adults at risk for type 2 diabetes: A pilot randomized, placebo-controlled trial. *PLoS ONE* **2014**, *9*, e109607. [CrossRef] [PubMed]
45. Oosterwerff, M.M.; Eekhoff, E.M.; Van Schoor, N.M.; Boeke, A.J.P.; Nanayakkara, P.; Meijnen, R.; Knol, D.L.; Kramer, M.H.; Lips, P. Effect of moderate-dose vitamin D supplementation on insulin sensitivity in vitamin D-deficient non-Western immigrants in the Netherlands: A randomized placebo-controlled trial. *Am. J. Clin. Nutr.* **2014**, *100*, 152–160. [CrossRef] [PubMed]
46. Salehpour, A.; Shidfar, F.; Hosseinpanah, F.; Vafa, M.; Razaghi, M.; Amiri, F. Does vitamin D3 supplementation improve glucose homeostasis in overweight or obese women? A double-blind, randomized, placebo-controlled clinical trial. *Diabet. Med.* **2013**, *30*, 1477–1481. [CrossRef] [PubMed]
47. Tuomainen, T.-P.; Virtanen, J.K.; Voutilainen, S.; Nurmi, T.; Mursu, J.; de Mello, V.D.F.; Schwab, U.; Hakumaki, M.; Pulkki, K.; Uusitupa, M. Glucose Metabolism Effects of Vitamin D in Prediabetes: The VitDmet Randomized Placebo-Controlled Supplementation Study. *J. Diabetes Res.* **2015**, *2015*, 672653. [CrossRef] [PubMed]
48. Wagner, H.; Alvarsson, M.; Mannheimer, B.; Degerblad, M.; Ostenson, C.-G. No Effect of High-Dose Vitamin D Treatment on beta-Cell Function, Insulin Sensitivity, or Glucose Homeostasis in Subjects With Abnormal Glucose Tolerance: A Randomized Clinical Trial. *Diabetes Care* **2016**, *39*, 345–352. [CrossRef]
49. Von Hurst, P.R.; Stonehouse, W.; Coad, J. Vitamin D supplementation reduces insulin resistance in South Asian women living in New Zealand who are insulin resistant and vitamin D deficient—A randomised, placebo-controlled trial. *Br. J. Nutr.* **2010**, *103*, 549. [CrossRef]
50. Mitri, J.; Dawson-Hughes, B.; Hu, F.B.; Pittas, A.G. Effects of vitamin D and calcium supplementation on pancreatic beta cell function, insulin sensitivity, and glycemia in adults at high risk of diabetes: The Calcium and Vitamin D for Diabetes Mellitus (CaDDM) randomized controlled trial. *Am. J. Clin. Nutr.* **2011**, *94*, 486–494. [CrossRef]

51. Manson, J.E.; Cook, N.R.; Lee, I.-M.; Christen, W.; Bassuk, S.S.; Mora, S.; Gibson, H.; Gordon, D.; Copeland, T.; D'Agostino, D.; et al. Vitamin D Supplements and Prevention of Cancer and Cardiovascular Disease. *N. Engl. J. Med.* **2018**, *380*, 33–44. [CrossRef]
52. Rafiq, S.; Jeppesen, P.B. Body mass index, vitamin d, and type 2 diabetes: A systematic review and meta-analysis. *Nutrients* **2018**, *10*, 1182. [CrossRef]
53. Tang, H.; Li, D.; Li, Y.; Zhang, X.; Song, Y.; Li, X. Effects of Vitamin D Supplementation on Glucose and Insulin Homeostasis and Incident Diabetes among Nondiabetic Adults: A Meta-Analysis of Randomized Controlled Trials. *Int. J. Endocrinol.* **2018**, *2018*, 7908764. [CrossRef] [PubMed]
54. LeBlanc, E.S.; Pratley, R.E.; Dawson-Hughes, B.; Staten, M.A.; Sheehan, P.R.; Lewis, M.R.; Peters, A.; Kim, S.H.; Chatterjee, R.; Aroda, V.R.; et al. Baseline Characteristics of the Vitamin D and Type 2 Diabetes (D2d) Study: A Contemporary Prediabetes Cohort That Will Inform Diabetes Prevention Efforts. *Diabetes Care* **2018**, *41*, 1590–1599. [CrossRef] [PubMed]
55. Belenchia, A.M.; Tosh, A.K.; Hillman, L.S.; Peterson, C.A. Correcting vitamin D insufficiency improves insulin sensitivity in obese adolescents: A randomized controlled trial. *Am. J. Clin. Nutr.* **2013**, *97*, 774–781. [CrossRef] [PubMed]
56. Jorde, R.; Sneve, M.; Torjesen, P.; Figenschau, Y. No improvement in cardiovascular risk factors in overweight and obese subjects after supplementation with vitamin D3 for 1 year. *J. Intern. Med.* **2010**, *267*, 462–472. [CrossRef] [PubMed]
57. Pittas, A.G.; Lau, J.; Hu, F.B.; Dawson-Hughes, B. The Role of Vitamin D and Calcium in Type 2 Diabetes. A Systematic Review and Meta-Analysis. *J. Clin. Endocrinol. Metab.* **2007**, *92*, 2017–2029. [CrossRef]
58. Ojuka, E.O. Role of calcium and AMP kinase in the regulation of mitochondrial biogenesis and GLUT4 levels in muscle. *Proc. Nutr. Soc.* **2004**, *63*, 275–278. [CrossRef] [PubMed]
59. Milner, R.D.G.; Hales, C.N. The role of calcium and magnesium in insulin secretion from rabbit pancreas studied in vitro. *Diabetologia* **1967**, *3*, 47–49. [CrossRef]
60. Zemel, M.B. Nutritional and endocrine modulation of intracellular calcium: Implications in obesity, insulin resistance and hypertension. *Mol. Cell. Biochem.* **1998**, *188*, 129–136. [CrossRef]
61. Dunlop, T.W.; Väisänen, S.; Frank, C.; Molnár, F.; Sinkkonen, L.; Carlberg, C. The Human Peroxisome Proliferator-activated Receptor δ Gene is a Primary Target of 1α,25-Dihydroxyvitamin D3 and its Nuclear Receptor. *J. Mol. Biol.* **2005**, *349*, 248–260. [CrossRef]
62. Mozaffarian, D.; Cao, H.; King, I.B.; Lemaitre, R.N.; Song, X.; Siscovick, D.S.; Hotamisligil, G.S. *Trans*-Palmitoleic Acid, Metabolic Risk Factors, and New-Onset Diabetes in U.S. Adults. *Ann. Intern. Med.* **2010**, *153*, 790. [CrossRef] [PubMed]
63. Mozaffarian, D.; de Oliveira Otto, M.C.; Lemaitre, R.N.; Fretts, A.M.; Hotamisligil, G.; Tsai, M.Y.; Siscovick, D.S.; Nettleton, J.A. trans-Palmitoleic acid, other dairy fat biomarkers, and incident diabetes: The Multi-Ethnic Study of Atherosclerosis (MESA). *Am. J. Clin. Nutr.* **2013**, *97*, 854–861. [CrossRef] [PubMed]
64. Kratz, M.; Baars, T.; Guyenet, S. The relationship between high-fat dairy consumption and obesity, cardiovascular, and metabolic disease. *Eur. J. Nutr.* **2013**, *52*, 1–24. [CrossRef] [PubMed]
65. Alhazmi, A.; Stojanovski, E.; McEvoy, M.; Garg, M.L. Macronutrient Intakes and Development of Type 2 Diabetes: A Systematic Review and Meta-Analysis of Cohort Studies. *J. Am. Coll. Nutr.* **2012**, *31*, 243–258. [CrossRef] [PubMed]
66. Givens, D.I.; Beswick, A.D.; Fehily, A.M.; Pickering, J.E.; Gallacher, J. The Survival Advantage of Milk and Dairy Consumption: An Overview of Evidence from Cohort Studies of Vascular Diseases, Diabetes and Cancer AU—Elwood, Peter C. *J. Am. Coll. Nutr.* **2008**, *27*, 723S–734S.
67. Tong, X.; Dong, J.-Y.; Wu, Z.-W.; Li, W.; Qin, L.-Q. Dairy consumption and risk of type 2 diabetes mellitus: A meta-analysis of cohort studies. *Eur. J. Clin. Nutr.* **2011**, *65*, 1027. [CrossRef]
68. Soedamah-Muthu, S.S.; Masset, G.; Verberne, L.; Geleijnse, J.M.; Brunner, E.J. Consumption of dairy products and associations with incident diabetes, CHD and mortality in the Whitehall II study. *Br. J. Nutr.* **2013**, *109*, 718–726. [CrossRef] [PubMed]
69. Struijk, E.A.; Heraclides, A.; Witte, D.R.; Soedamah-Muthu, S.S.; Geleijnse, J.M.; Toft, U.; Lau, C.J. Dairy product intake in relation to glucose regulation indices and risk of type 2 diabetes. *Nutr. Metab. Cardiovasc. Dis.* **2013**, *23*, 822–828. [CrossRef]

70. Fumeron, F.; Lamri, A.; Abi Khalil, C.; Jaziri, R.; Porchay-Baldérelli, I.; Lantieri, O.; Vol, S.; Balkau, B.; Marre, M. Dairy Consumption and the Incidence of Hyperglycemia and the Metabolic Syndrome. *Diabetes Care* **2011**, *34*, 813–817. [CrossRef] [PubMed]
71. Sluijs, I.; Forouhi, N.G.; Beulens, J.W.J.; van der Schouw, Y.T.; Agnoli, C.; Arriola, L.; Balkau, B.; Barricarte, A.; Boeing, H.; Bueno-de-Mesquita, H.B.; et al. The amount and type of dairy product intake and incident type 2 diabetes: Results from the EPIC-InterAct Study. *Am. J. Clin. Nutr.* **2012**, *96*, 382–390.
72. Pittas, A.G.; Dawson-Hughes, B.; Li, T.; Van Dam, R.M.; Willett, W.C.; Manson, J.E.; Hu, F.B. Vitamin D and calcium intake in relation to type 2 diabetes in women. *Diabetes Care* **2006**, *29*, 650–656. [CrossRef] [PubMed]
73. Van Dam, R.M.; Hu, F.B.; Rosenberg, L.; Krishnan, S.; Palmer, J.R. Dietary calcium and magnesium, major food sources, and risk of type 2 diabetes in U.S. black women. *Diabetes Care* **2006**, *29*, 2238–2243. [CrossRef] [PubMed]
74. Villegas, R.; Gao, Y.-T.; Dai, Q.; Yang, G.; Cai, H.; Li, H.; Zheng, W.; Shu, X.O. Dietary calcium and magnesium intakes and the risk of type 2 diabetes: The Shanghai Women's Health Study. *Am. J. Clin. Nutr.* **2009**, *89*, 1059–1067. [CrossRef]
75. Kirii, K.; Mizoue, T.; Iso, H.; Takahashi, Y.; Kato, M.; Inoue, M.; Noda, M.; Tsugane, S. Calcium, vitamin D and dairy intake in relation to type 2 diabetes risk in a Japanese cohort. *Diabetologia* **2009**, *52*, 2542–2550. [CrossRef] [PubMed]
76. Oh, J.M.; Woo, H.W.; Kim, M.K.; Lee, Y.-H.; Shin, D.H.; Shin, M.-H.; Choi, B.Y. Dietary total, animal, vegetable calcium and type 2 diabetes incidence among Korean adults: The Korean Multi-Rural Communities Cohort (MRCohort). *Nutr. Metab. Cardiovasc. Dis.* **2017**, *27*, 1152–1164. [CrossRef] [PubMed]
77. Gagnon, C.; Lu, Z.X.; Magliano, D.J.; Dunstan, D.W.; Shaw, J.E.; Zimmet, P.Z.; Sikaris, K.; Grantham, N.; Ebeling, P.R.; Daly, R.M. Serum 25-hydroxyvitamin D, calcium intake, and risk of type 2 diabetes after 5 years: Results from a national, population-based prospective study (the Australian diabetes, obesity and lifestyle study). *Diabetes Care* **2011**, *34*, 1133–1138. [CrossRef]
78. Reyes-Garcia, R.; Mendoza, N.; Palacios, S.; Salas, N.; Quesada-Charneco, M.; Garcia-Martin, A.; Fonolla, J.; Lara-Villoslada, F.; Muñoz-Torres, M. Effects of Daily Intake of Calcium and Vitamin D-Enriched Milk in Healthy Postmenopausal Women: A Randomized, Controlled, Double-Blind Nutritional Study. *J. Women's Heal.* **2018**, *27*, 561–568. [CrossRef]
79. Grantham, N.M.; Magliano, D.J.; Hodge, A.; Jowett, J.; Meikle, P.; Shaw, J.E. The association between dairy food intake and the incidence of diabetes in Australia: The Australian Diabetes Obesity and Lifestyle Study (AusDiab). *Public Health Nutr.* **2013**, *16*, 339–345. [CrossRef]
80. Malik, V.S.; Sun, Q.; van Dam, R.M.; Rimm, E.B.; Willett, W.C.; Rosner, B.; Hu, F.B. Adolescent dairy product consumption and risk of type 2 diabetes in middle-aged women1–3. *Am. J. Clin. Nutr.* **2011**, *94*, 854–861. [CrossRef]
81. Dehghan, M.; Mente, A.; Rangarajan, S.; Sheridan, P.; Mohan, V.; Iqbal, R.; Gupta, R.; Lear, S.; Wentzel-Viljoen, E.; Avezum, A.; et al. Association of dairy intake with cardiovascular disease and mortality in 21 countries from five continents (PURE): A prospective cohort study. *Lancet* **2018**, *392*, 2288–2297. [CrossRef]
82. Rideout, T.C.; Marinangeli, C.P.F.; Martin, H.; Browne, R.W.; Rempel, C.B. Consumption of low-fat dairy foods for 6 months improves insulin resistance without adversely affecting lipids or bodyweight in healthy adults: A randomized free-living cross-over study. *Nutr. J.* **2013**, *12*, 56. [CrossRef] [PubMed]
83. Aune, D.; Norat, T.; Romundstad, P.; Vatten, L.J. Dairy products and the risk of type 2 diabetes: A systematic review and dose-response meta-analysis of cohort studies. *Am. J. Clin. Nutr.* **2013**, *98*, 1066–1083. [CrossRef] [PubMed]
84. Krebs-Smith, S.M.; Guenther, P.M.; Subar, A.F.; Kirkpatrick, S.I.; Dodd, K.W. Americans do not meet federal dietary recommendations. *J. Nutr.* **2010**, *140*, 1832–1838. [CrossRef]
85. Liu, A.-D.; Zhang, B.; DU, W.-W.; Wang, H.-J.; Su, C.; Zhai, F.-Y. Milk consumption and its changing trend of Chinese adult aged 18–44 in nine provinces (autonomous region) from 1991 to 2006. *Zhonghua Yu Fang Yi Xue Za Zhi* **2011**, *45*, 304–309. [PubMed]
86. NIH Consensus conference. Optimal calcium intake. NIH Consensus Development Panel on Optimal Calcium Intake. *JAMA* **1994**, *272*, 1942–1948. [CrossRef]
87. Ross, A.C.; Taylor, C.L.; Yaktine, A.L.; Del Valle, H.B. (Eds.) *Dietary Reference Intakes for Calcium and Vitamin D*; National Academies Press: Washington, DC, USA, 2012; Volume 130, ISBN 978-0-309-16394-1.

88. Rosen, C.J.; Abrams, S.A.; Aloia, J.F.; Brannon, P.M.; Clinton, S.K.; Durazo-Arvizu, R.A.; Gallagher, J.C.; Gallo, R.L.; Jones, G.; Kovacs, C.S.; et al. IOM Committee Members Respond to Endocrine Society Vitamin D Guideline. *J. Clin. Endocrinol. Metab.* **2012**, *97*, 1146–1152. [CrossRef] [PubMed]
89. Scragg, R. Emerging Evidence of Thresholds for Beneficial Effects from Vitamin D Supplementation. *Nutrients* **2018**, *10*, 561. [CrossRef] [PubMed]

5

Dietary Approaches for Japanese Patients with Diabetes

Satoru Yamada [1,*], Yusuke Kabeya [2] and Hiroshi Noto [3]

1. Diabetes Center, Kitasato Institute Hospital, 5-9-1 Shirokane, Minato-ku, Tokyo 108-8642, Japan
2. Department of Home Care Medicine, Saiyu Clinic, 3-217-1 Sagamicho, Koshigaya-shi, Saitama 343-0823, Japan; ykabeyan@yahoo.co.jp
3. Endocrinology Department, St. Luke's International Hospital, 9-1 Akashicho, Chuo-ku, Tokyo 104-8560, Japan; noto-tky@umin.net

* Correspondence: yamada-s@insti.kitasato-u.ac.jp

Abstract: This study aimed to elucidate the effect of an energy restricted and carbohydrate restricted diet on the management of Japanese diabetes patients. Several databases including MEDLINE, EMBASE, and the Japan Medical Abstracts Society were searched for relevant articles published prior to June 2017. The articles identified were systematically reviewed. We identified 286 articles on an energy restricted diet, assessed seven and included two studies in our review. On a carbohydrate restricted diet, 75 articles were extracted, seven articles assessed and three included in the review, of which two were the studies that were selected for the energy restricted diet group, since they compared energy restricted diets with carbohydrate restricted diets. All selected studies were on Japanese patients with type 2 diabetes. No studies for type 1 diabetes were found in our search. Two randomized controlled trials on an energy restricted diet were also included in the three studies for a carbohydrate restricted diet. All the three randomized controlled trials showed better glucose management with the carbohydrate restricted diet. Our study revealed that there is very little evidence on diets, particularly in Japanese patients with diabetes, and that the energy restricted diet, which has been recommended by the Japan Diabetes Society in the sole dietary management approach, is not supported by any scientific evidence. Our findings suggest that the carbohydrate restricted diet, but not the energy restricted diet, might have short term benefits for the management of diabetes in Japanese patients. However, since our analysis was based on a limited number of small randomized controlled trials, large scale and/or long term trials examining the dietary approaches in these patients are needed to confirm our findings.

Keywords: energy restricted diet; low energy diet; carbohydrate restricted diet; low carbohydrate diet; diabetes; Japanese

---

1. Introduction

Nutrition therapy plays an integral role in the management of diabetes [1]. Several dietary approaches such as the Mediterranean diet, dietary approaches to stop hypertension (DASH), a vegetarian diet, and a carbohydrate restricted diet have been recommended by the American Diabetes Association (ADA) and reviewed by Ley et al. in *The Lancet* [2,3]. On the other hand, the Japan Diabetes Society (JDS) has officially recommended only an energy restricted diet since 1965 [4], as it believes that the pathophysiology and food preferences of Japanese patients with diabetes are unique when compared to patients in Western countries [5]. As per the JDS guidelines, energy restriction was calculated based on the ideal body weight as follows: total energy intake (kcal) = ideal body weight (kg = height (m) × height (m) × 22) × physical activity index (obese, 20–25; non-obese sedentary, 25–30; non-obese normal intensity active, 30–35; non-obese high intensity active, 35 and above). In fact, a recent study of the trajectory of body mass index (BMI) in Japanese patients with diabetes has shown it to be continuously normal (approximately 24.4) and not obese [6]. The BMI of Japanese individuals is very different from that of Americans [7] and Europeans [8], suggesting that there must be differences in the pathophysiology as well. However, because the European Association for the Study of Diabetes (EASD) mentioned that energy restriction is not needed in patients whose BMI is lower than 25 [9], the discrepancy in the position of energy restriction between the JDS and the Western countries seems more problematic. Although the JDS guidelines [4] on the dietary recommendations are reportedly based on 86 studies, none of those references support the JDS recommended an energy restriction diet. Eighty-three of these papers were not studies on dietary approach for Japanese patients with type 2 diabetes. The remaining three references were on dietary approaches for Japanese diabetic patients, where one is the 'eating vegetables before carbohydrate' diet [10], one is the before-after study on exercise and energy restriction diet which instructed a deficit of 140 kcal/d from the baseline for subjects with metabolic syndrome [11], and the last is the carbohydrate restriction diet [12]. Thus, it is evident that the JDS guidelines are not based on any supportive evidence for energy restriction in diabetic patients with normal BMI, despite the fact that energy restriction is the basis of the consensus in preparing the guidelines by the writing committee [4]. However, since the JDS recognizes that an evaluation of the effectiveness and safety of dietary approaches is needed in their recommendation [5], in this study we have tried to evaluate the effectiveness of the energy restricted diet in Japanese patients with diabetes. Furthermore, in recent years, emerging evidence has suggested that a restricted carbohydrate diet improves glycemic control [13], although it is not yet conclusive, especially in long term follow-ups [1,14]. We have, therefore, evaluated the effectiveness of the carbohydrate restricted diet as well.

2. Materials and Methods

2.1. Study Search

Searches of MEDLINE, EMBASE, and Japan Medical Abstracts Society (JAMAS) databases from their inception (MEDLINE 1966, EMBASE 1947, AND JAMAS 1964) until 30 June 2017, were performed. To identify studies related to an energy restricted diet, we used a combination of the following keywords: "low-energy" or "energy-restriction" or "low-calorie" or "caloric-restriction" and "diabetes," and "Japanese" in the MEDLINE and EMBASE databases. Similarly, for articles related to a carbohydrate restricted diet, we used the terms "low-carbohydrate" or "carbohydrate-restriction," and "diabetes," and "Japanese" in the MEDLINE and EMBASE databases. In the JAMAS database, we used the same combination of keywords in Japanese. Other dietary approaches such as, the Mediterranean diet, DASH (dietary approaches to stop hypertension), fat restriction (low fat) diet, low glycemic index (low GI) diet, vegetarian diet, and high-protein diet were excluded because preliminary searches by one author (S.Y.) found no relevant study in Japanese (partly presented in 60th JDS annual meeting in 2017, Nagoya by S.Y.).

2.2. Study Selection

The following exclusion criteria were applied: (1) non-Japanese data, (2) non-diabetic patient data, (3) other dietary approaches, (4) unpublished data (including abstracts presented only in scientific meetings), and (5) studies not appropriate for our evaluation such as case series and case reports.

After each search, based on the title and abstract, two authors (S.Y. and Y.K.) extracted relevant reports independently. One author (S.Y.) collected the papers for a full-text evaluation by two independent authors (S.Y and Y.K). Disagreements were primarily resolved through discussions and by consulting a third author (H.N.). We did not perform any quantitative data analysis because our search found few studies that were not enough to perform a meta-analysis.

2.3. Validity and Quality Assessment

The risk of bias was assessed against the key criteria: random sequence generation; allocation concealment; blinding of participants, personnel, and assessors; incomplete outcome data; selective outcomes reporting; and other sources of bias, in accordance with the recommendations of the Medical Information Network Distribution Service (Minds) [15].

2.4. Data Abstraction

We reviewed each full-text report to determine its eligibility and extracted and tabulated all the relevant data independently. The extracted data included the characteristics of the subjects (including age, gender), the study design, publication year, follow-up period, and risk parameters. Any disagreement was resolved by consensus among the investigators.

3. Results

We identified a total of 286 articles related to an energy restricted diet, of which seven [16–22] were assessed for their eligibility for inclusion in our review (Figure 1). All were studies on patients with type 2 diabetes. No study was identified for type 1 diabetes. There were no articles outlining the adverse effects of energy restriction. Five articles were excluded from the systematic review because (a) counseling [16], (b) meal delivery [17], and (c) periodization [18] were evaluated under the same level of energy restriction in three studies; one study assessed the effects of very strict energy restriction under hospitalization (1000 kcal/day) [19]; while another did not evaluate an energy restricted diet [20]. After excluding these five studies, the remaining two randomized controlled trials (RCTs) were appraised in our systematic review [21,22]. The two selected articles were moderately homogeneous in terms of the level of energy restriction. Both studies adopted a carbohydrate restricted diet as the control group. The sample sizes in these two studies were 24 [21] and 66 [22].

Both studies were also selected in the carbohydrate restricted diet section. To avoid redundancy, we created a summary table that included the two studies each on a carbohydrate restricted diet and an energy restricted diet, and an energy restricted diet was used as the control group (Table 1). In both studies, the energy restricted diet (Table 1, control group) had inferior effects on HbA1c improvement when compared to the carbohydrate restriction group (Table 1, intervention group). However, a review of dietary energy in one study [21] revealed that the levels of energy intake were similar in both the energy and carbohydrate restriction groups. In the other study [22], the levels of energy intake were higher in the energy restriction group compared to those in the carbohydrate restriction group. Thus, we concluded that the net effect of energy restriction on glycemic control could not be assessed in both studies (Table 2).

We identified a total of 75 articles related to a carbohydrate restricted diet, of which seven were assessed for their eligibility to be included in our review (Figure 2) [19–25]. All were studies on patients with type 2 diabetes. No studies were identified for type 1 diabetes. There were no articles that showed adverse effects of carbohydrate restriction. Four articles were excluded from the study because the same levels of carbohydrate restriction were recommended for all participants, and a longitudinal change in glycemic control was observed in two studies [20,23]. One study evaluated the effect of very strict energy restriction under hospitalization (1000 kcal/day) [19]. In one study, carbohydrate restriction was prescribed only on a single day (admission day 8) [24]. After excluding these four studies, the remaining three RCTs were appraised in our systematic review [21,22,25]. The three selected articles were moderately homogeneous in terms of the level of carbohydrate restriction. Among these studies, two had an energy restricted diet as the control groups and were the same studies selected for the energy restricted diet analysis [21,22], while the third study had a carbohydrate-rich diet with similar energy intake [25]. The sample sizes in these three studies were 24 [21], 66 [22], and 15 [25].

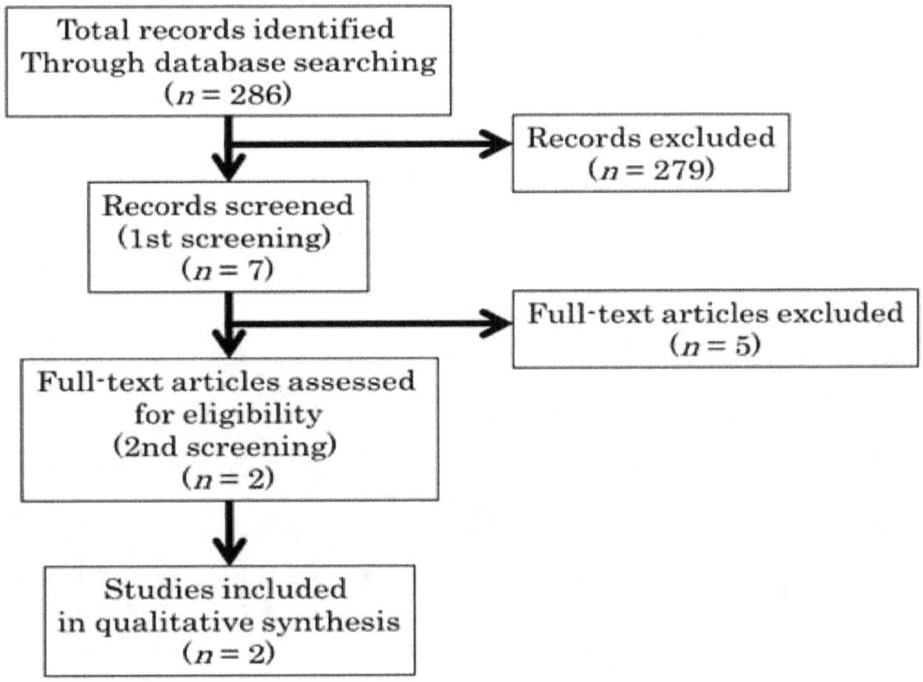

Figure 1. Flow diagram of selecting the energy restriction studies included in our study. Two randomized controlled trials were appraised in our systematic review.

Table 1 shows the summary of each study. A carbohydrate restricted diet had superior effects on improvement of HbA1c [21,22] or the postprandial glucose levels as determined by continuous glucose monitoring [25] compared to the control group in all three studies. However, in one study the energy intake was lower in the intervention (carbohydrate restriction) group than in the control (energy restriction) group [22] (Table 2). Thus, we concluded that a carbohydrate restriction diet was supported by limited evidence in Japanese patients with type 2 diabetes.

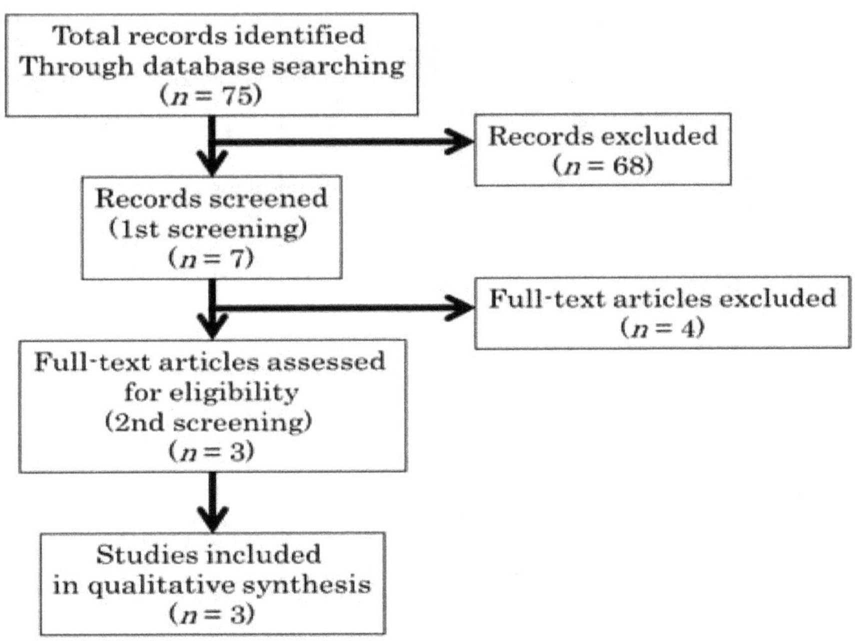

Figure 2. Flow diagram of selecting the carbohydrate studies included in our study. Three randomized controlled trials were appraised in our systematic review.

Table 1. Summary table of studies on carbohydrate restriction diet (including energy restriction studies as control group [21,22]).

Study ID (Reference Number)	Setting	Study Design	Patients					Intervention	Control	Primary Outcome	Results		
			Number of Participants	Number of Dropouts	Age	Sex (M/F)	Duration of Diabetes (Years)				Intervention	Control	Median Difference
Yamada et al., 2014 [21]	Outpatient University Hospital	RCT	24	C: 0 E: 0	C: 63.3 ± 13.5 E: 63.2 ± 10.2	C: 7/5 E: 5/7	C: 8.9 ± 3.6 E: 9.5 ± 4.8	Carbohydrate: 70–130 g/day	IBW (kg) ×25 kcal/day	HbA1c change after 6 month	−0.6 ± 0.48	−0.2 ± 0.68	−0.40
Sato et al., 2017 [22]	Outpatient University Hospital	RCT	66	C: 1 E: 3	C: 60.5 ± 10.5 E: 58.4 ± 10.0	C: 23/7 E: 24/8	(median) C: 14.0 E: 13.0	Carbohydrate 130 g/day	IBW (kg) x 28 kcal/day	HbA1c change after 6 month	(median)-0.65	(median) 0.00	−0.65
Yabe et al., 2017 [25]	Meal test 2 Medical Institutions	RCT	15	C: 0 H: 0	C: 56.9 ± 7.3 H: 54.3 ± 5.2	C: 7/0 E: 5/3	C: 7.6 ± 4.3 E: 4.4 ± 3.3	Carbohydrate 180 g/day, Energy 1800 kcal/d	Carbohydrate 247.5 g/day, Energy 1800 kcal/day	CGM data during 5–7 days	130.32 ± 27.72	142.92 ± 39.6	n.a.

C: carbohydrate restriction group = intervention group, E: energy restriction group = control group [21,22], H: high carbohydrate group=control group, RCT: randomized controlled trials. M = male, F = female. IBW: ideal body weight. n.a.; not available.

Table 2. Methodological quality and risk of bias of carbohydrate restriction studies (including energy restriction studies as control group [21,22]).

Study ID [Reference Number]	Sample Size Calculation	Risk of Bias								Indirectness				
		Random Sequence Generation	Allocation Concealment *	Blinding of Participants and Personnel *	Blinding of Outcome Assessment *	Incomplete Outcome Data	Selective Reporting	Other Source of Bias	Study free from total biases *	Subjects	Intervention	Control	Outcome	Total Indirectness
Yamada et al., 2014 [21]	Yes	Yes	Low	Unclear	Unclear	Low	Low	Unclear	Unclear	No	No	No	No	No
Sato et al., 2017 [22]	Yes	Yes	Low	Unclear	Unclear	Low	Low	Unclear	Unclear	Yes **	Yes ***	No	No	No
Yabe et al., 2017 [25]	n.a.	Yes	Low	Unclear	Unclear	Low	Low	Unclear	Unclear	Yes **	Yes ****	Yes ****	No	Yes

* In dietary study, blinding and concealment are impossible. Thus, no dietary study is unbiased. ** In these studies [22,25], female/male ratio was different between intervention and control group. *** In this study [22], energy intake is strictly restricted to the intervention group. **** This study [25] used test meals supplied by Nichirei Foods Inc. (Tokyo, Japan).

4. Discussion

The present study was an attempt to elucidate the effects of an energy restricted diet and carbohydrate restricted diet on the management of diabetes in Japanese patients by reviewing previous studies from available databases. The first and most important finding of our study is that there is very little evidence on diets in Japanese patients with diabetes.

Our second finding was that an energy restricted diet, which has been recommended by the JDS as the sole dietary management approach, is not supported by any scientific evidence so far. The two studies in our review were not appropriate to judge the effects of an energy restricted diet on glycemic control because the levels of energy intake in the energy restriction group were not lower than those in the control group [21,22]. While in one study the energy restriction group showed a non-significant reduction of HbA1c (from 7.7 $\pm$ 0.6 to 7.5 $\pm$ 1.0%, $p = 0.45$) [18], no change was seen in HbA1c in another study [22], indicating that an energy restricted diet is not supported by scientific evidence in Japan. The available data on the effects of an energy restricted diet are very limited, which results in difficulties in the evaluation and recommendation of such a diet. Furthermore, the CALERIE (Comprehensive Assessment of Long term Effects of Reducing Intake of Energy) study revealed that energy restriction in non-obese subjects leads to loss of bone mineral density [26] and lean body mass [27] in a two year period. In light of these findings, a multi-faceted evaluation might be required for patients with diabetes in terms of examining the effects and safety of energy restriction. If the JDS continues to adopt dietary guidelines [4] different from those in Western countries, it should be backed by sufficient evidence that can be critically evaluated. Well-designed, multi-centered RCTs to establish dietary evidence should be actively encouraged.

The third finding of our study was that as a short-term management approach a carbohydrate restricted diet is more effective than an energy restricted diet. All three RCTs in our review were small but well-designed [21,22,25]. Although observational studies have presented safety concerns regarding the carbohydrate restricted diet in Western countries [28,29], a similar study in Japan was in favor of carbohydrate restriction [30]. Furthermore, recently the PURE (Prospective Urban and Rural Epidemiological) study, which was held in 18 countries, showed that carbohydrate intake was positively correlated with mortality [31], suggesting the safety of carbohydrate restriction.

Regarding the long-term effects of carbohydrate restriction, Sato et al. have recently reported that the statistical superiority of a carbohydrate restricted diet receded in an 18-month follow-up study. In their cohort, the median HbA1c level changed from 8.3% at baseline to 8.2% at 18 months in the energy restriction group and from 8.0% to 7.7% in the carbohydrate restriction group [32]. Hence, Sato et al. concluded that well-constructed nutrition therapy, including both energy and carbohydrate restricted diets, might be equally effective in improving HbA1c levels in the long term [32]. However, improvement in HbA1c have not yet been observed with energy restricted diets. Furthermore, although it was a non-RCT, Haimoto et al. [33] have previously shown that the carbohydrate restriction group had better HbA1c, BMI, and tapering of sulfonylureas during a 24-month period. Sanada et al. [34] have reported that a carbohydrate restriction diet was effective during a 36-month period. Thus, we cannot exclude the possibility that a carbohydrate restricted diet is effective in the long term. Unlike other carbohydrate restriction studies, the study by Sato et al. [22,32], showed that the carbohydrate restriction group consumed less energy than the energy restriction group. This reduced energy intake in the energy non-restricted group may explain the rebound in the carbohydrate restriction group in the study by Sato et al. [32]. Our findings therefore point towards the possibility that a carbohydrate restricted diet could potentially be an option as a first line dietary approach for Japanese patients with diabetes. However, longer-term and larger RCTs are needed to confirm this hypothesis.

Our study has some limitations. First, all three studies included in our review were small and short term. Second, the included studies all have a potential performance bias because the subjects and healthcare providers were not blinded. However, it might be difficult to solve this problem in studies evaluating dietary effects on glycemic control under actual clinical situations.

5. Conclusions

Our systematic review revealed that there are only a few dietary studies in Japanese patients with diabetes. Large-scale trials are needed to more fully evaluate the risks and benefits of an energy restricted diet, which is recommended by JDS. On the other hand, the effectiveness of a carbohydrate restricted diet is supported by limited evidence, at least in the short term. Well-designed and more sophisticated trials are needed to establish evidence-based dietary approaches specifically for these patients.

Author Contributions: Conceptualization, S.Y., Y.K. and H.N.; Methodology, S.Y., Y.K. and H.N.; Data curation, S.Y. and Y.K.; Formal Analysis, S.Y. and Y.K.; Writing-Original Draft Preparation, S.Y.; Supervision, H.N.

Acknowledgments: Our study was supported by the Kitasato Institute Hospital Study Grant. The funders had no role in the design of the study; in the collection, analyses, or interpretation of data; in the writing of the manuscript, and in the decision to publish the results. We would like to thank Editage (https://www.editage.com/) for editing and reviewing this manuscript for English language.

References

1. American Diabetes Association. Lifestyle management: Standards of Medical Care in Diabetes—2018. *Diabetes Care* **2018**, *41*, S38–S50. [CrossRef] [PubMed]
2. Evert, A.B.; Boucher, J.L.; Cypress, M.; Dunbar, S.A.; Franz, M.J.; Mayer-Davis, E.J.; Neumiller, J.J.; Nwankwo, R.; Verdi, C.L.; Urbanski, P.; et al. Nutrition therapy recommendations for the management of adults with diabetes. *Diabetes Care* **2013**, *36*, 3821–3824. [CrossRef] [PubMed]
3. Ley, S.H.; Hamdy, O.; Mohan, V.; Hu, F.B. Prevention and management of type 2 diabetes: Dietary components and nutritional strategies. *Lancet* **2014**, *383*, 1999–2007. [CrossRef]
4. The Japan Diabetes Society. Diet therapy. In *Practice Guideline for the Treatment for Diabetes in Japan*; Nankodo: Tokyo, Japan, 2016; pp. 37–66. (In Japanese)
5. The Japan Diabetes Society. Recommendation of Diet Therapy for Japanese Patients with Diabetes. Available online: http://www.jds.or.jp/modules/important/index.php?page=article&storyid=40 (accessed on 30 December 2017).
6. Heianza, Y.; Arase, Y.; Kodama, S.; Tsuji, H.; Tanaka, S.; Saito, K.; Hara, S.; Sone, H. Trajectory of body mass index before the development of type2 diabetes in japanese men: Toranomon hospital health management center study 15. *J. Diabetes Investig.* **2015**, *6*, 289–294. [CrossRef] [PubMed]
7. Looker, H.C.; Knowler, W.C.; Hanson, R.L. Changes in bmi and weight before and after the development of type 2 diabetes. *Diabetes Care* **2001**, *24*, 1917–1922. [CrossRef] [PubMed]
8. De Fine Olivarius, N.; Richelsen, B.; Siersma, V.; Andreasen, A.H.; Beck-Nielsen, H. Weight history of patients with newly diagnosed type 2 diabetes. *Diabet. Med.* **2008**, *25*, 933–941. [CrossRef] [PubMed]
9. Mann, J.I.; De Leeuw, I.; Hermansen, K.; Karamanos, B.; Karlström, B.; Katsilambros, N.; Riccardi, G.; Rivellese, A.A.; Rizkalla, S.; Slama, G.; et al. Diabetes and Nutrition Study Group (DNSG) of the European Association. Evidence-based nutritional approaches to the treatment and prevention of diabetes mellitus. *Nutr. Metab. Cardiovasc. Dis.* **2004**, *14*, 373–394. [CrossRef]
10. Imai, S.; Matsuda, M.; Hasegawa, G.; Fukui, M.; Obahashi, H.; Ozasa, N.; Kajiyama, S. A simple meal plan of 'eating vegetables before carbohydrate' was more effective for achieving glycemic control than an exchange-based meal plan in Japanese patients with type 2 diabetes. *Asia Pac. J. Clin. Nutr.* **2011**, *20*, 161–168. [PubMed]
11. Muramoto, A.; Yamamoto, N.; Nakamura, M.; Koike, J.; Numata, T.; Tamakoshi, A.; Tsushita, K. Effect of intensive lifestyle intervention programs on metabolic syndrome and obesity. *Himan Kenkyuu* **2010**, *16*, 182–187.
12. Nanri, A.; Mizoue, T.; Kurotani, K.; Goto, A.; Oba, S.; Noda, M.; Sawada, N.; Tsugane, S. Low-carbohydrate diet and type 2 diabetes risk in japanese men and women: The japan public health center-based prospective study. *PLoS ONE* **2015**, *10*, e0118377. [CrossRef] [PubMed]

13. Feinman, R.D.; Pogozelski, W.K.; Astrup, A.; Bernstein, R.K.; Fine, E.J.; Westman, E.C.; Accurso, A.; Frassetto, L.; Gower, B.A.; McFarlane, S.I.; et al. Dietary carbohydrate restriction as the first approach in diabetes management: Critical review and evidence base. *Nutrition* **2015**, *31*, 1–13. [CrossRef] [PubMed]
14. Snorgaard, O.; Poulsen, G.M.; Andersen, H.K.; Astrup, A. Systematic review and meta-analysis of dietary carbohydrate restriction in patients with type 2 diabetes. *BMJ Open Diabetes Res. Care* **2017**, *5*, e000354. [CrossRef] [PubMed]
15. Fukui, T.; Yamaguchi, N. Systematic Review. In *Minds Guide to Establish Clinical Guideline*; Igakushoin: Tokyo, Japan, 2014; pp. 29–50.
16. Noda, K.; Zhang, B.; Iwata, A.; Nishikawa, H.; Ogawa, M.; Nomiyama, T.; Miura, S.; Sako, H.; Matsuo, K.; Yahiro, E.; et al. Lifestyle changes through the use of delivered meals and dietary counseling in a single-blind study. STYLIST study. *Circ. J.* **2012**, *76*, 1335–1344. [CrossRef] [PubMed]
17. Yamanouchi, T.; Isobe, K.; Terashima, H.; Hayashi, T.; Hiroshima, Y.; Hosaka, A. Intervention with delivered meals changes lifestyle and improves weight and glycemic control in patients with impaired glucose tolerance. *J.J.C.L.A.* **2017**, *42*, 26–30. (In Japanese)
18. Enosawa, N.; Inoue, M.; Sato, T.; Suzuki, S. New trial in diet therapy for weight reduction in obese type 2 diabetic patients. *J. Jap. Diab. Soc.* **2004**, *47*, 635–641. (In Japanese)
19. Miyashita, Y.; Itoh, Y.; Hashiguchi, S.; Shirai, K. Effect of low carbohydrate content of low calorie diet for obese non-insulin-dependent diabetes mellitus patients on glucose and lipid metabolism. *J. Jap. Diab. Soc.* **1998**, *41*, 885–890. (In Japanese)
20. Sato, A.; Ueno, K.; Sugimoto, I. Diet therapy in diabetes mellitus. *Nippon. Byouinkai Zasshi* **2012**, *59*, 314–316. (In Japanese)
21. Yamada, Y.; Uchida, J.; Izumi, H.; Tsukamoto, Y.; Inoue, G.; Watanabe, Y.; Irie, J.; Yamada, S. A non-calorie-restricted low-carbohydrate diet is effective as an alternative therapy for patients with type 2 diabetes. *Intern. Med.* **2014**, *53*, 13–19. [CrossRef] [PubMed]
22. Sato, J.; Kanazawa, A.; Makita, S.; Hatae, C.; Komiya, K.; Shimizu, T.; Ikeda, F.; Tamura, Y.; Ogihara, T.; Mita, T.; et al. A randomized controlled trial of 130 g/day low-carbohydrate diet in type 2 diabetes with poor glycemic control. *Clin. Nutr.* **2017**, *36*, 992–1000. [CrossRef] [PubMed]
23. Okada, K.; Ito, Y.; Kitagawa, M.; Maeda, K.; Nakamura, R. The effect of low carbohydrate diet for type 2 diabetic patients. *Nippon Rinsho Eiyougakkai Zasshi* **2013**, *35*, 103–113. (In Japanese)
24. Nishimura, R.; Omiya, H.; Sugio, K.; Ubukata, M.; Sakai, S.; Samukawa, Y. Sodium-glucose cotransporter 2 inhibitor luseogliflozin improves glycaemic control, assessed by continuous glucose monitoring, even on a low-carbohydrate diet. *Diabetes Obes. Metab.* **2016**, *18*, 702–706. [CrossRef] [PubMed]
25. Yabe, D.; Iwasaki, M.; Kuwata, H.; Haraguchi, T.; Hamamoto, Y.; Kurose, T.; Sumita, K.; Yamazato, H.; Kanada, S.; Seino, Y. Sodium-glucose co-transporter-2 inhibitor use and dietary carbohydrate intake in japanese individuals with type 2 diabetes: A randomized, open-label, 3-arm parallel comparative, exploratory study. *Diabetes Obes. Metab.* **2017**, *19*, 739–743. [CrossRef] [PubMed]
26. Villareal, D.T.; Fontana, L.; Das, S.K.; Redman, L.; Smith, S.R.; Saltzman, E.; Bales, C.; Rochon, J.; Pieper, C.; Huang, M.; et al. Effect of two-year caloric restriction on bone metabolism and bone mineral density in non-obese younger adults: A randomized clinical trial. *J. Bone Miner. Res.* **2016**, *31*, 40–51. [CrossRef] [PubMed]
27. Das, S.K.; Roberts, S.B.; Bhapkar, M.V.; Villareal, D.T.; Fontana, L.; Martin, C.K.; Racette, S.B.; Fuss, P.J.; Kraus, W.E.; Wong, W.W.; et al. Body-composition changes in the comprehensive assessment of long-term effects of reducing intake of energy (calerie)-2 study: A 2-y randomized controlled trial of calorie restriction in nonobese humans. *Am. J. Clin. Nutr.* **2017**, *105*, 913–927. [CrossRef] [PubMed]
28. Fung, T.T. Low-carbohydrate diets and all-cause and cause-specific mortality. *Ann. Intern. Med.* **2010**, *153*, 289. [CrossRef] [PubMed]
29. Noto, H.; Goto, A.; Tsujimoto, T.; Noda, M. Low-carbohydrate diets and all-cause mortality: A systematic review and meta-analysis of observational studies. *PLoS ONE* **2013**, *8*, e55030. [CrossRef] [PubMed]
30. Nakamura, Y.; Okuda, N.; Okamura, T.; Kadota, A.; Miyagawa, N.; Hayakawa, T.; Kita, Y.; Fujiyoshi, A.; Nagai, M.; Takashima, N.; et al. Low-carbohydrate diets and cardiovascular and total mortality in japanese: A 29-year follow-up of nippon data80. *Columbia J. Nutr.* **2014**, *112*, 916–924. [CrossRef] [PubMed]

31. Dehghan, M.; Mente, A.; Zhang, X.; Swaminathan, S.; Li, W.; Mohan, V.; Iqbal, R.; Kumar, R.; Wentzel-Viljoen, E.; Rosengren, A.; et al. Associations of fats and carbohydrate intake with cardiovascular disease and mortality in 18 countries from five continents (PURE): A prospective cohort study. *Lancet* **2017**, *390*, 2050–2062. [CrossRef]
32. Sato, J.; Kanazawa, A.; Hatae, C.; Makita, S.; Komiya, K.; Shimizu, T.; Ikeda, F.; Tamura, Y.; Ogihara, T.; Mita, T.; et al. One year follow-up after a randomized controlled trial of a 130g/day low-carbohydrate diet in patients with type 2 diabetes mellitus and poor glycemic control. *PLoS ONE* **2017**, *12*, e0188892. [CrossRef] [PubMed]
33. Haimoto, H.; Iwata, M.; Wakai, K.; Umegaki, H. Long-term effects of a diet loosely restricting carbohydrates on HbA1c levels, BMI and tapering of sulfonylureas in type 2 diabetes: A 2-year follow-up study. *Diabetes Res. Clin. Pract.* **2008**, *79*, 350–356. [CrossRef] [PubMed]
34. Sanada, M.; Kabe, C.; Hata, H.; Uchida, J.; Inoue, G.; Tsukamoto, Y.; Yamada, Y.; Irie, J.; Tabata, S.; Tabata, M.; et al. Efficacy of a moderate low carbohydrate diet in a 36-month observational study of Japanese patients with type 2 diabetes. *Nutrients* **2018**, *10*, 528. [CrossRef] [PubMed]

6

Leucine Supplementation Differently Modulates Branched-Chain Amino Acid Catabolism, Mitochondrial Function and Metabolic Profiles at the Different Stage of Insulin Resistance in Rats on High-Fat Diet

Rui Liu, Hui Li, Wenjuan Fan, Qiu Jin, Tingting Chao, Yuanjue Wu, Junmei Huang, Liping Hao and Xuefeng Yang *

Department of Nutrition and Food Hygiene, Hubei Key Laboratory of Food Nutrition and Safety, MOE Key Laboratory of Environment and Health, School of Public Health, Tongji Medical College, Huazhong University of Science and Technology, Wuhan 430030, Hubei, China; amicable123lr@163.com (R.L.); 15032280368@163.com (H.L.); fanwenjuan0706@163.com (W.F.); 15927486696@163.com (Q.J.); weikeccs@sina.com (T.C.); wuyuanjue@hust.edu.cn (Y.W.); huangjunmeihust@163.com (J.H.); haolp@mails.tjmu.edu.cn (L.H.)

* Correspondence: xxyxf@mails.tjmu.edu.cn

Abstract: The available findings concerning the association between branched-chain amino acids (BCAAs)—particularly leucine—and insulin resistance are conflicting. BCAAs have been proposed to elicit different or even opposite effects, depending on the prevalence of catabolic and anabolic states. We tested the hypothesis that leucine supplementation may exert different effects at different stages of insulin resistance, to provide mechanistic insights into the role of leucine in the progression of insulin resistance. Male Sprague-Dawley rats were fed a normal chow diet, high-fat diet (HFD), HFD supplemented with 1.5% leucine, or HFD with a 20% calorie restriction for 24 or 32 weeks. Leucine supplementation led to abnormal catabolism of BCAA and the incompletely oxidized lipid species that contributed to mitochondrial dysfunction in skeletal muscle in HFD-fed rats in the early stage of insulin resistance (24 weeks). However, leucine supplementation induced no remarkable alternations in BCAA catabolism, but did enhance mitochondrial biogenesis with a concomitant improvement in lipid oxidation and mitochondrial function during the hyperglycaemia stage (32 weeks). These findings suggest that leucine trigger different effects on metabolic signatures at different stages of insulin resistance, and the overall metabolic status of the organisms should be carefully considered to potentiate the benefits of leucine.

Keywords: leucine; BCAAs; BCAA catabolism; insulin resistance; metabolomic; mitochondria

---

1. Introduction

Branched-chain amino acids (BCAAs), comprising leucine, isoleucine and valine, are essential amino acids and important nutrient signals that have direct and indirect effects on metabolism. Substantial evidence indicates that increased dietary intake of BCAAs, particularly leucine, has positive effects on the regulation of body weight, muscle protein synthesis, glucose homeostasis, lipid metabolism, and the ageing process [1–4]. Nevertheless, the idea that BCAAs or their supplementation might have a positive role in glucose metabolism and insulin resistance remains controversial. In other studies, leucine supplementation has no effect, or leads to deterioration in insulin sensitivity [5,6]. Along with these effects on metabolic health, it has long been recognized that elevated levels of circulating BCAAs and related metabolites are strongly associated with obesity and insulin resistance and are predictive of future type 2 diabetes mellitus (T2DM) in humans and in some rodent models [7–10]. The mechanisms underlying these paradoxical findings are not completely understood.

BCAAs modulate insulin resistance via multiple mechanisms. Generally, BCAAs have been shown to induce insulin resistance by phosphorylation of serine IRS-1 via activating mammalian targets of the rapamycin complex 1 (mTORC1) signaling pathway, and lead to a negative feedback loop of insulin signaling [11]. However, several previous studies, including a study conducted in our laboratory, have indicated that BCAA–associated mTORC1 activation is not required or sufficient to elicit insulin resistance [12,13]. Alternatively, the Lynch group have observed that abnormal tissue-specific BCAA metabolism in obesity results in the accumulation of BCAAs and related toxic metabolites, thereby triggering "anaplerotic stress" and mitochondrial dysfunction associated with insulin resistance and type 2 diabetes mellitus (T2DM) [14,15]. In contrast, BCAAs supplementation has been shown to promote mitochondrial biogenesis and extend the lifespan of yeast and middle-aged mice [16]. Recently, BCAAs and leucine have been hypothesised to elicit different or even opposing effects, depending on the catabolic and anabolic states of the organism [17]. Development of T2DM is a time-dependent process accompanied with different metabolic characteristics [18]. Notably, during the progression of insulin resistance to T2DM, the predominantly anabolic processes transition to predominantly catabolic processes, with the loss of insulin activity. This complexity introduces interpretive limitations, when using data derived from a static time point, on understanding how BCAAs affect the progression of insulin resistance [19].

In the present study, we performed comprehensive metabolic and physiological profiling to investigate dynamic alterations in BCAA catabolism, mitochondrial function, and metabolic responses to long-term leucine supplementation in rats with hyperinsulinaemia or hyperglycaemia induced by a high-fat diet (HFD). We aimed to provide mechanistic insights into the role of leucine in insulin resistance progression. Furthermore, we compared the effects of leucine with those of calorie restriction (CR), a well-known approach for improving insulin sensitivity.

2. Materials and Methods

2.1. Animals, Diets and Treatments

Male Sprague-Dawley rats at six weeks of age (160–180 g) were obtained from Sino-British Sipper/BK Lab Animal Co., Ltd. (Shanghai, China) and housed in a temperature- and humidity-controlled environment on a 12 h light/dark cycle with free access to food and water. After acclimation, the rats were randomly divided into four groups (n = 20 per group) based on body weight and fed a normal chow diet (ND; D12450B, Research Diet Inc., New Brunswick, NJ, USA), HFD (D12451, Research Diet Inc., New Brunswick, NJ, USA), HFD supplemented with 1.5% leucine (HFD + Leu) or HFD with 20% CR (HFD + CR). The administered leucine dose was determined in our preliminary experiments [12] and nearly doubled the total daily leucine intake from food. The diet of the HFD + Leu group was also supplemented with small amounts of valine and isoleucine to prevent valine and isoleucine deficiencies. The HFD was rendered isonitrogenous and isocalorie to the HFD + Leu diet by the addition of a mixture of non-essential amino acids (alanine, glycine, proline, aspartate and serine in isomolar amounts) (Table 1). Food intake was monitored daily, and that of HFD controls was used as a reference to calculate the amount of food provided to the rats subjected to CR (80% of food consumption of controls). Half of the rats in each group were killed at week 24, and the other half were killed at week 32 after overnight fasting. Blood samples were obtained and centrifuged at 4000× g for 20 min. The serum was then collected and stored in a freezer at −80 °C until further analysis. Tissues were rapidly excised, weighed, flash-frozen in liquid nitrogen and then stored at −80 °C until use. All animal studies were conducted in accordance with the National Institutes of Health guide for the Care and Use of Laboratory Animals and approved by the Institutional Animal

Care and Use Committee of Tongji Medical College, Huazhong University of Science and Technology (IACUC No. 417, Date: 2015.3.28).

Table 1. Composition of the experimental diets (/100g).

	ND	HFD	HFD + Leu
	Macronutrients (g)		
Protein	20.3	20.3	20.3
Carbohydrate	64.5	44.6	44.6
Fat	4.5	24.4	24.4
Fiber	5.0	5.0	5.0
Minerals	3.0	3.0	3.0
Calories (kcal)	379.7	479.2	479.2
Fat (energy %)	10.7	45.8	45.8
Protein (energy %)	21.3	17.0	17.0
Carbohydrate (energy %)	68.0	37.2	37.2
	Amino acids (g)		
Leucine	1.3	1.5	2.9
Isoleucine	0.6	0.7	1.0
Valine	0.7	0.9	1.1
Alanine	0.8	0.8	0.5
Aspartic acid	1.5	1.6	1.2
Glycine	0.7	0.5	0.3
Threonine	0.7	0.7	0.7
Serine	0.8	1.0	0.8
Glutamic acid	3.4	3.2	3.2
Tyrosine	0.5	0.7	0.6
Phenylalanine	0.7	0.8	0.8
Lysine	1.1	1.2	1.2
Histidine	0.5	0.5	0.4
Proline	1.2	1.7	1.6
Arginine	1.0	0.5	0.6
Methionine	0.4	0.3	0.4
Serine	0.8	1.0	0.8

ND: Normal chow diet; HFD: High fat diet.

2.2. Insulin Sensitivity Analysis

After 24 or 32 weeks on the respective diets, the fasting serum glucose levels were determined by colorimetric assay (Nanjing Jiancheng Bioengineering Institute, Nanjing, China), and insulin levels were assessed using a commercial ELISA kit (Mercodia AB, Uppsala, Sweden), according to the manufacturer's instructions. The HOMA-IR index was calculated using the following formula: HOMA-IR = [fasting glucose levels (mmol/L)] × [fasting serum insulin (mU/L)]/22.5. The glucose tolerance test (GTT) and insulin tolerance test (ITT) were performed following intragastric glucose administration and intraperitoneal insulin injection, respectively, after overnight starvation of the rats. Blood samples were collected from the tail vein at 0, 15, 30, 60 and 120 min, and the glucose levels were measured with a Glucose Meter (Roche Diagnostics, Shanghai, China).

2.3. Western Blot Analysis

Frozen gastrocnemius muscle, liver and adipose tissues were lysed in RIPA buffer (Beyotime Biotechnology, Shanghai, China) supplemented with phosphatase inhibitors and PMSF (Roche, Ltd., Basel, Switzerland) before use. For the total MitoProfile Oxidative phosphorylation complexes (OXPHOS) analysis, mitochondrial proteins were extracted from the gastrocnemius muscle according to the manufacturer's instructions (Nanjing Jiancheng Bioengineering Institute, Nanjing, China). Protein concentrations were assayed using a bicinchoninic acid (BCA) kit (Beyotime Biotechnology, Shanghai, China). A total of 20–50 μg of protein were resolved on SDS-PAGE gels and then transferred to polyvinylidene difluoride (PVDF) membranes. Information regarding the primary antibodies used in this study is provided in Table S1. Protein bands were visualized with Molecular Imager VersaDoc MP 4000 System (Bio-Rad, Berkeley, CA, USA).

2.4. Transmission Electron Microscopy

The mitochondrial morphology was investigated using electron microscopy. Briefly, gastrocnemius muscles were isolated and fixed with 2.5% glutaraldehyde for 1 day. The muscles were washed and cut longitudinally into 0.5 mm thick strips. Following osmification with 2% osmium tetroxide and 1% uranyl acetate en bloc, the stained tissue was routinely dehydrated in a methanol gradient and embedded in Eponate-12. After polymerization, the ultrastructural features of the mitochondria were observed and photographed using a Tecnai G2 12 transmission electron microscope (FEI Company, Holland, The Netherlands).

2.5. Quantitative Real-Time PCR Analysis

Total RNA was extracted from gastrocnemius muscles with Trizol reagent (Invitrogen, New York, NY, USA) and reverse transcribed into cDNA using a high-capacity cDNA archive kit (Takara, Dalian, China). Real-time PCR was performed using the StepOnePlus^{TM} Real-Time PCR System (Applied Biosystems, Grand Island, NY, USA) with the cDNA templates, gene-specific primers and the SYBR Green qPCR Master mix (Takara, Dalian, China). Calculations were performed using a comparative method ($2^{-\Delta\Delta Ct}$), with GAPDH as the internal control. Total DNA was extracted from the gastrocnemius muscles using acommercial kit (Tiangen Biotech Co., Ltd., Beijing, China), according to the manufacturer's instructions. The mitochondrial DNA (mtDNA) content was assessed using RT-PCR by measuring the threshold cycle ratio of a mitochondria-encoded gene (COXII) to a nucleus-encoded gene (β-globin). All RT-PCR experiments were performed in triplicate using the same sample. The primer pairs for each gene are shown in Table S2.

2.6. Statistical Analysis

Unless otherwise stated, data are presented as means $\pm$ SD. Statistical analyses were performed using the SPSS 15.0 software package (SPSS, Inc., Chicago, IL, USA). Significant differences were assessed by student t test or one-way ANOVA followed by the Student-Newman-Keuls test. $p < 0.05$ were considered statistically significant.

2.7. Serum Preparation and Metabolite Profiling

A targetedLC-MS/MSbased analysis was performed in the State Key Laboratory of Quality Research in Chinese Medicine at Macau University of Science and Technology and Beijing Mass Spectrometry Medical Research Co., Ltd. Broad metabolite profiling of serum was performed using LC-MS/MS (ACQUITYTM ultra-Performance LC (Waters, Milford, MA, USA) equipped with an AB 4000 Q-TRAP mass spectrometer (Applied Biosystems, Grand Island, NY, USA). Serum (200 μL) was mixed with 200 μL of n-Ethylmaleimide (10 mol/L) in PBS buffer and 1000 μL of methanol containing the internal standard L-phenylalanine-d5 (Phe-d5) at a concentration of 10 ng/mL. The mixture was incubated at -20 °C for 20 min and centrifuged at 12,000 rpm for 10 min at 4 °C. The supernatant was evaporated under a vacuum, and the dry residue was reconstituted with distilled water in preparation for analysis.

In addition to the internal standards used for quality control, a quality control (QC) sample was prepared and analyzed after every 10 serum samples. The blank serum used for QC was prepared from serum that had been stripped of endogenous materials by adding 6 g of charcoal activated powder (Sigma-Aldrich, St. Louis, MO, USA) to 100 mL of serum. This suspension was stirred at room temperature for 2 h and centrifuged at 13,500 rpm for 20 min at 4 °C. Then, the supernatant was filtered using a Millipore Express PES Membrane (Merck Millipore, Ltd., Hesse, Germany). The obtained blank serumwas confirmed to be free of biomarkers using LC-MS/MS.

For quantitative amino acid profiling, the LC-MS/MS analysis was performed on an UltiMate3000 (Dionex, Sunnyvale, CA, USA) equipped with an API 3200 Q TRAP MS System (Applied Biosystems, Grand Island, NY, USA). The samples were thawed, extracted and derivatized before analysis. In detail, after dilution with 80 μL of water, the sample was extracted with 500 μL of a mixture of methanol and acetonitrile (1:9, *v*/*v*). The extraction procedure was performed at −20 °C for 10 min after 2 min of vortexing and 1 min of ultrasonication. Then, the residue was re-dissolved in 100 μL of a mixture of methanol and water (1:1, *v*/*v*) with 1 μg/mL of L-2-chlorophenylalanine, and the same steps were repeated (vortexing, ultrasonication and centrifugation). The supernatant (80 μL) was transferred into the sample vial for the analysis.

2.8. Metabolomics Data Processing and Multivariate Analysis

The pre-processed LC-MS/MS data were log-transformed, and the resulting data were analyzed by orthogonal partial least squares projection to latent structure-discriminant analysis (OPLS-DA) using SIMCA-P version 14.0 (Umetrics, Umea, Sweden). OPLS-DA was also used to identify and rank signature metabolites that discriminated the different groups. Qualities of the OPLS-DA models were assessed by R2 indicative of variation described by all components in the model and by Q2, measuring the model ability to predict class membership.

Variables with a variable importance in the projection (VIP) score >1 were considered relevant for group discrimination. Serum metabolite concentrations in HFD + Leu and HFD + CR rats at different time points were compared with their age-matched HFD controls and significantly changed metabolites were analyzed by One-way ANOVA. p value < 0.05 was considered statistically significant. In addition, metabolic pathway interpretation of differential metabolites were performed using the MetaboAnalyst 3.0 and KEGG database.

3. Results

3.1. Body Weight and Calorie Intake

As expected, HFD-fed rats exhibited a higher body weight than controls. However, HFD-induced weight gain was significantly attenuated by CR or leucine supplementation from 3 or 13 weeks, respectively. The rats supplemented with leucine had significantly higher body weight when compared to CR rat from 7 weeks (Figure S1A). Consistent with our experimental design, the total calorie intake of CR rats was reduced by 20% over the 32-week feeding period compared with that of HFD-fed rats. Leucine addition to the high fat diet did not significantly alter calorie intake across all time points, with the exception of a slight decrease during week 3 (Figure S1B). The average daily leucine intake in ND, HFD, HFD + CR and HFD + Leu-fed rats were 0.68 g, 0.69 g, 0.54 g and 1.28 g, respectively.

3.2. Insulin Sensitivity

As shown in Figure 1A,B, the 24-week HFD did not alter fasting blood glucose but significantly increased fasting serum insulin. Leucine addition to the HFD for 24 weeks had no obvious effects on fasting serum glucose or insulin, but CR prevented the HFD-induced increase in fasting insulin. Accordingly, the HOMA-IR index was unchanged in leucine-supplemented rats, but was decreased in CR rats (Figure 1C). CR rats had lower insulin level and HOMA-IR than HFD + Leu rats at 24 weeks (Figure 1B,C). After 32 weeks, both fasting blood glucose and insulin were elevated in HFD-fed rats compared with ND-fed rats. HFD + Leu diet induced no significant effect on fast serum glucose and insulin levels. CR largely prevented HFD-induced hyperglycaemia and hyperinsulinaemia (Figure 1A,B). The HOMA-IR index was lower in rats treated with either leucine or CR than that in the corresponding HFD-fed controls (Figure 1C), while the CR rats had lower glucose than HFD + Leu rats at 32 weeks (Figure 1A). The results of the OGTT and ITT confirmed that CR or leucine-supplemented rats were significantly more glucose-tolerant and insulin-sensitive than HFD-fed rats (Figure 1D–I) at the two time points. As expected, insulin-stimulated Protein kinase B (PKB/AKT) phosphorylation in the skeletal muscle was increased in CR rats compared with the HFD-fed controls at both time points (Figure 1J). However, leucine-induced AKT phosphorylation was only observed at 32 weeks. The insulin-stimulated AKT phosphorylation protein expression in CR rats was higher than HFD + Leu rats at week 24 (Figure 1J).

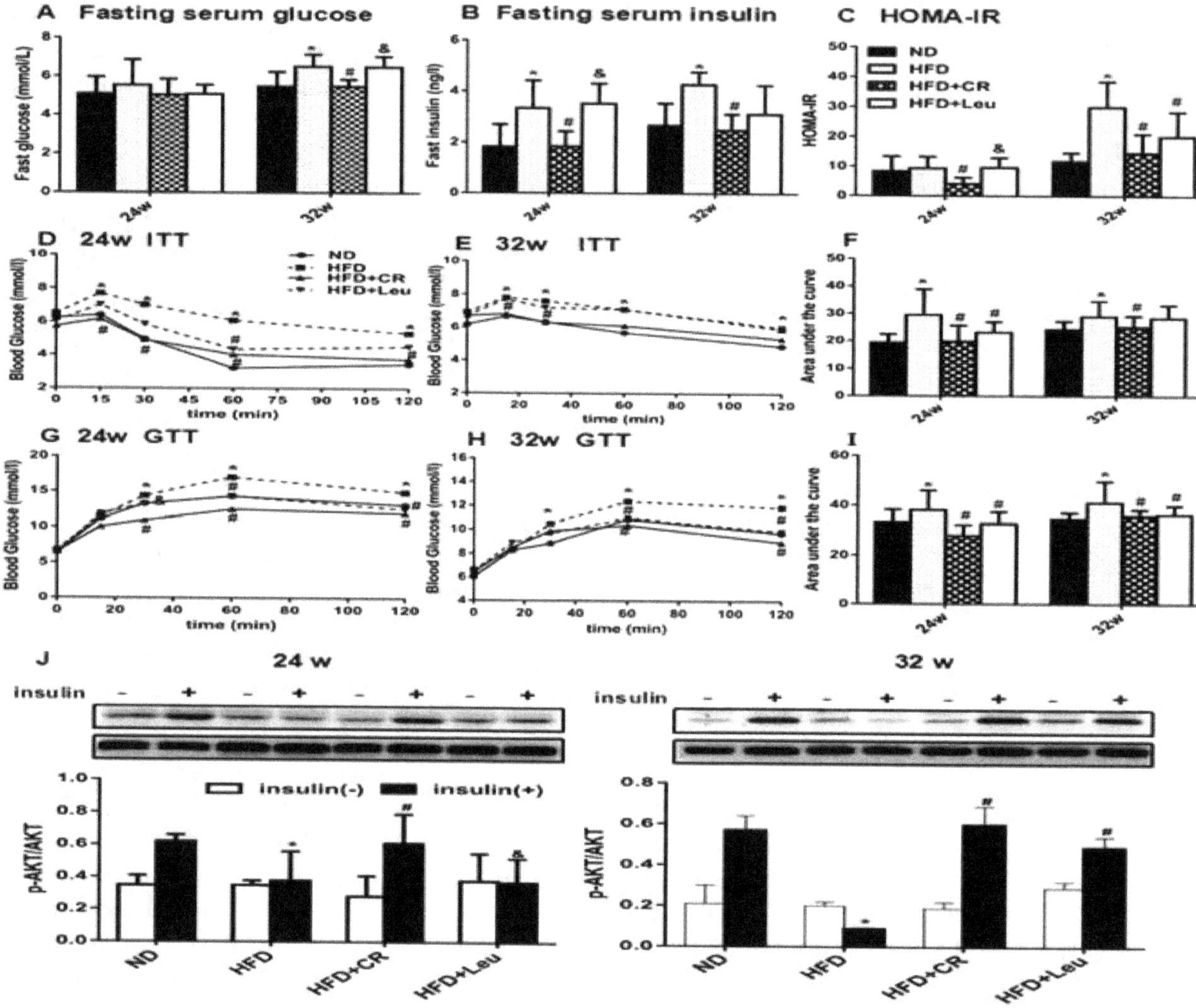

Figure 1. Leucine supplementation improved insulin sensitivity in HFD-fed rats. (**A**) Serum glucose and (**B**) insulin levels were measured after overnight fasting. (**C**) HOMA-IR indices were calculated from fasting glucose and insulin levels. (**D,E**) The intraperitoneal ITT (0.8 IU/kg.bw) and (**G,H**) OGTT (2 g/kg.bw) were performed after overnight fasting at the end of 24 and 32 weeks, respectively. (**F,I**) The area under the curve was calculated (n = 8). The results are presented as the mean ± SD. (**J**) AKT and phospho-AKT (Ser473) protein levels in skeletal muscle before (insulin−) and after (insulin+) 2 IU/kg insulin stimulation for 15 min were determined by immunoblotting (n = 3–6). * $p < 0.05$ versus ND-fed rats, # $p < 0.05$ versus HFD-fed rats, & $p < 0.05$ versus HFD + CR rats. HFD: High fat diet; ND: Normal chow diet; CR: Calorie restriction; ITT: Insulin tolerance test; OGTT: Oral glucose tolerance test; AKT: Protein kinase B.

3.3. Serum Amino Acid Profiles

Over 24 weeks of feeding, serum concentrations of BCAAs (valine and leucine), glucogenogenic amino acids (alanine, asparagine and glutamate), and gluconeogenic and ketogenic amino acids (phenylalanine and tryptophan) were significantly lower in HFD-fed rats relative to ND control, While the ketogenic amino acids (lysine) was significantly increased (Table 2). However, BCAA (except for isoleucine) concentrations were significantly elevated after leucine supplementation for 24 weeks compared with those in HFD-fed rats. The concentrations of other amino acids, such as aromatic amino acids (phenylalanine and tryptophan) and several gluconeogenic amino acids (asparagine, proline and alanine), were also significantly elevated (Table 3).

Table 2. Amino acids profile in HFD rats.

Parameter	24 weeks	32 weeks
BCAAs		
isoleucine	1.01 (0.93, 1.09)	0.97 (0.89, 1.06)
valine	0.62 (0.55, 0.70) *	1.04 (0.96, 1,11)
leucine	0.70 (0.56, 0.84) *	0.92 (0.84, 1.01)
Glucogenogenic amino acids		
alanine	0.48 (0.37, 0.59) *	1.02 (0.89, 1.16)
asparagine	0.72 (0.65, 0.80) *	1.36 (1.14, 1.59) *
aspartic acid	1.01 (0.60, 1.43)	1.01 (0.83, 1.20)
cysteine	1.06 (0.92, 1.20)	1.33 (1.24, 1.42) *
glutamate	0.79 (0.69, 0.90) *	1.65 (1.38, 1.92) *
glutamine	1.04 (0.98, 1.10)	1.08 (1.02, 1.14)
glycine	1.46 (1.24, 1.68)	0.94 (0.83, 1.05)
histidine	1.02 (0.95, 1.09)	0.83 (0.77, 0.88) *
methionine	1.01 (0.93, 1.08)	1.09 (0.94, 1.24)
proline	0.91 (0.84, 0.99)	1.23 (1.06, 1.41) *
serine	1.23 (1.04, 1.42)	1.08 (1.02, 1.15)
arginine	1.19 (1.06, 1.32)	0.95 (0.83, 1.08)
Gluconeogenic and ketogenic amino acids		
phenylalanine	0.54 (0.48, 0.59) *	1.10 (0.94, 1.25)
threonine	1.05 (0.95, 1.15)	1.34 (1.25, 1.42) *
tryptophan	0.76 (0.68, 0.85) *	0.90 (0.83, 0.98)
tyrosine	1.12 (0.95, 1.29)	0.89 (0.82, 0.96)
Ketogenic amino acids		
lysine	1.37 (1.20, 1.54) *	1.46 (1.21, 1.71) *

Data were expressed as mean fold difference (95% CI) of HFD-fed rats relative to their corresponding ND-fed controls at week 24 and 32, respectively ($n = 8$). * $p < 0.05$ versus age-matched ND controls. HFD: High-fat diet; ND: Normal chow diet; CR: Calorie restriction; BCAAs, branched-chain amino acids.

At week 32, serum BCAA levels were not significantly changed in HFD rats compared to corresponding controls, but glucogenogenic amino acids (asparagine, cysteine, glutamate and proline), gluconeogenic and ketogenic amino acids (threonine) and ketogenic amino acid lysine were significantly increased (Table 2). However, after 32 weeks of leucine treatment, serum BCAA and aromatic amino acid levels did not significantly differ, whereas asparagine and glycine were significantly reduced and proline was increased. The concentrations of most amino acids in CR rats were reduced at week 24 compared with those in HFD controls, but the observed differences were not statistically significant (except for leucine, isoleucine, alanine, phenylalanine and lysine). However, CR-induced alterations in serum amino acid concentrations were not remarkable at 32 weeks, but alanine and proline were significantly increased (Table 3).

Table 3. Amino acids profile.

Parameter	24 weeks CR	24 weeks HFD + Leu	32 weeks CR	32 weeks HFD + Leu
BCAAs				
isoleucine	0.82 (0.76, 0.88) *	0.91 (0.84, 0.98)	0.88 (0.79, 0.96)	0.94 (0.77, 1.11)
valine	0.91 (0.86, 0.96)	1.38 (1.18, 1.58) *	0.94 (0.85, 1.03)	0.95 (0.74, 1.15)
leucine	0.85 (0.79, 0.91) *	1.43 (1.02, 1.84) *	0.91 (0.84, 0.98)	0.98 (0.69, 1.27)
Glucogenogenic amino acids				
alanine	0.79 (0.71, 0.87) *	1.49 (1.34, 1.65) *	1.29 (1.02, 1.56) *	0.92 (0.71, 1.12)
asparagine	0.91 (0.76, 1.06)	1.49 (1.25, 1.72) *	0.90 (0.73, 1.06)	0.79 (0.60, 0.98) *
aspartic acid	0.93 (0.82, 1.03)	0.91 (0.74, 1.08)	1.08 (0.96, 1.20)	1.14 (0.97, 1.31)
cysteine	1.19 (1.08, 1.30) *	0.96 (0.85, 1.08)	1.09 (0.93, 1.25)	0.93 (0.77, 1.08)
glutamate	0.93 (0.80, 1.07)	1.07 (0.92, 1.23)	1.08 (0.86, 1.31)	1.00 (0.83, 1.17)
glutamine	0.93 (0.85, 1.01)	0.92 (0.84, 1.00)	1.03 (0.88, 1.18)	1.06 (0.91, 1.21)
glycine	0.96 (0.90, 1.03)	0.95 (0.91, 0.99)	0.89 (0.81, 0.98)	0.82 (0.71, 0.93) *
histidine	0.98 (0.90, 1.05)	0.97 (0.83, 1.11)	1.09 (0.98, 1.20)	1.05 (0.92, 1.18)
methionine	0.94 (0.86, 1.03)	1.01 (0.94, 1.08)	0.94 (0.86, 1.02)	0.97 (0.89, 1.04)
proline	1.04 (0.80, 1.29)	1.28 (1.00, 1.57) *	1.24 (1.00, 1.49) *	1.27 (1.02, 1.52) *
serine	0.98 (0.91, 1.04)	0.92 (0.85, 0.98)	1.08 (0.98, 1.18)	0.95 (0.84, 1.05)
arginine	0.86 (0.82, 0.91)	0.98 (0.84, 1.12)	1.08 (1.00, 1.15)	1.16 (0.96, 1.36)
Gluconeogenic and ketogenic amino acids				
phenylalanine	0.89 (0.83, 0.95) *	1.35 (1.20, 1.50) *	0.94 (0.90, 0.97)	1.07 (0.91, 1.21)
threonine	1.17 (1.05, 1.29)	0.92 (0.81, 1.02)	1.08 (0.92, 1.25)	1.09 (0.97, 1.21)
tryptophan	1.00 (0.69, 1.31)	1.43 (1.17, 1.69) *	1.22 (0.94, 1.50)	0.97 (0.77, 1.16)
tyrosine	0.87 (0.71, 1.04)	1.00 (0.87, 1.14)	1.08 (0.92, 1.25)	1.09 (0.97, 1.21)
Ketogenic amino acids				
lysine	0.82 (0.74, 0.90) *	0.65 (0.55, 0.74) *	0.90 (0.75, 1.06)	0.99(0.79, 1.19)

Data were expressed as mean fold difference (95% CI) of HFD + Leu and HFD + CR rats relative to their corresponding HFD control at week 24 and 32, respectively ($n = 8$). * $p < 0.05$ versus age-matched HFD controls. HFD: High-fat diet; CR: Calorie restriction.

3.4. Serum Metabolic Profiles

An LC-MS/MS-based metabolic approach was used to obtain more insights into the mechanisms underlying the different effects of leucine supplementation on insulin resistance. OPLS-DA model was carried out for ND, HFD, HFD + Leu and HFD + CR groups at week 24 and 32, respectively, and the R2 and Q2 values confirmed good qualities for all models (Figure 2A,B). The score plots for each model showed clear separation among the different groups suggesting they had different metabolic features at different pathological stages of HFD induced insulin resistance.

The metabolites detected in the serum were almost decreased in HFD-fed rats compared to the ND controls at week 24. Prominent decreases were observed for metabolites from amino acids including aromatic amino acid catabolites (5-hydroxytryptophan, 4,6-dihydroxyquinoline, and L-kynurenine), methionine catabolites (spermidine and S-adenosylhomocysteine) and nitrogenous compounds derived from amino acid catabolism (creatinine, Creatine, and uridine), fatty acid metabolites (3-hydroxybutyric, Acetylcarnitine and Carnitine), tricarboxylic acid (TCA) cycle intermediates (Fumaric acid and a-Ketoglutaric acid), bile acid metabolites (Ursodeoxycholic acid, Glycochenodeoxycholic acid) and some lysophosphatidylcholines (LPCs). However, fatty acid metabolism (palmitic acid) and TCA intermediate (malic acid) were marked elevated (Table 4). The serum metabolites that discriminated between leucine-supplemented and HFD-fed rats were primarily involved in the TCA cycle, fatty acid, bile acid and amino acid metabolism (Table 5). Specifically, the serum levels ofTCA intermediates (fumaric acid, malic acid and α-ketoglutarate) and metabolites related to lipid metabolism (acylcarnitine, palmitoyl-L-carnitine, carnitine, palmitic acid and 3-hydroxybutyrate) were markedly higher in leucine-treated rats than in HFD-fed controls at week 24.

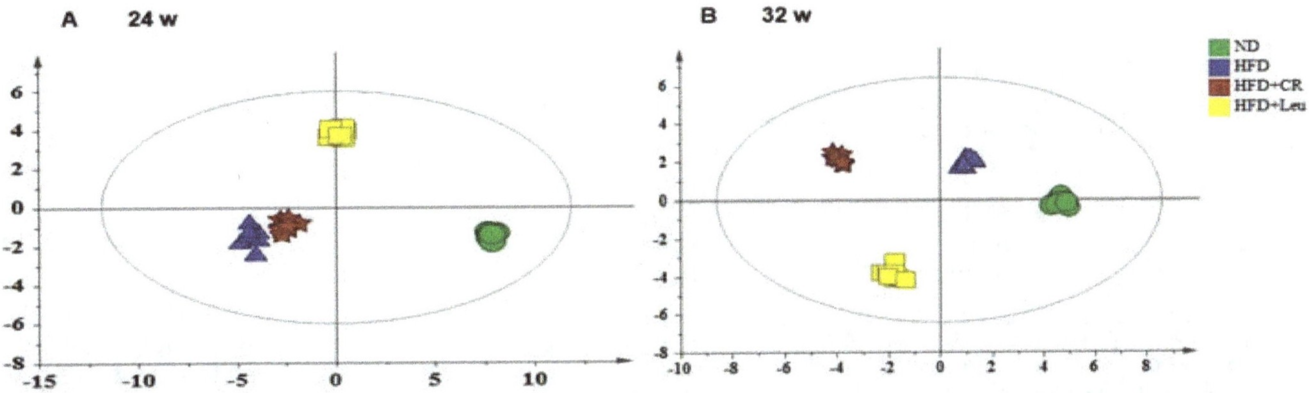

Figure 2. Orthogonal partial least squares projection to latent structure-discriminant analysis (OPLS-DA) score plots displaying the separation of the ND-fed, HFD-fed, Calorie-restricted and HFD + leurats after (**A**) 24 and (**B**) 32 weeks of treatment. Model parameters: (**A**) R2X = 0.944, Q2 = 0.424; (**B**) R2X = 0.938, Q2 = 0.652.HFD: High-fat diet; ND: Normal chow diet.

Table 4. Fold difference of serum metabolites significantly changed in HFD rats relative to the corresponding ND controls.

Metabolites	24 weeks	32 weeks
Amino acids derivatives		
L-Kynurenine	0.72 (0.64, 0.79) *	1.09 (0.87, 1.31)
5-hydroxytryptophan	0.55 (0.44, 0.66) *	1.11 (0.93, 1.29) *
Spermidine	0.52 (0.48, 0.57) *	1.26 (1.10, 1.42)
2-hydroxyisobutyrate	0.86 (0.77, 0.95)	2.23 (1.87, 2.59) *
2-hydroxyglutarate	0.55 (0.47, 0.62) *	1.37 (1.20, 1.54) *
S-(adenosyl)-L-homocysteine	0.49 (0.41, 0.58) *	1.28 (0.96, 1.60)
4,6-dihydroxyquinoline	0.55 (0.49, 0.62) *	1.20 (0.93, 1.46)
Creatinine	0.43 (0.33, 0.54) *	1.19 (0.98, 1.40)
Creatine	0.41 (0.31, 0.52) *	1.34 (1.04, 1.64) *
Uridine	0.39 (0.25, 0.52) *	1.36 (1.17, 1.54) *
Fatty acid metabolism		
3-hydroxybutyric	0.77 (0.70, 0.85) *	1.92 (1.56, 2.27) *
Palmitic acid	3.92 (3.25, 4.59) *	1.53 (0.93, 2.12)
Acetylcarnitine	0.70 (0.64, 0.77) *	1.02 (0.84, 1.19)
Palmitoyl-L-carnitine	0.91 (0.75, 1.08)	1.48 (1.11, 1.86)
Carnitine	0.46 (0.38, 0.54) *	1.04 (0.68, 1.41)
Phospholipids		
Lysophosphatidylcholine (C18:1)	0.50 (0.43, 0.57) *	1.18 (0.99, 1.37)
Lysophosphatidylcholine (C16:1)	0.38 (0.34, 0.41) *	0.99 (0.82, 1.16)
Lysophosphatidylcholine (C16:0)	0.65 (0.58, 0.72) *	0.97 (0.83, 1.12)
Lysophosphatidylcholine (C20:4)	0.16 (0.12, 0.20) *	1.21 (0.94, 1.48)
TCA cycle intermediates		
Fumaric acid	0.82 (0.74, 0.89) *	1.12 (0.93, 1.31)
Malic acid	3.54 (2.81, 4.27) *	1.23 (1.07, 1.39) *
Citric acid	0.91 (0.80, 1.03)	1.22 (1.10, 1.34) *
a-Ketoglutaric acid	0.52 (0.45, 0.59) *	1.13 (0.98, 1.29)

Table 4. *Cont.*

Metabolites	24 weeks	32 weeks
Bile acid metabolism		
Ursodeoxycholic acid	0.28 (0.19, 0.38) *	1.15 (0.73, 1.56)
Glycochenodeoxycholic acid	0.32 (0.28, 0.35) *	0.73 (0.60, 0.86)
Glycocholic acid	0.71 (0.13, 1.28)	0.65 (0.22, 1.08)
Purine metabolism		
Xanthosine	0.71 (0.46, 0.96)	0.93 (0.71, 1.16)
Allantoin	0.42 (0.33, 0.50) *	1.00 (0.85, 1.14)
Uric acid	0.88 (0.77, 0.98)	1.10 (0.95, 1.25)
Xanthine	0.83 (0.56, 1.09)	1.00 (0.71, 1.29)

Data were expressed as mean fold difference (95% Confidence Interval) of HFD-fed rats relative to their corresponding ND controls at week 24 and 32, respectively ($n = 8$). * $p < 0.05$ versus age-matched ND controls. HFD: High fat diet; ND: Normal chow diet; TCA, tricarboxylic acid.

Table 5. Fold difference of serum metabolites significantly changed in HFD + CR or HFD + Leu rats relative to the corresponding HFD-fed controls.

	24 weeks		32 weeks	
Metabolites	HFD + CR	HFD + Leu	HFD + CR	HFD + Leu
Amino acids derivatives				
L-Kynurenine	1.30 (0.66, 1.95)	1.70 (1.23, 2.19) *	1.10 (0.43, 1.78)	1.10 (0.81, 1.39)
5-hydroxytryptophan	1.10 (0.96, 1.25)	1.58 (1.16, 1.92) *	1.29 (0.82, 1.76)	1.43 (1.07, 1.79) *
Spermidine	1.17 (1.02, 1.33) *	1.43 (1.26, 1.60) *	1.18 (1.04, 1.32) *	1.05 (0.89, 1.21)
2-hydroxyisobutyrate	0.90 (0.70, 1.10)	1.54 (1.26, 1.81) *	0.82 (0.56, 1.09)	0.67 (0.38, 0.95) *
2-hydroxyglutarate	0.88 (0.73, 1.03)	1.71 (1.50, 1.92) *	1.07 (0.86, 1.28)	1.01 (0.86, 1.16)
S-(adenosyl)-L-homocysteine	1.24 (0.87, 1.60)	1.57 (1.28, 1.86) *	1.51 (1.20, 1.83) *	1.34 (1.03, 1.66) *
4,6-dihydroxyquinoline	1.54 (1.21, 1.87) *	1.81 (1.56, 2.06) *	1.50 (1.17, 1.82) *	0.90(0.75, 1.05)
Creatinine	1.31 (1.19, 1.43) *	1.50 (1.36, 1.64) *	1.14 (0.91, 1.37)	1.16 (0.91, 1.40)
Creatine	0.91 (0.76, 1.06)	1.33 (0.99, 1.68)	1.04 (0.70, 1.37)	1.71 (1.34, 2.08) *
Uridine	1.32 (0.93, 1.72)	1.61 (1.37, 1.85*	1.02 (0.88, 1.17)	0.92 (0.68, 1.17)
Fatty acid metabolism				
3-hydroxybutyric	0.92 (0.71, 1.13)	1.36 (1.13, 1.59) *	0.92 (0.60, 1.24)	0.91 (0.48, 1.33)
Palmitic acid	1.28 (1.03, 1.53) *	1.81 (1.47, 2.15) *	1.55 (1.17, 1.94) *	0.54 (0.38, 0.70) *
Acetylcarnitine	1.12 (0.96, 1.30)	1.34 (1.21, 1.48) *	1.15 (0.92, 1.39)	0.87 (0.67, 1.07)
Palmitoyl-L-carnitine	1.17 (0.97, 1.37)	1.90 (1.54, 2.26) *	0.99 (0.59, 1.40)	0.49 (0.39, 0.58) *
Carnitine	1.29 (1.09, 1.48) *	1.86 (1.46, 2.26) *	1.28 (1.09, 1.47)	1.04 (0.93, 1.15)
Phospholipids				
Lysophosphatidylcholine (C18:1)	1.35 (1.13, 1.56) *	1.42 (1.19, 1.65) *	1.55 (1.19, 1.90) *	1.49 (1.14, 1.83) *
Lysophosphatidylcholine (C16:1)	1.40 (1.15, 1.64) *	1.42 (1.23, 1.60) *	1.41 (1.00, 1.83) *	0.91 (0.71, 1.10)
Lysophosphatidylcholine(C16:0)	1.20 (1.05, 1.36) *	1.34 (1.18, 1.49) *	1.31 (1.13, 1.48) *	1.21 (1.03, 1.40) *
Lysophosphatidylcholine (C20:4)	1.06 (0.87, 1.25)	1.04 (0.77, 1.30)	0.87 (0.50, 1.24)	3.82 (3.23, 4.41) *
TCA cycle intermediates				
Fumaric acid	1.09 (0.93, 1.24)	1.23 (1.08, 1.38) *	1.09 (0.96, 1.22)	0.82 (0.72, 0.93) *
Malic acid	0.87 (0.74, 1.00)	1.33 (1.11, 1.55) *	0.97 (0.48, 1.47)	0.15 (0.09, 0.22) *
Citric acid	1.02 (0.90, 1.15)	1.18 (0.97, 1.39)	0.94 (0.77, 1.11)	0.86 (0.74, 0.97) *
a-Ketoglutaric acid	0.95 (0.80, 1.09)	1.32 (1.13, 1.50) *	1.23 (1.00, 1.47)	1.05 (0.85, 1.25)
Bile acid metabolism				
Ursodeoxycholic acid	1.57 (0.96, 2.19)	2.58 (1.91, 3.24) *	1.37 (1.06, 1.68) *	1.35 (1.08, 1.61) *
Glycochenodeoxycholic acid	1.45 (1.19, 1.71) *	1.26 (0.92, 1.60)	1.63 (1.13, 2.13) *	1.43 (1.19, 1.66) *
Glycocholic acid	2.20 (1.04, 3.36) *	4.17 (0.60, 7.74)	3.17 (1.08, 5.27) *	3.76 (1.45, 6.07) *
Purine metabolism				
Xanthosine	0.90 (0.63, 1.18)	1.20 (0.77, 1.62)	1.49 (1.13, 1.85) *	1.05 (0.90, 1.19)
Allantoin	1.05 (0.86, 1.24)	1.33 (1.00, 1.66) *	1.27 (1.04, 1.50) *	1.41 (1.23, 1.59) *
Uric acid	0.91 (0.77, 1.05)	1.24 (1.07, 1.41) *	1.08 (0.93, 1.23)	0.90 (0.83, 0.96)
Xanthine	1.05 (0.55, 1.55)	1.26 (0.76, 1.76)	1.71(1.38, 2.02) *	1.12 (0.96, 1.27)

Data were expressed as mean fold difference (95% Confidence Interval) of HFD + Leu and HFD + CR rats relative to their corresponding HFD controls at week 24 and 32, respectively ($n = 8$). * $p < 0.05$ versus age-matched HFD controls. HFD: High fat diet; CR: Calorie restriction.

The amino acid derivatives (5-hydroxytryptophan, 2-hydroxyisobutyrate, 2-hydroxyglutarate, Creatine and Uridine), fatty acid metabolites (3-hydroxybutyric), TCA cycle intermediates (Malic acid, Citric acid) were significantly elevated after 32 weeks of HFD feeding relative to the age-matched ND control (Table 4). Notably, we observed sharp decreases in the levels of TCA intermediates (fumaric acid, malic acid and citric acid) and lipid-related metabolites (palmitoyl-L-carnitine and palmitic acid) at week 32 relative to HFD-fed controls (Table 5).

In addition, leucine supplementation for 24 weeks contributed to the accumulation of metabolites associated with amino acid catabolism, including aromatic amino acid catabolites (5-hydroxytryptophan, 4,6-dihydroxyquinoline, and L-kynurenine), methionine catabolites (spermidine and S-adenosylhomocysteine) and nitrogenous compounds derived from amino acid catabolism (creatinine, uric acid, and uridine).In contrast, at week 32, the levels of amino acid catabolites that discriminated the leucine group from the HFD-fed controls were reduced. Moreover, prominentincreases in bile acid metabolites and some lysophosphatidylcholines (LPCs) were detected at both 24 and 32 weeks (Table 5).

Metabolites related to lipid metabolism (palmitic acid and LPCs), bile acid metabolism (glycochenodeoxycholic acid and glycocholic acid) and some amino acid catabolites were significantly elevated at week 24 and 32 in CR rats compared with the corresponding HFD-fed controls (Table 5).

3.5. BCAA Catabolizing Enzymes and Metabolites

HFD feeding for 24 weeks, the levels of transamination products of BCAAs— branched-chain α-keto acids (BCKAs)—did not change significantly compared with ND-fed control at 24 weeks (Figure 3B). Mitochondrial branched-chain aminotransferase (BCATm) protein expression in skeletal muscle and adipose tissue were both significantly increased. Branched-chain α-keto acid dehydrogenase kinase (BCKDK) protein expression in HFD rats was lower in skeletal muscle, while higher in adipose tissue than ND controls (Figure 4A–C). BCATm protein expression was significantly increased in skeletal muscle and adipose tissue, concurrent with a significant increase in BCKDKandno change in branched-chain α-keto acid dehydrogenase E1 α (BCKDHE1α) in skeletal muscles, livers and adipose tissues of leucine-supplemented rats, compared with those of HFD-fed controls at week 24 (Figure 4A–C). Furthermore, the levels of transamination products of leucine (α-Ketoisocaproate, KIC) were also increased (Figure 3B).

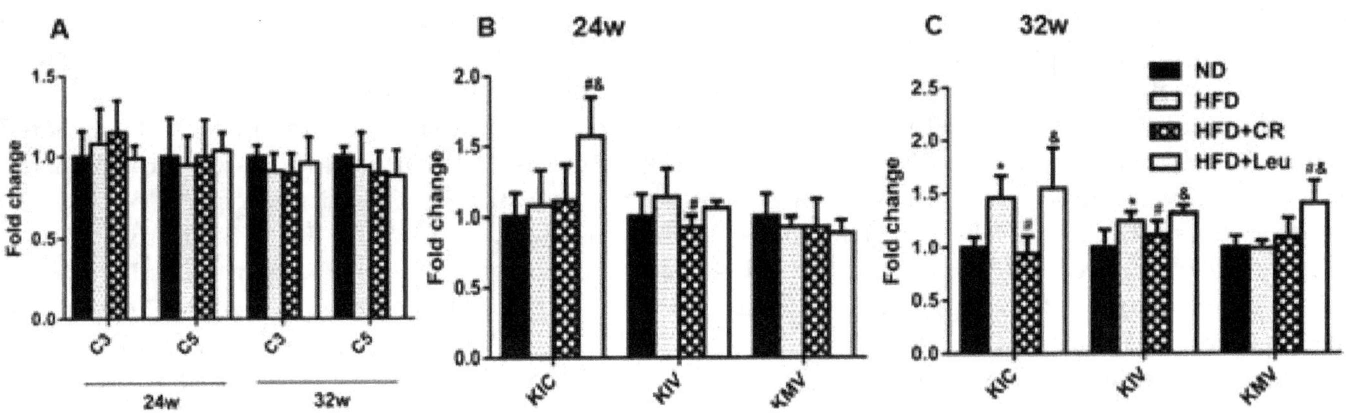

Figure 3. Leucine supplementation-induced alterations in the levels of BCAA derivatives. (**A**) Serum levels of short-chain acylcarnitines (C3 and C5) and (**B**,**C**) Branched-chain α-keto acids (BCKAs) ($n = 8$). The results are presented as means ± SD. * $p < 0.05$ versus ND-fed rats, # $p < 0.05$ versus HFD-fed rats, & $p < 0.05$ versus HFD + CR rats. HFD: High fat diet; ND: Normal chow diet; CR: Calorie restriction.

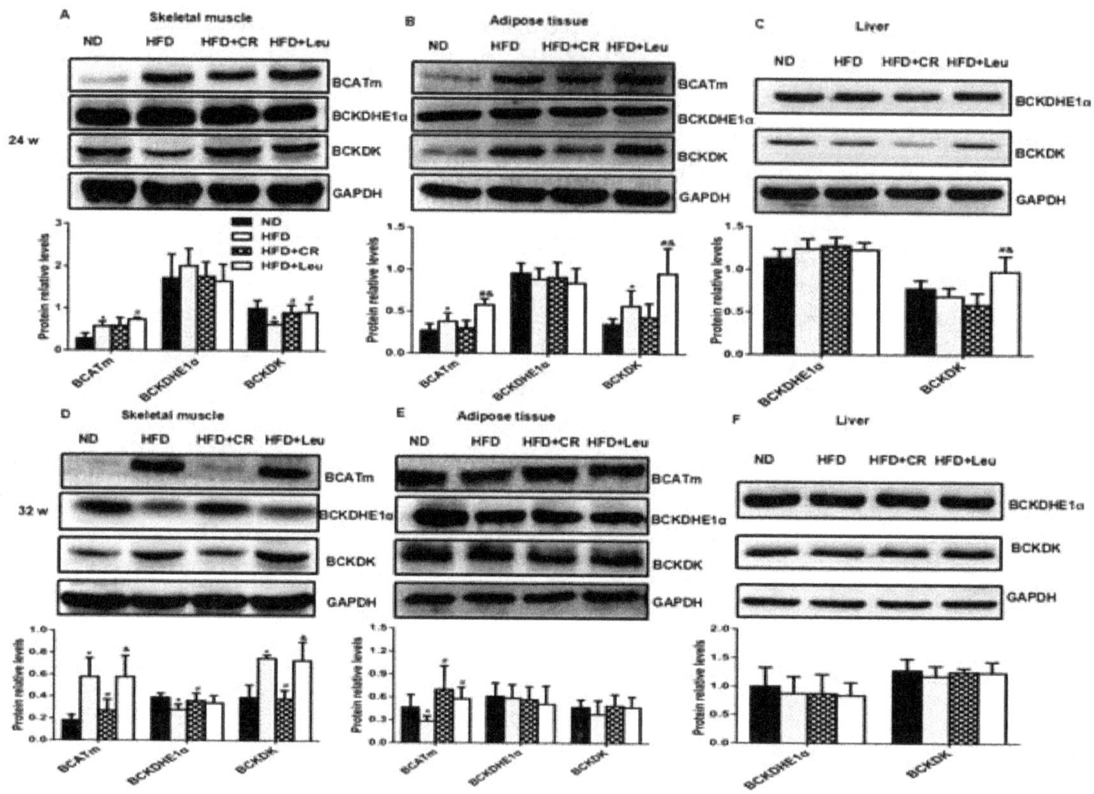

Figure 4. Leucine supplementation-induced alterations in BCAA catabolic enzyme protein expression. Representative immunoblots of total mBCAT, BCKDHE1α and BCKDK protein levels in skeletal muscle (**A**,**D**), adipose tissue (**B**,**E**) and liver (**C**,**F**); $n = 6$. The results are presented as the mean ± SD. * $p < 0.05$ versus ND-fed rats, # $p < 0.05$ versus HFD-fed rats, & $p < 0.05$ versus HFD + CR rats. mBCAT: Mitochondrial branched-chain aminotransferase; BCKDHE1α: Branched-chain α-keto acid dehydrogenase E1 α; BCKDK: Branched-chain α-keto acid dehydrogenase kinase, HFD: High fat diet; ND: Normal chow diet; CR: Calorie restriction.

However, HFD feeding for 32 weeks led to significantly increase in the levels of transamination products of leucine (α-Ketoisocaproate, KIC) and transamination products of valine (α-Ketoisovalerate, KIV) compared to corresponding ND control (Figure 3C). BCATm and BCKDK protein expression were significantly elevated, but BCKDHE1αprotein expression was significantly decreased in skeletal muscle. In addition, BCATm protein expression in adipose tissue was significantly decreased compared with ND-fed control at 32 weeks (Figure 4D–F). In contrast, the only changes observed in the levels of BCAA catabolizing enzymes and metabolites were an increased expression of BCATm in adipose tissue (Figure 4D–F) and increased isoleucine-derived KMV (α-Keto-β-methylvalerate, KMV) levels compared to the HFD-fed controls after 32 weeks of leucine supplementation (Figure 3C). BCAA-catabolizing enzyme protein expression did not significantly differ between CR rats and HFD-fed controls at week 24 (Figure 4A–C). However, BCATm and BCKDK protein expression was significantly decreased, whereas BCKDHE1α expression was significantly increased in skeletal muscle in CR rats at week 32 compared to the HFD-fed controls (Figure 4D–F). Notably, neither leucine supplementation nor CR had a significant impact on serum BCAA-derived short-chain acylcarnitine (C3 and C5) levels throughout the experiment (Figure 3A).

3.6. Mitochondrial Properties

Long-term HFD feeding-induced mitochondrial structural damage was exacerbated by leucine supplementation at 24 weeks (Figure 5A). Mitochondrial function was also impaired, as indicated by the reduced expression of enzymes involved in OXPHOSand serum ATP production (Figure 5B,D).

The expression of genes controlling mitochondrial biogenesis, including mitochondrial transcription factor A (TFAM), peroxisome proliferator-activated receptor γ coactivator-1-α (PGC-1α) and sirtuin 1 (SIRT1), were greatly decreased (Figure 5F) in HFD + Leurats at this time point. In contrast, HFD-induced mitochondrial damage was partially restored by leucine supplementation at 32 weeks (Figure 5A), accompanied by increases in the mtDNA content (Figure 5E), the expression of genes involved in mitochondrial biogenesis (TFAM) (Figure 5G) and ATP production (Figure 5D). As expected, CR ameliorated HFD-induced mitochondrial damage at both time points. At week 24, CR enhanced expression of enzymes involved in OXPHOS, and the gene expression related to mitochondrial biogenesis (TFAM, NRF-1, PGC-1α and SIRT1) (Figure 5B,F). At week 32, CR-induced mitochondrial biogenesis was not greatly changed, but ATP production was significantly increasedcompared to HFD controls (Figure 5D,E,G). CR exhibited better effects on improving HFD-induced mitochondrial damage at week 24 as demonstrated by increases in OXPHOS protein levels (Figure 5B), ATP production (Figure 5D), and mitochondrial biogenesis compared to leucine supplementation (Figure 5F).

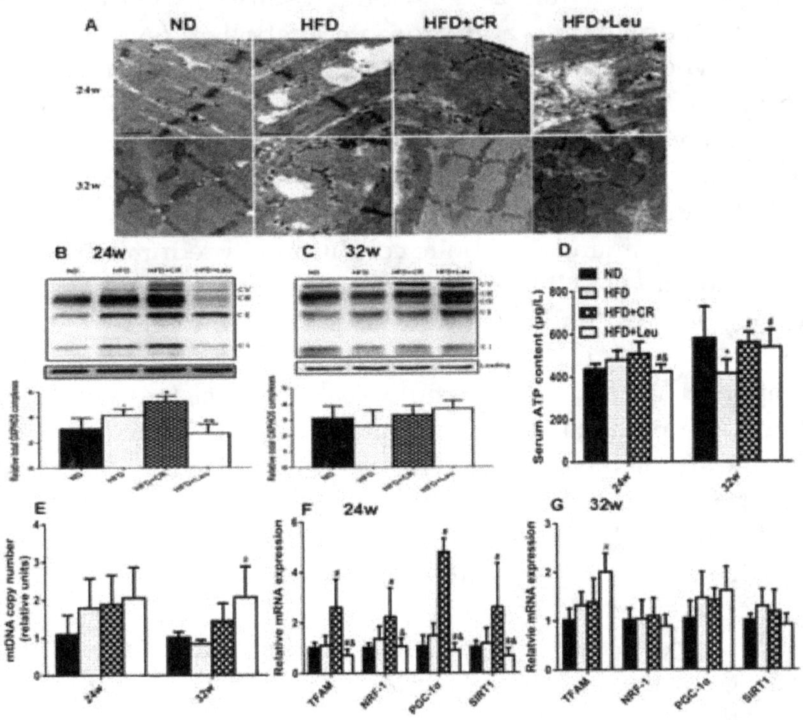

Figure 5. Leucine supplementation-induced alterations in mitochondrial properties. (**A**) Transmission electronic microscopy (×20,000) of the mitochondrial ultrastructure in skeletal muscle (n = 4). (**B**,**C**) Protein expression of Oxidative phosphorylation complexes (OXPHOS) complexes I to V in the electron transport chain in skeletal muscle were analyzed by western blotting (n = 6). (**D**) Serum ATP levels (n = 8). (**E**) Mitochondrial DNA (mtDNA) copy number (n = 6). (**F**,**G**) Expression of mitochondrial biogenesis-related genes (n = 6). The results are presented as the mean ± SD. * $p < 0.05$ versus ND-fed rats, # $p < 0.05$ versus HFD-fed rats, & $p < 0.05$ versus HFD + CR rats. ND: Normal chow diet; HFD: High fat diet; CR: Calorie restriction.

4. Discussion and Conclusions

The effects of BCAA (especially leucine) supplementation on insulin resistance remains elusive. Numerous studies have shown that leucine supplementation may prevent HFD-induced obesity [1,2,20], modulate glucose metabolism [21,22] and improve insulin sensitivity in rodent models. However, Newgard et al. suggested that excess BCAAs could contribute to development of insulin resistance, at least under conditions of high fat feeding or elevated tissue fatty acid availability [7]. The underlying mechanisms contributing to these inconsistent results are incompletely understood.

Exactly how leucine exerts effects on insulin resistance is complex, and may depend on the study design, dietary composition, the animal models typically used and the BCAA concentrations, duration and form of administration. Recently, it has been supposed that BCAAs can trigger different and even opposite effects, depending on the catabolic and anabolic state of the organisms [17]. Given the different metabolic signature in the progression of T2DM, and leucine's ability to stimulate both anabolic and catabolic processes [23], we applied an integrative, time-resolved approach to gain a deeper understanding the effects of leucine supplementation in the complexity of the disease on BCAA metabolism, mitochondrial properties and metabolic profiling. Several interesting and important findings were obtained.

In the present study, HFD feeding induced hyperinsulinaemia at 24 weeks. During this period, the rats became increasingly obese, and exhibited lower concentrations of amino acids and related metabolites, fatty acid metabolites and TCA intermediates compared to corresponding ND controls. Studies have shown that insulin signaling functions at an increased basal level in the presence of insulin resistance and hyperinsulinaemia [24,25]. Compensatory increased insulin secretion response to overnutrition may slow fat oxidation and promote anabolism (syntheses of glycogen, proteins, and fats), leading to body weight gain and glucose homeostasis. In contrast, after HFD feeding for 32 weeks, the rats progressively developed hyperglycaemia. The increased insulin level could not maintain glucose at normal levels, and was accompanied by elevated levels of amino acids and related metabolites, fatty acid metabolites and TCA intermediates relative to corresponding ND-fed rats. These data suggested that at this stage the anabolic response to hyperinsulinaemia was blunted, HFD rats were transition from predominantly anabolic condition to predominantly catabolic condition.

The effect of supplementation of HFD with leucine was examined in these two different metabolic conditions, respectively. Our results indicated that doubling dietary leucine globally improved HFD-induced insulin resistance but caused different changes in BCAA catabolism in rats with hyperinsulinaemia or hyperglycaemia. These results seem inconsistent with the finding that elevated circulation of BCAAs and related metabolites promotes insulin resistance, particularly in response to HFD feeding [5,7]. Leucine supplementation ameliorated HFD-induced insulin resistance to different extents at the two time points, as indicated by the improved HOMA-IR values, insulin tolerance and glucose tolerance. Interestingly, this leucine-induced elevation in insulin sensitivity may not be correlated with changes in serum BCAAs, which were increased in HFD + Leu rats at 24 weeks and unaltered at 32 weeks compared with those in HFD-fed rats.

Recent metabolomic, proteomic and genomic studies have suggested that altered BCAA catabolism contributes to elevated BCAAs [14,26,27]. The enzymes involved in the first two steps of the BCAA catabolic pathway, BCATm and Branched-chain α-keto acid dehydrogenase (BCKDH), were examined in the present study. Leucine supplementation increased BCATm protein expression in adipose tissue and skeletal muscle at 24 weeks, suggesting a substrate-induced effect of increased dietary BCAAs (~70% increase for three BCAAs) compared with that in HFD-fed rats. No differences were observed in protein expression of BCKDHE1α, whereas that of BCKDK, a kinase that inactivates BCKDH by phosphorylating the subunit E1α, was increased in observed tissues, including skeletal muscle, liver and adipose tissues. BCKDK participates in a key mechanism for the nutritional and hormonal regulation of BCAA oxidative flux [28,29], and its expression is increased by insulin [30]. This potentially impaired BCKD activity may contribute to the accumulation of BCKAs, such as KIC, in leucine-supplemented rats during the early stage of insulin resistance, which was characterized by hyperinsulinaemia in the present study. Following the progression of insulin resistance to hyperglycaemia, no significant leucine-induced alterations were observed in serum BCAAs or BCAA-catabolizing enzyme levels, with the exception of increased BCATm in adipose tissue. This tight regulation of BCAA catabolism suggests that an elegant method exists for increasing the degradation of BCAAs when they are present in excess and sparing them [31] when they are needed for anabolic or other necessary processes during the different stages of insulin resistance.

In addition to alterations in BCAA catabolism, we identified several leucine-associated changes in TCA cycle intermediates, lipids and other amino acid metabolites in rats with hyperinsulinaemia or hyperglycaemia. Leucine-induced alterations in serum amino acid concentrations at 24 weeks included increased aromatic amino acid (phenylalanine and tryptophan), alanine and asparagine levels, which may have occurred because BCAAs share a competitive transport system with aromatic amino acids [32]. In addition, BCAA transamination provides a nitrogen source for the synthesis of other dispensable amino acids. The levels of almost all amino acid catabolites investigated in the present study were increased in leucine-supplemented rats at 24 weeks, but were unaltered or decreased at 32 weeks, compared with those in HFD-fed controls. It is noteworthy that various factors affect serum amino acid concentrations, including protein turnover (protein synthesis and degradation), and the metabolism of individual amino acids. The exact mechanisms by which leucine supplementation affect the levels of amino acids and their metabolites at different stage of insulin resistance are still unknown, and warrant further study.

Acylcarnitines are intermediates of fatty acid oxidation, and accumulate as a consequence of the metabolic dysfunction resulting from the insufficient integration between β-oxidation and the TCA cycle [33–35]. Elevated BCAAs in a lipotoxic environment have been proposed to induce the accumulation of BCAA-derived acylcarnitines and incompletely oxidized lipid species [5,7]. In HFD-induced hyperinsulinaemic rats in the present study, leucine supplementation caused increases in acylcarnitine species (carnitine, acylcarnitine and palmitoyl-L-carnitine), but no remarkable changes in BCAA-derived short-chain acylcarnitines (C3 and C5). However, TCA cycle intermediates were significantly elevated, reflecting an early compensatory response to substrate overload. Accumulated by-products of BCAA transamination are catabolized to BCAA-related acetyl-CoAs, ketones and other intermediates, leading to competitive inhibition of lipid-derived acetyl-CoA entry into the TCA cycle [36–38]; in turn, this process may reduce fatty acid oxidation and induce acylcarnitine accumulation and ketogenesis, as indicated by the results (Table 3). Interestingly, as insulin resistance progressed, leucine promoted reductions in the accumulation of serum acylcarnitine species and levels of multiple TCA cycle intermediates at 32 weeks compared with those in age-matched HFD-fed controls.Skeletal muscle serves as a major reservoir of free carnitine and is thought to be a principal contributor to the serum acylcarnitine pool. The accumulation of acylcarnitine species is mitotoxic and promotes mitochondrial dysfunction. The above-mentioned alterations in the metabolic phenotype might be correlated with changes in skeletal muscle mitochondrial properties. Consistent with this hypothesis, the HFD + Leu treatment caused increased mitochondrial damage, accompanied by decreases in mitochondrial biogenesis, ATP production and mitochondrial oxidative enzyme levels in skeletal muscle compared with those in HFD-fed controls.These data were seemingly in conflict with the favorable effects of leucine on overall insulin sensitivity at this stage. It is well-known that insulin resistance is associated with mitochondrial dysfunction, but the causality of this association is controversial. More recent findings suggest that mitochondrial dysfunction is not an early event in the development of insulin resistance [39], but rather an adaptation to excess nutrients [40,41]. Skeletal muscle is the initial site for most BCAA catabolism and major insulin-target tissue. Thus, at this stage, improved insulin sensitivity by leucine supplementation may facilitate both the anabolic effects of insulin and the adaptive catabolic effects of "nutrient overload" in skeletal muscle under the background of a HFD, leading to an impaired mitochondrial function. Notably, the HFD-induced mitochondrial damage was relieved and mitochondrial biogenesis was increased by leucine supplementation after 32 weeks. These results are consistent with previous studies reporting that leucine supplementation increases mitochondrial biogenesis while simultaneously enhancing lipid oxidation [42–44], leading to the reduced accumulation of acylcarnitine species. Therefore, we speculate that BCAAs are primarily used for anabolism at this stage; thus, BCAAs and their derivatives that flow into the mitochondria are decreased. This hypothesis is consistent with our observations of decreased levels of TCA cycle intermediates and no obvious changes in BCAAs and amino acids related catabolites concentrations in circulation. The reduced mitochondrial load occurred simultaneously with improved mitochondrial function, leading to increased ATP production. Thus, altered mitochondrial function may partly account for the improvement in skeletal muscle insulin sensitivity. Moreover, Li et al. observed that in HFD-induced obese mice, leucine supplementation prevented obesity and insulin resistance in association with attenuation of mitochondrial dysfunction [45].

Taken together, these results indicated that abnormal BCAA metabolism induced by dietary supplementation coupled with HFD intake might lead to the accumulation of BCKAs and incompletely oxidized lipid species, which contributed to mitochondrial dysfunction in skeletal muscle during the early stage of insulin resistance (24 weeks). In contrast, during the hyperglycaemic stage (32 weeks), when catabolic processes predominate, leucine supplementation enhanced mitochondrial biogenesis, with concomitantly improved lipid oxidation and mitochondrial function in skeletal muscle (Figure 6).

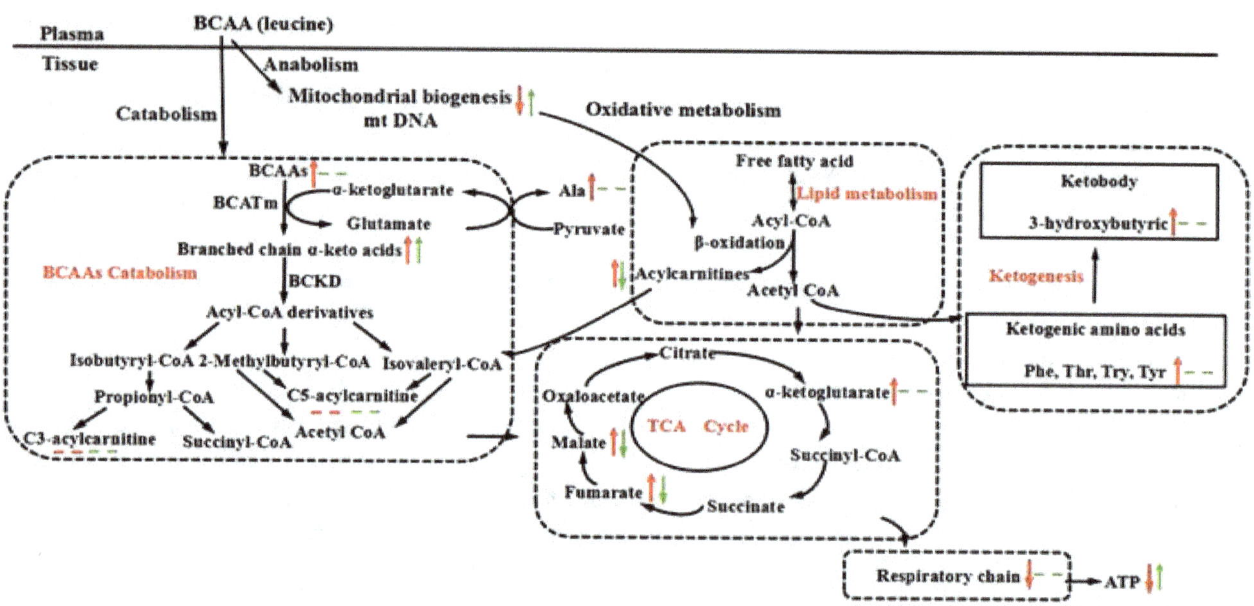

Figure 6. Summary of the possible metabolic alterations induced by leucine supplementation at the different stage of insulin resistance in high-fat diet-fed rats. The red arrows indicate the changes observed at 24 weeks, whereas the blue arrows represent the changes observed at 32 weeks compared with the age-matched high-fat diet-fed controls. The up-arrows indicate an increase in concentration; the down-arrows indicate a decrease in concentration; the dotted lines indicate no significant change in concentration.

CR without malnutrition has long been considered an effective strategy for protecting againstage-associated disorders by modulating mitochondrial biogenesis and activating the reactive oxygen species defense system [46–48]. However, long-term CR is hard for compliance and its possible disadvantages remain to be determined, particularly in the elderly [49]. There has been a growing interest in developing dietary strategies that mimic the beneficial effects of CR. Dietary supplementation with BCAAs has been shown to improve mitochondrial biogenensis and prevent oxidative damage in middle-aged mice [4,16]. In this study, both CR and leucine supplementation improved HFD-induced insulin resistance, but they differently modulated mitochondrial properties at the different stage of insulin resistance. At the hyperinsulinaemia stage, CR improved skeletal muscle mitochondrial biogenesis and function in HFD rats. However, leucine supplementation increased metabolic overload in mitochondria of skeletal muscle accompanied by impaired mitochondrial biogenesis and function. Interestingly, at the hyperglycaemic stage, both CR and leucine supplementationalleviate the HFD-induced mitochondrial damage, whereas HFD + Leu showed a more pronounced effect on mitochondrial biogenesis than CR.

Our study has several limitations. First, T2DM progression and development are long-term processes, with different metabolic characteristics at different stages. Our animal studies only revealed alterations at two time points; thus, they may not reflect the total metabolic changes associated with leucine supplementation. Second, the metabolites detected in our study were limited and we only observed the skeletal muscle's response to leucine supplementation, further investigation should use untargeted metabolomic analysis to capture a large number of differences in metabolite levels and metabolic responses in multiple organs to improve our understanding of the relevant mechanisms. Third, our data demonstrated that the effects of leucine supplementation on insulin resistance were associated with the metabolic condition of the organisms, but the metabolic conditions of HFD rats in the progression of insulin resistance were mainly estimated by the serum metabolites in the present study;this should be further verified by other experiments.

To our knowledge, this study is the first to report that leucine exerts different effects during different stages of insulin resistance in a diet-induced animal model, depending on the prevalence of catabolic and anabolic signals in the organism [17]. During the early stage of insulin resistance, increased insulin levels to maintain normal blood glucose by promoting anabolism (glycogen, protein and fat synthesis) and suppressing fat oxidation [50–52]. Thus, strategies that improve insulin sensitivity may facilitate both the anabolic effects of insulin and the adaptive catabolic effects of "nutrient overload" in the context of a HFD, leading to an adverse metabolic phenotype and mitochondrial dysfunction. Leucine supplementation may not be beneficial if calorie intake is not restricted at this stage. However, as insulin resistance progresses and insulin loses its effectiveness, the condition is characterized by a catabolic state. BCAA or leucine supplementation improves insulin sensitivity, mitochondrial function and other metabolic outcomes, as demonstrated in many conditions, including muscle sarcopaenia, burns, trauma and T2DM in elderly patients [53–55]. The findings of this study help explain the conflicting results reported by different studies and indicate that the patients' overall metabolic status should be carefully considered to potentiate the health benefits of leucine or BCAAs in each clinical setting.

Acknowledgments: We thank Ying Xie and Zhongwen Yuan at Macau University of Science and Technology and Xude Zhang at Beijing Mass Spectrometry Medical Research Co., Ltd. for expert technical support. This study was supported by The National Natural Science Foundation of China (NSFC) Grant No. 81373006 (to X.Y.).

Author Contributions: R.L. and X.Y. designed the study, analyzed the data and drafted the article. R.L., H.L., W.F., Q.J., T.C., Y.W., J.H. and L.H. contributed to the animal studies and acquisition of data. All authors interpreted the data, revised the manuscript critically for important intellectual content and approved the final version to be published. X.Y. is the guarantor of the article.

References

1. Zhang, Y.; Guo, K.; LeBlanc, R.E.; Loh, D.; Schwartz, G.J.; Yu, Y.H. Increasing dietary leucine intake reduces diet-induced obesity and improves glucose and cholesterol metabolism in mice via multimechanisms. *Diabetes* **2007**, *56*, 1647–1654. [CrossRef] [PubMed]
2. Eller, L.K.; Saha, D.C.; Shearer, J.; Reimer, R.A. Dietary leucine improves whole-body insulin sensitivity independent of body fat in diet-induced obese Sprague-Dawley rats. *J. Nutr. Biochem.* **2013**, *24*, 1285–1294. [CrossRef] [PubMed]
3. Nagata, C.; Nakamura, K.; Wada, K.; Tsuji, M.; Tamai, Y.; Kawachi, T. Branched-chain amino acid intake and the risk of diabetes in a japanese community: The takayama study. *Am. J. Epidemiol.* **2013**, *178*, 1226–1232. [CrossRef] [PubMed]
4. Valerio, A.; D'Antona, G.; Nisoli, E. Branched-chain amino acids, mitochondrial biogenesis, and healthspan: An evolutionary perspective. *Aging (Albany NY)* **2011**, *3*, 464–478. [CrossRef] [PubMed]
5. Newgard, C.B.; An, J.; Bain, J.R.; Muehlbauer, M.J.; Stevens, R.D.; Lien, L.F.; Haqq, A.M.; Shah, S.H.; Arlotto, M.; Slentz, C.A.; et al. A branched-chain amino acid-related metabolic signature that differentiates obese and lean humans and contributes to insulin resistance. *Cell Metab.* **2009**, *9*, 311–326. [CrossRef] [PubMed]
6. Nairizi, A.; She, P.; Vary, T.C.; Lynch, C.J. Leucine supplementation of drinking water does not alter susceptibility to diet-induced obesity in mice. *J. Nutr.* **2009**, *139*, 715–719. [CrossRef] [PubMed]

7. Newgard, C.B. Interplay between lipids and branched-chain amino acids in development of insulin resistance. *Cell Metab.* **2012**, *15*, 606–614. [CrossRef] [PubMed]
8. Wang, T.J.; Larson, M.G.; Vasan, R.S.; Cheng, S.; Rhee, E.P.; McCabe, E.; Lewis, G.D.; Fox, C.S.; Jacques, P.F.; Fernandez, C.; et al. Metabolite profiles and the risk of developing diabetes. *Nat. Med.* **2011**, *17*, 448–453. [CrossRef] [PubMed]
9. Batch, B.C.; Shah, S.H.; Newgard, C.B.; Turer, C.B.; Haynes, C.; Bain, J.R.; Muehlbauer, M.; Patel, M.J.; Stevens, R.D.; Appel, L.J.; et al. Branched chain amino acids are novel biomarkers for discrimination of metabolic wellness. *Metabolism* **2013**, *62*, 961–969. [CrossRef] [PubMed]
10. Shah, S.H.; Crosslin, D.R.; Haynes, C.S.; Nelson, S.; Turer, C.B.; Stevens, R.D.; Muehlbauer, M.J.; Wenner, B.R.; Bain, J.R.; Laferrere, B.; et al. Branched-chain amino acid levels are associated with improvement in insulin resistance with weight loss. *Diabetologia* **2012**, *55*, 321–330. [CrossRef] [PubMed]
11. Sengupta, S.; Peterson, T.R.; Sabatini, D.M. Regulation of the mTOR complex 1 pathway by nutrients, growth factors, and stress. *Mol. Cell* **2010**, *40*, 310–322. [CrossRef] [PubMed]
12. Li, X.; Wang, X.; Liu, R.; Ma, Y.; Guo, H.; Hao, L.; Yao, P.; Liu, L.; Sun, X.; He, K.; et al. Chronic leucine supplementation increases body weight and insulin sensitivity in rats on high-fat diet likely by promoting insulin signaling in insulin-target tissues. *Mol. Nutr. Food Res.* **2013**, *57*, 1067–1079. [CrossRef] [PubMed]
13. Houde, V.P.; Brule, S.; Festuccia, W.T.; Blanchard, P.G.; Bellmann, K.; Deshaies, Y.; Marette, A. Chronic rapamycin treatment causes glucose intolerance and hyperlipidemia by upregulating hepatic gluconeogenesis and impairing lipid deposition in adipose tissue. *Diabetes* **2010**, *59*, 1338–1348. [CrossRef] [PubMed]
14. Herman, M.A.; She, P.; Peroni, O.D.; Lynch, C.J.; Kahn, B.B. Adipose tissue branched chain amino acid (BCAA) metabolism modulates circulating bcaa levels. *J. Biol. Chem.* **2010**, *285*, 11348–11356. [CrossRef] [PubMed]
15. Lynch, C.J.; Adams, S.H. Branched-chain amino acids in metabolic signalling and insulin resistance. *Nat. Rev. Endocrinol.* **2014**, *10*, 723–736. [CrossRef] [PubMed]
16. D'Antona, G.; Ragni, M.; Cardile, A.; Tedesco, L.; Dossena, M.; Bruttini, F.; Caliaro, F.; Corsetti, G.; Bottinelli, R.; Carruba, M.O.; et al. Branched-chain amino acid supplementation promotes survival and supports cardiac and skeletal muscle mitochondrial biogenesis in middle-aged mice. *Cell Metab.* **2010**, *12*, 362–372. [CrossRef] [PubMed]
17. Bifari, F.; Nisoli, E. Branched-chain amino acids differently modulate catabolic and anabolic states in mammals: A pharmacological point of view. *Br. J. Pharmacol.* **2016**. [CrossRef] [PubMed]
18. Kleemann, R.; van Erk, M.; Verschuren, L.; van den Hoek, A.M.; Koek, M.; Wielinga, P.Y.; Jie, A.; Pellis, L.; Bobeldijk-Pastorova, I.; Kelder, T.; et al. Time-resolved and tissue-specific systems analysis of the pathogenesis of insulin resistance. *PLoS ONE* **2010**, *5*, e8817. [CrossRef] [PubMed]
19. Adams, S.H. Emerging perspectives on essential amino acid metabolism in obesity and the insulin-resistant state. *Adv. Nutr.* **2011**, *2*, 445–456. [CrossRef] [PubMed]
20. Macotela, Y.; Emanuelli, B.; Bang, A.M.; Espinoza, D.O.; Boucher, J.; Beebe, K.; Gall, W.; Kahn, C.R. Dietary leucine—An environmental modifier of insulin resistance acting on multiple levels of metabolism. *PLoS ONE* **2011**, *6*, e21187. [CrossRef] [PubMed]
21. Binder, E.; Bermudez-Silva, F.J.; Elie, M.; Leste-Lasserre, T.; Belluomo, I.; Clark, S.; Duchampt, A.; Mithieux, G.; Cota, D. Leucine supplementation modulates fuel substrates utilization and glucose metabolism in previously obese mice. *Obesity (Silver Spring)* **2014**, *22*, 713–720. [CrossRef] [PubMed]
22. Guo, K.; Yu, Y.H.; Hou, J.; Zhang, Y. Chronic leucine supplementation improves glycemic control in etiologically distinct mouse models of obesity and diabetes mellitus. *Nutr. Metab. (Lond.)* **2010**, *7*, 57. [CrossRef] [PubMed]
23. Gannon, N.P.; Vaughan, R.A. Leucineinduced anabolic-catabolism: Two sides of the same coin. *Amino Acids* **2016**, *48*, 321–336. [CrossRef] [PubMed]
24. Kim, B.; McLean, L.L.; Philip, S.S.; Feldman, E.L. Hyperinsulinemia induces insulin resistance in dorsal root ganglion neurons. *Endocrinology* **2011**, *152*, 3638–3647. [CrossRef] [PubMed]
25. Kim, B.; Sullivan, K.A.; Backus, C.; Feldman, E.L. Cortical neurons develop insulin resistance and blunted akt signaling: A potential mechanism contributing to enhanced ischemic injury in diabetes. *Antioxid. Redox Signal.* **2011**, *14*, 1829–1839. [CrossRef] [PubMed]

26. Tai, E.S.; Tan, M.L.; Stevens, R.D.; Low, Y.L.; Muehlbauer, M.J.; Goh, D.L.; Ilkayeva, O.R.; Wenner, B.R.; Bain, J.R.; Lee, J.J.; et al. Insulin resistance is associated with a metabolic profile of altered protein metabolism in Chinese and Asian-Indian men. *Diabetologia* **2010**, *53*, 757–767. [CrossRef] [PubMed]
27. She, P.; Van Horn, C.; Reid, T.; Hutson, S.M.; Cooney, R.N.; Lynch, C.J. Obesity-related elevations in plasma leucine are associated with alterations in enzymes involved in branched-chain amino acid metabolism. *Am. J. Physiol. Endocrinol. Metab.* **2007**, *293*, E1552–E1563. [CrossRef] [PubMed]
28. Harris, R.A.; Joshi, M.; Jeoung, N.H. Mechanisms responsible for regulation of branched-chain amino acid catabolism. *Biochem. Biophys. Res. Commun.* **2004**, *313*, 391–396. [CrossRef] [PubMed]
29. Shimomura, Y.; Obayashi, M.; Murakami, T.; Harris, R.A. Regulation of branched-chain amino acid catabolism: Nutritional and hormonal regulation of activity and expression of the branched-chain alpha-keto acid dehydrogenase kinase. *Curr. Opin. Clin. Nutr. Metab. Care* **2001**, *4*, 419–423. [CrossRef] [PubMed]
30. Nellis, M.M.; Doering, C.B.; Kasinski, A.; Danner, D.J. Insulin increases branched-chain alpha-ketoacid dehydrogenase kinase expression in clone 9 rat cells. *Am. J. Physiol.Endocrinol. Metab.* **2002**, *283*, E853–E860. [CrossRef] [PubMed]
31. Brosnan, J.T.; Brosnan, M.E. Branched-chain amino acids: Enzyme and substrate regulation. *J. Nutr.* **2006**, *136*, 207S–211S. [PubMed]
32. Fernstrom, J.D. Branched-chain amino acids and brain function. *J. Nutr.* **2005**, *135*, 1539S–1546S. [PubMed]
33. Koves, T.R.; Ussher, J.R.; Noland, R.C.; Slentz, D.; Mosedale, M.; Ilkayeva, O.; Bain, J.; Stevens, R.; Dyck, J.R.; Newgard, C.B.; et al. Mitochondrial overload and incomplete fatty acid oxidation contribute to skeletal muscle insulin resistance. *Cell Metab.* **2008**, *7*, 45–56. [CrossRef] [PubMed]
34. Aguer, C.; McCoin, C.S.; Knotts, T.A.; Thrush, A.B.; Ono-Moore, K.; McPherson, R.; Dent, R.; Hwang, D.H.; Adams, S.H.; Harper, M.E. Acylcarnitines: Potential implications for skeletal muscle insulin resistance. *FASEB J.* **2015**, *29*, 336–345. [CrossRef] [PubMed]
35. Adams, S.H.; Hoppel, C.L.; Lok, K.H.; Zhao, L.; Wong, S.W.; Minkler, P.E.; Hwang, D.H.; Newman, J.W.; Garvey, W.T. Plasma acylcarnitine profiles suggest incomplete long-chain fatty acid beta-oxidation and altered tricarboxylic acid cycle activity in type 2 diabetic African-American women. *J. Nutr.* **2009**, *139*, 1073–1081. [CrossRef] [PubMed]
36. Hutson, S.M.; Sweatt, A.J.; Lanoue, K.F. Branched-chain [corrected] amino acid metabolism: Implications for establishing safe intakes. *J. Nutr.* **2005**, *135*, 1557S–1564S. [PubMed]
37. White, P.J.; Lapworth, A.L.; An, J.; Wang, L.; McGarrah, R.W.; Stevens, R.D.; Ilkayeva, O.; George, T.; Muehlbauer, M.J.; Bain, J.R.; et al. Branched-chain amino acid restriction in zucker-fatty rats improves muscle insulin sensitivity by enhancing efficiency of fatty acid oxidation and acyl-glycine export. *Mol. Metab.* **2016**, *5*, 538–551. [CrossRef] [PubMed]
38. Lerin, C.; Goldfine, A.B.; Boes, T.; Liu, M.; Kasif, S.; Dreyfuss, J.M.; De Sousa-Coelho, A.L.; Daher, G.; Manoli, I.; Sysol, J.R.; et al. Defects in muscle branched-chain amino acid oxidation contribute to impaired lipid metabolism. *Mol. Metab.* **2016**, *5*, 926–936. [CrossRef] [PubMed]
39. Di Meo, S.; Iossa, S.; Venditti, P. Skeletal muscle insulin resistance: Role of mitochondria and other ROS sources. *J. Endocrinol.* **2017**, *233*, R15–R42. [CrossRef] [PubMed]
40. Affourtit, C. Mitochondrial involvement in skeletal muscle insulin resistance: A case of imbalanced bioenergetics. *Biochim. Biophys. Acta* **2016**, *1857*, 1678–1693. [CrossRef] [PubMed]
41. Liesa, M.; Shirihai, O.S. Mitochondrial dynamics in the regulation of nutrient utilization and energy expenditure. *Cell Metab.* **2013**, *17*, 491–506. [CrossRef] [PubMed]
42. Vaughan, R.A.; Garcia-Smith, R.; Gannon, N.P.; Bisoffi, M.; Trujillo, K.A.; Conn, C.A. Leucine treatment enhances oxidative capacity through complete carbohydrate oxidation and increased mitochondrial density in skeletal muscle cells. *Amino Acids* **2013**, *45*, 901–911. [CrossRef] [PubMed]
43. Sun, X.; Zemel, M.B. Leucine modulation of mitochondrial mass and oxygen consumption in skeletal muscle cells and adipocytes. *Nutr. Metab. (Lond.)* **2009**, *6*, 26. [CrossRef] [PubMed]
44. Vaughan, R.A.; Mermier, C.M.; Bisoffi, M.; Trujillo, K.A.; Conn, C.A. Dietary stimulators of the PGC-1 superfamily and mitochondrial biosynthesis in skeletal muscle. A mini-review. *J. Physiol. Biochem.* **2014**, *70*, 271–284. [CrossRef] [PubMed]
45. Li, H.; Xu, M.; Lee, J.; He, C.; Xie, Z. Leucine supplementation increases sirt1 expression and prevents mitochondrial dysfunction and metabolic disorders in high-fat diet-induced obese mice. *Am. J. Physiol. Endocrinol. Metab.* **2012**, *303*, E1234–E1244. [CrossRef] [PubMed]

46. Lopez-Lluch, G.; Hunt, N.; Jones, B.; Zhu, M.; Jamieson, H.; Hilmer, S.; Cascajo, M.V.; Allard, J.; Ingram, D.K.; Navas, P.; et al. Calorie restriction induces mitochondrial biogenesis and bioenergetic efficiency. *Proc. Natl. Acad. Sci. USA* **2006**, *103*, 1768–1773. [CrossRef] [PubMed]
47. Guarente, L. Mitochondria—A nexus for aging, calorie restriction, and sirtuins? *Cell* **2008**, *132*, 171–176. [CrossRef] [PubMed]
48. Nisoli, E.; Tonello, C.; Cardile, A.; Cozzi, V.; Bracale, R.; Tedesco, L.; Falcone, S.; Valerio, A.; Cantoni, O.; Clementi, E.; et al. Calorie restriction promotes mitochondrial biogenesis by inducing the expression of enos. *Science* **2005**, *310*, 314–317. [CrossRef] [PubMed]
49. Ingram, D.K.; Roth, G.S. Glycolytic inhibition as a strategy for developing calorie restriction mimetics. *Exp. Gerontol.* **2011**, *46*, 148–154. [CrossRef] [PubMed]
50. Liu, H.Y.; Hong, T.; Wen, G.B.; Han, J.; Zuo, D.; Liu, Z.; Cao, W. Increased basal level of akt-dependent insulin signaling may be responsible for the development of insulin resistance. *Am. J. Physiol. Endocrinol. Metab.* **2009**, *297*, E898–E906. [CrossRef] [PubMed]
51. Cao, W.; Ning, J.; Yang, X.; Liu, Z. Excess exposure to insulin is the primary cause of insulin resistance and its associated atherosclerosis. *Curr. Mol. Pharmacol.* **2011**, *4*, 154–166. [CrossRef] [PubMed]
52. Nolan, C.J.; Ruderman, N.B.; Kahn, S.E.; Pedersen, O.; Prentki, M. Insulin resistance as a physiological defense against metabolic stress: Implications for the management of subsets of type 2 diabetes. *Diabetes* **2015**, *64*, 673–686. [CrossRef] [PubMed]
53. Solerte, S.B.; Fioravanti, M.; Locatelli, E.; Bonacasa, R.; Zamboni, M.; Basso, C.; Mazzoleni, A.; Mansi, V.; Geroutis, N.; Gazzaruso, C. Improvement of blood glucose control and insulin sensitivity during a long-term (60 weeks) randomized study with amino acid dietary supplements in elderly subjects with type 2 diabetes mellitus. *Am. J. Cardiol.* **2008**, *101*, 82E–88E. [CrossRef] [PubMed]
54. Leenders, M.; van Loon, L.J. Leucine as a pharmaconutrient to prevent and treat sarcopenia and type 2 diabetes. *Nutr. Rev.* **2011**, *69*, 675–689. [CrossRef] [PubMed]
55. Kawaguchi, T.; Nagao, Y.; Matsuoka, H.; Ide, T.; Sata, M. Branched-chain amino acid-enriched supplementation improves insulin resistance in patients with chronic liver disease. *Int. J. Mol. Med.* **2008**, *22*, 105–112. [CrossRef] [PubMed]

Glycemia Lowering Effect of an Aqueous Extract of *Hedychium coronarium* Leaves in Diabetic Rodent Models

Ling-Shan Tse [1], Po-Lin Liao [2], Chi-Hao Tsai [1,3], Ching-Hao Li [4], Jiunn-Wang Liao [5], Jaw-Jou Kang [2] and Yu-Wen Cheng [1,*]

1 School of Pharmacy, College of Pharmacy, Taipei Medical University, Taipei 110, Taiwan; zoetsels@gmail.com (L.-S.T.); d01447001@ntu.edu.tw (C.-H.T.)
2 Institute of Food Safety and Health Risk Assessment, School of Pharmaceutical Sciences, National Yang-Ming University, Taipei 112, Taiwan; plliao0825@gmail.com (P.-L.L.); jjkang@ym.edu.tw (J.-J.K.)
3 Institute of Toxicology, College of Medicine, National Taiwan University, Taipei 100, Taiwan
4 Department of Physiology, School of Medicine, Graduate Institute of Medical Sciences, College of Medicine, Taipei Medical University, Taipei 110, Taiwan; bros22@tmu.edu.tw
5 Graduate Institute of Veterinary Pathobiology, National Chung Hsing University, Taichung 402, Taiwan; jwliao@dragon.nchu.edu.tw
* Correspondence: ywcheng@tmu.edu.tw

Abstract: *Hedychium coronarium* has a long history of use worldwide as a food and in folk medicine. In this study, we aimed to investigate the effect of an aqueous extract of *H. coronarium* leaves (HC) on type 2 diabetes mellitus (T2DM). Two types of animal models were used in this study: Streptozotocin (STZ)-induced T2DM (Wistar rats; $N = 8$) and C57BKSdb/db mice ($N = 5$). After treatment with HC for 28 days, glucose tolerance improved in both of the diabetic animal models. As significant effects were shown after 14 days of treatment in the STZ-induced T2DM model, we carried out the experiments with it. After 28 days of treatment with HC, the levels of cholesterol, triglyceride, high-density lipoprotein, and low-density lipoprotein were significantly improved in the STZ-induced T2DM model. The lesions degree of islet β-cells was decreased after the HC treatment. Although the insulin level increased moderately, the aldosterone level was significantly decreased in the HC-treated groups, suggesting that aldosterone might play an important role in this effect. In summary, HC is a natural product and it is worth exploring its effect on T2DM.

Keywords: *Hedychium coronarium*; type 2 diabetes; aldosterone; streptozotocin; metabolic syndrome; folk medicine

1. Introduction

Diabetes is a chronic progressive disease and one of the ten leading causes of death worldwide [1]. In the past three decades, the prevalence of type 2 diabetes mellitus (T2DM) has increased dramatically in countries of all income levels. Over time, diabetes causes various complications: It starts by damaging blood vessels, reducing the blood flow, with sequelae that may be macrovascular (heart attack, stroke, and heart failure) [2–4], or microvascular (blindness [5–7] and kidney failure [8]), or causing neuropathies (lower limb amputation). When diabetes is not controlled, not only is the patient quality of life affected and present a burden on medical resources, but the condition may also lead to death. In 2015, the World Health Organization (WHO) declared diabetes as one of the four priority noncommunicable diseases (NCDs) and established a diabetes program to reduce the impact of diabetes by 2020. The management of diabetes consists of two main steps: Preventing (decreasing the possible risk factors) and stabilizing the disease progress (early diagnosis, medication, and intake management) [9]. To stabilize the disease, it is crucial to adopt effective measures for surveillance and treatment strategies (pharmacologic and non-pharmacologic interventions) [10,11]. In addition to the development of novel drugs, the use of traditional medicine and food supplements for the treatment of T2DM should be investigated.

Traditional medicine (also known as folk medicine) has been used globally for centuries. Although the medicinal properties of resources such as mollusks and plants rely on the inheritance of experience, they have been gradually accepted in modern medicine. A food supplement is a dosed formulation of food and herbs, and provides medical benefits through its biologically active components [12]. Therefore, both traditional medicine and food supplements can be part of the treatment strategies for diabetes.

Extensive research has focused on the rhizome of *Hedychium coronarium*. However, the pharmacological benefits of *H. coronarium* leaf appear overlooked. *H. coronarium* is highly accessible and its leaf is a common vegetable in Taiwan. Therefore, in this study, two types of animal models were used to evaluate the lowering blood glucose level benefits of an aqueous extract of *H. coronarium* leaves (HC). A new supplement was developed, called SugarOut (SO), which contained 15% red yeast rice (RYR) and 7.2% *H. coronarium*. Red yeast rice (RYR) is a fermentation product that is traditionally used in East Asia to dye and preserve food. Its main pharmacologically active compound is monacolin-K (also called lovastatin).

H. coronarium (also called ginger lily), a plant approximately 1–3 m in height and has a long history of use in food and traditional folk medicine. For example, it is used in beauty products in Hawaii and Japan, as an essential oil in Vietnam, and as a vegetable in Malaysia. It can help ease indigestion, inflammation, insomnia, and pain in the muscles, joints, and abdomen [13,14]. In Brazil, *H. coronarium* leaf is considered a diuretic [15] and is used for the treatment of hypertension [16]. In India, the rhizome is used for the treatment of diabetes [17]. Many different bioactive compounds have been isolated from *H. coronarium* and their pharmacological effects have been established. For example, diterpenoids and a diarylheptanoid showed anti-angiogenic activity and suppressed the growth of different cancer cell types [18]. Coronarin D shows active resistance to Gram-positive bacteria and fungi [19], induces G2/M arrest, apoptosis, and autophagy [20]. Hedychilactones A, B, and C inhibit increases in nitric oxide (NO) production and the induction of inducible NO synthase [21]. Quercetin-3-*O*-glucuronide (Q3GA) has been reported to show beneficial effects in the reduction and prevention of various diseases, including neurodegenerative diseases, and to exert anti-inflammatory and antioxidant activities [22].

2. Material and Methods

2.1. Preparation of Aqueous Extract of Hedychium coronarium and SugarOut

The HC (containing 1.4% Q3GA) was a deep brown powder. Fresh overground parts (leaves and stems) of *H. coronarium* were collected in Pingtung, Taiwan. The dried leaves and stems of *H. coronarium* (100 kg) were extracted in 100% water at room temperature (25–35 °C). The 100% water extracts were concentrated in vacuo and then lyophilized to obtain a dark brown powder (8.4% yield).

SO was a prototype supplement (dark red powder) developed from *H. coronarium* that assisted with blood glucose regulation. It contained two main extracts: The RYR extract (15%) and the HC (7.2%). The two main bioactive compounds were monacolin K 1.8 mg (±20%) and Q3GA 0.6 mg (±20%).

Both test substances were provided by Vinovo Inc. The HC was stored at 4 °C and the SO was stored at room temperature. Both test substances were freshly dissolved in distilled water and administered by oral gavage daily to all rodents in the morning.

2.2. *Animal Study*

The Streptozotocin (STZ)-induced T2DM model was established in Wistar rats obtained from BioLASCO Ltd. (Taipei, Taiwan) and C57BKS$^{db/db}$ mice (termed db/db here) were obtained from the National Laboratory Animal Center (Taipei, Taiwan). All procedures involving the use of animals were in compliance with the Guide for the Care and Use of Laboratory Animals (Press, 1996) and approved by the Institutional Animal Care and Use Committee at our institution (Approval no. LAC-2016-0168). The preliminary data suggested that the effective dose of SO was 246 mg/kg in the db/db model. As bioavailability differs between rodent species, based on FDA Guidance, the conversion factors for the rat Wistar STZ model and the mouse db/db model were 6.2 and 12.3, respectively [23]. Therefore, 124 mg/kg SO was administered to the STZ-T2DM rats and 246 mg/kg was administered to the C57BKS$^{db/db}$ mice by oral gavage.

2.2.1. C57BKS$^{db/db}$ Mice (db/db Model)

The C57BKS$^{db/db}$ mouse is a model of diabetes with a spontaneous mutation (Lepr^{db}) resulting in morbid obesity, chronic hyperglycemia, pancreatic beta cell atrophy, and low insulin [24]. The diabetes model is determined to be well-established when the blood glucose level is >230 mg/dL after 18 h fasting. Fifteen male mice (25–30 g) were divided into the following three groups (N = 5): Control (treated with distilled water); HC (17.71 mg/kg); and SO (246 mg/kg) [23] (Figure 1).

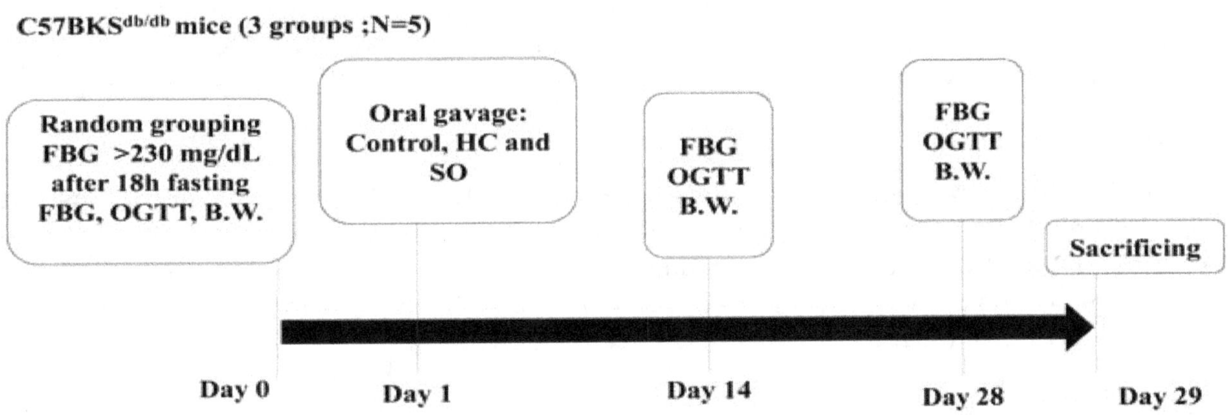

Figure 1. Study procedure for the C57BKS$^{db/db}$ mice (termed db/db here). Fifteen male db/db mice were randomly divided into three groups (N = 5): Control, treatment with *Hedychium coronarium* leaves (HC), or SugarOut (SO) supplement. FBG, fasting blood glucose; OGTT, oral glucose tolerance test; B.W., Body Weight.

2.2.2. STZ-Induced Type 2 Diabetes Model

T2DM was induced in 24 6-week-old male Wistar rats by the administration of 65 mg/kg STZ in 0.1 M citrate solution 15 min after nicotinamide injection (230 mg/kg in saline; intraperitoneally) [25–28]. The rats were caged (two animals per cage) in a controlled environment (12 h light/dark cycle, 23 ± 1 °C, and 39–43% relative humidity). The fasting glucose level was measured 1 week after the injections. The T2DM model was determined to be well-established when the blood glucose level was >230 mg/dL after 18 h of fasting. After T2DM was established, the rats were randomly divided into three groups of eight rats: Control; HC (8.928 mg/kg); and SO (124 mg/kg). An additional eight Wistar rats were used as the sham control (Figure 2).

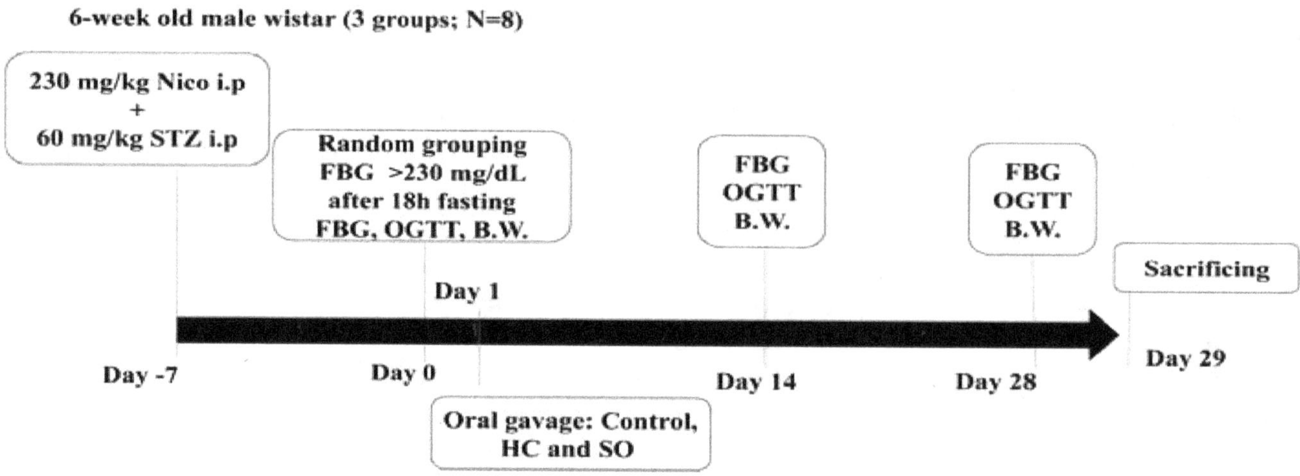

Figure 2. Study procedure for Streptozotocin (STZ)-induced type 2 diabetes rats. Diabetes was induced in 24 male Wistar rats, which were then randomly divided into three groups (Control, HC, and SO; *N* = 8).

2.3. Fasting Blood Glucose and Oral Glucose Tolerance Test

All rodents were administered the test substances daily. The body weight and fasting blood glucose (FBG) was measured on day 0, 14, and 28. The oral glucose tolerance test (OGTT) was performed on day 14 and 28. Each rodent fasted for 16 h before the FBG measurement. The test substances were administered 30 min before glucose challenge (1 g/kg), and then the blood glucose was tested 0, 30, 60, 90, and 120 min after the challenge by using IME-DC glucose test strips (IME-DC, Berlin, Germany).

2.4. Aldosterone and Insulin Levels

Serum samples were collected on day 29 after the T2DM rats were sacrificed. Insulin was quantified through the measurement of the optical density at 450 nm by using a Mercodia Ultrasensitive rat insulin ELISA kit (Mercodia AB, Uppsala, Sweden) and aldosterone was quantified through the measurement of the optical density at 405 nm corrected by the measurement at 590 nm by using an aldosterone ELISA kit (ab136933; Abcam, Cambridge, UK).

2.5. Histopathological Analysis

The pancreas was excised from T2DM rats after they were sacrificed on day 29. The samples were fixed in 10% neutral buffered formalin, and then prepared and examined by a professional pathologist from the Graduate Institute of Veterinary Pathobiology, National Chung Hsing University, Taichung, Taiwan. The severity of lesions in the islet β-cells of the pancreas was graded according to the methods described by Shackelford et al. [29]. The degree of lesions was graded from one to five, depending on severity: 1 = minimal (<1%); 2 = slight (1–25%); 3 = moderate (26–50%); 4 = moderately severe (51–75%); 5 = severe/high (76–100%).

2.6. Serum Biochemical Analysis

Blood samples from the T2DM rats were collected at the end of the 28-day oral administration period and then analyzed by using an Express Plus automatic clinical chemistry analyzer (Siemens Healthineers, Erlangen, Germany).

2.7. Statistical Analysis

All values are expressed as the mean ± standard deviation (SD) in tables and the mean ± standard error (SE) in figures. The comparisons between groups were performed by one-way analysis of variance (ANOVA) followed by Scheffe multiple comparison tests using SPSS Statistical Software (IBM, New York, NY, USA). Values of $p < 0.05$ were considered significant.

3. Results

3.1. HC Improved Fasting Blood Glucose and Glucose Tolerance in Both Diabetic Animal Models After 28 Days of Treatment

In the db/db model, after oral gavage of SO and HC, mice gained weight slower than the control group (Figure 3A). The HC decreased the FBG (Figure 3B) and increased the glucose tolerance after treatment for 14 days (Figure 3C); a significant difference was observed after treatment for 28 days (Figure 3D). SO also affected the FBG and glucose tolerance, however, the effects of SO were not as remarkable as those of the HC.

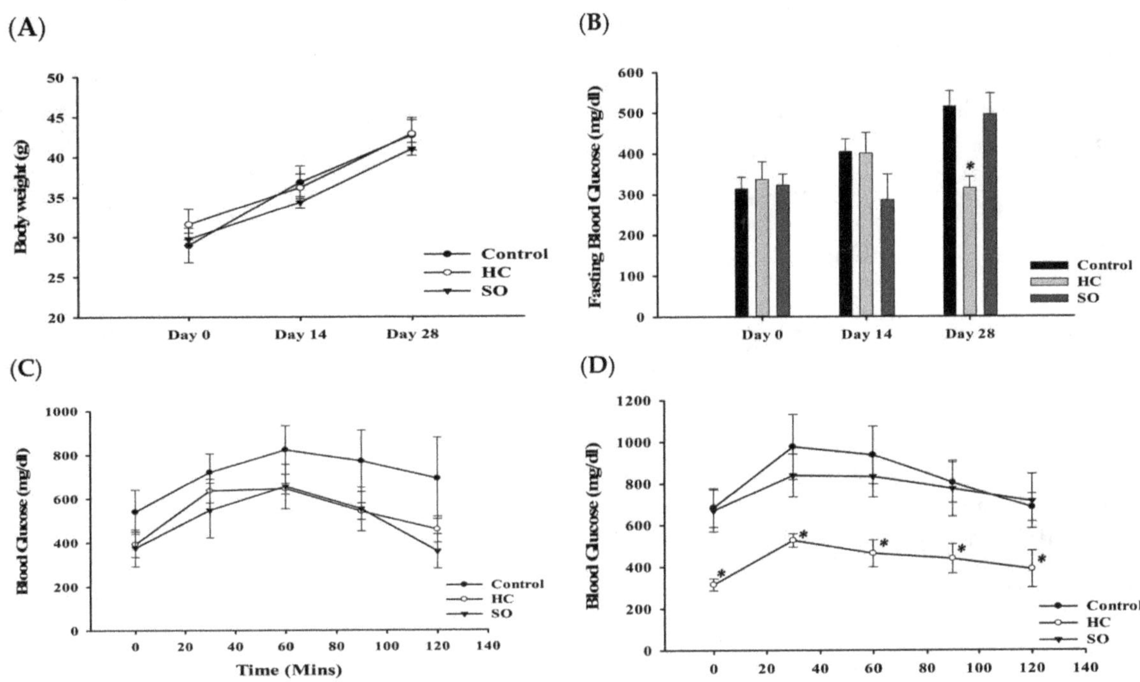

Figure 3. Effects of HC and SO in C57BKS$^{db/db}$ mice (N = 5). **(A)** Changes in body weight. **(B)** Changes in fasting blood glucose (FBG) after treatment with HC and SO for 14 days and 28 days. **(C)** Oral glucose tolerance test (OGTT) after administration of HC and SO for 14 days. **(D)** OGTT after administration of HC and SO for 28 days. Significant difference between the control-treated group at * $p < 0.05$, by one-way ANOVA.

In general, the STZ-induced T2DM model shows a significant weight reduction [30]. In this study, after oral gavage of SO and HC for 28 days, the body weights of mice receiving HC and SO was increased compared to that in the control group (Figure 4A) and the FBG was slightly lower in the SO group on day 28 (Figure 4B). After 14 days of oral administration of HC and SO, the blood glucose level in the HC and SO groups was significantly decreased compared with that in the control group at 60, 90, and 120 min after intake of 1 g/kg glucose (Figure 4C; p-value in Supplementary Table S1). After administration of HC and SO for 28 days (Figure 4D), the glucose level in the SO group was significantly lower than that in control group from 30 to 120 min after the intake of 1 g/kg glucose (p-value in Supplementary Table S1), however, the HC only resulted in a significant difference at 30 min after glucose intake. The area under the curve (AUC) of both the SO and HC groups was significantly lower than that of the control group (Table 1). These results suggested that HC could improve the FBG and glucose tolerance after 28 days in the db/db mice. A notable increase in glucose tolerance was observed in both the HC and SO groups after 14 days of administration, and a significant increase in glucose tolerance was observed after 28 days of administration in the T2DM model. Therefore, the following experiments focused on the STZ-induced T2DM model.

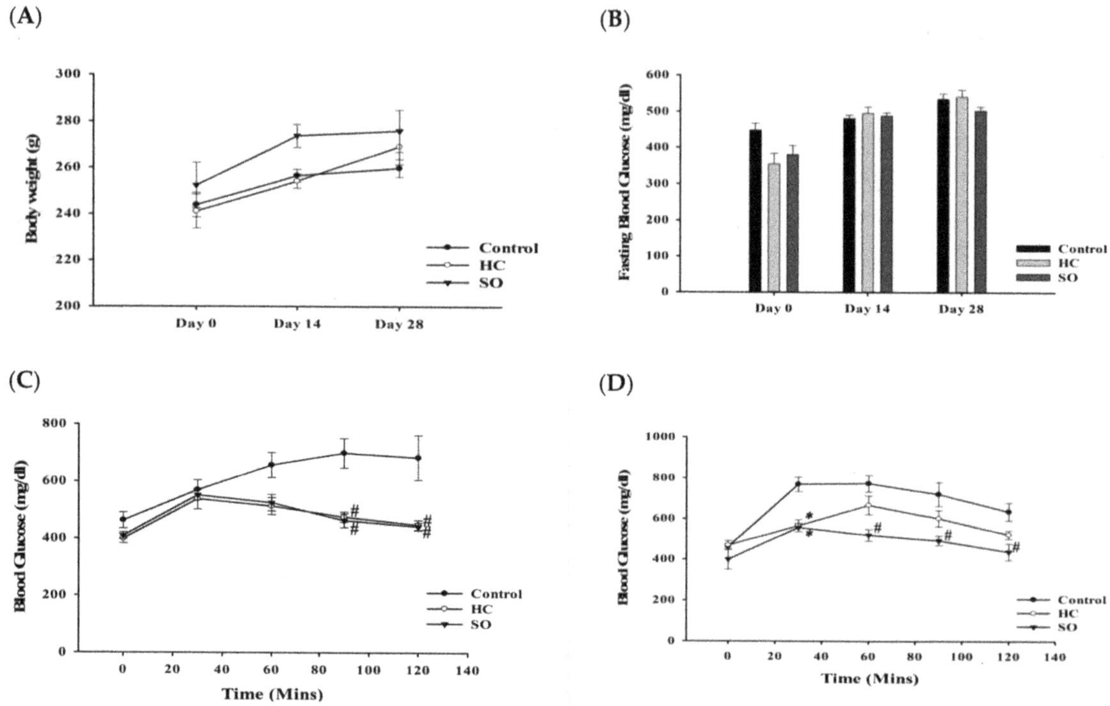

Figure 4. STZ-induced type 2 diabetes model (T2DM; $N = 8$) after the administration of HC and SO for 14 and 28 days. (**A**) Changes in body weight. (**B**) Changes in fasting blood glucose. (**C**) OGTT after administration of HC and SO for 14 days. (**D**) OGTT after administration of HC and SO for 28 days. Significant difference between control-treated group at * $p < 0.05$, # $p < 0.01$ by one-way ANOVA.

Table 1. Area under the curve (AUC) of blood glucose in the oral glucose tolerance test (OGTT).

AUC	14 Days	28 Days
Sham	8898.75 ± 1816.12	1666.88 ± 3399.66
Control	23,578.13 ± 9636.76	32,130.00 ± 8133.19
H. coronarium leaves (HC)	11,730.00 ± 5959.70	14,979.38 ± 5656.03 *
SugarOut (SO)	10,301.25 ± 5884.57	11,945.63 ± 13,782.89 **

Sham = wild-type Wistar rats treated with distilled water. $N = 8$ in each group. The data are expressed as the mean ± standard deviation (SD). Significant difference between the control-treated group at * $p < 0.05$, ** $p < 0.01$ by one-way ANOVA.

3.2. H. coronarium Attenuated STZ-Induced Pancreatic Damage and Ameliorated the Markers of Metabolic Syndrome

The levels of cholesterol, triglyceride, high-density lipoprotein (HDL), and low-density lipoprotein (LDL) were significantly decreased in the STZ-induced T2DM model compared with the control group. In the HC group, creatinine and blood urea nitrogen (BUN) were lower than the control group and similar to the sham group. The SO group did not show any significant differences compared with the control group, but the laboratory results tended to be similar to those in the sham group (Tables 2 and S2). STZ caused a severe decrease in islet β-cells (Figure 5B) and severe atrophy of acinar cells in the pancreas (Figure 5B; Figure 6B). Biopsy sections of the HC (Figure 5C; Figure 6C) and SO (Figure 5D; Figure 6D) groups showed that the morphology of the islet β-cells and acinar cells of the pancreas tended to be similar to the sham group (Figure 5A; Figure 6A). According to the degree of lesions (Table 3) after 28 days treatment, HC (0.79-fold) and SO (0.68-fold) prevented the decrease of islet cells and the atrophy of acinar cells (HC, 0.85-fold; SO 0.70-fold). HC and SO had moderate protective effects against the damage caused by STZ and regulated lipid markers (Table 2). However, the mechanism underlying the beneficial effects of HC on T2DM remains to be elucidated.

Table 2. Biochemical analysis of T2DM rat model after treatment with HC and SO for 28 days.

Group		Sham	Control	HC	SO
Number of Animals		8	8	8	8
Cholesterol	mg/dL	69.28 ± 25.71	161.50 ± 63.79	76.63 ± 15.30 **	111.63 ± 51.48
Triglycerides	mg/dL	58.13 ± 23.93	753.38 ± 434.92	105.13 ± 33.31 **	480.75 ± 410.14
HDL	mmol/L	27.13 ± 12.16	33.38 ± 13.23	42.75 ± 13.10	38.50 ± 12.31
LDL	mmol/L	7.63 ± 1.77	37.63 ± 19.83	10.50 ± 2.56 **	22.25 ± 21.02

HDL: low-density lipoproteins cholesterol; LDL: low-density lipoproteins cholesterol. Data are expressed as the mean ± SD. Significant difference between the control-treated group at ** $p < 0.01$ by one-way ANOVA.

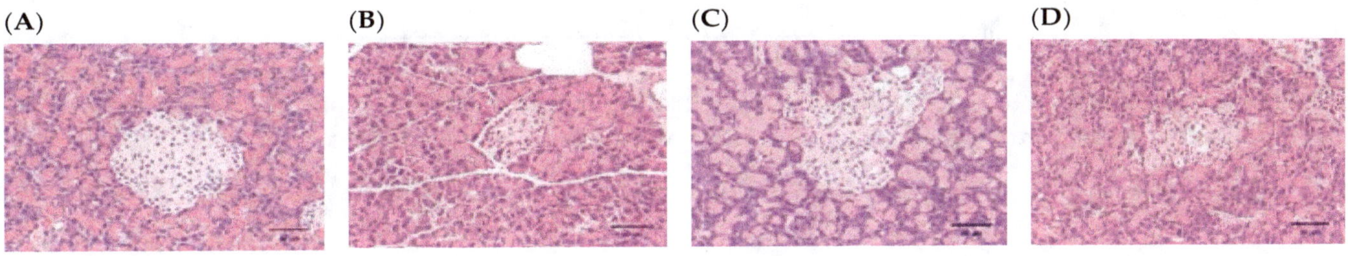

Figure 5. Histopathological changes by hemotoxylin and eosin (H & E) staining (400×) of the islets of the pancreas in rats with STZ-induced β-cell toxicity. (**A**) Sham control. Normal architecture of the β-cells in the islets of the pancreas. STZ induced a slight to moderate/severe decrease of β-cells in the islets of the pancreas in (**B**) T2DM control model. (**C**) T2DM model treated with HC for 28 days. (**D**) T2DM model treated with SO for 28 days. Scale bar = 50 μm.

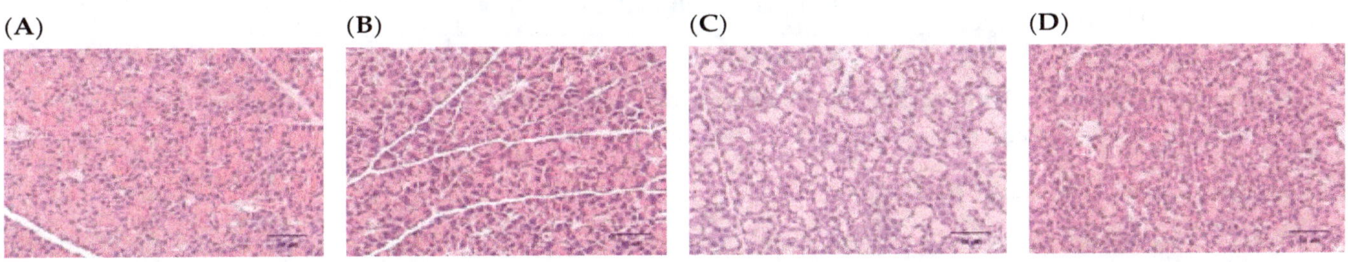

Figure 6. Histopathological changes (H & E staining, 400×) of the acinar cells in the pancreas in rats with STZ-induced β-cell toxicity. (**A**) Sham control. Normal architecture of the β-cells in the islets of the pancreas. STZ induced a slight to moderate/severe decrease of β-cells in the islets of the pancreas in (**B**) T2DM control model. (**C**) T2DM model treated with HC for 28 days. (**D**) T2DM model treated with SO for 28 days. Scale bar = 50 μm.

Table 3. Degree of lesions in the pancreas of the T2DM model animals after treatment with HC and SO for 28 days.

Pancreas	Control	HC	SO
Decrease, β-cell, islet, focal	3.80 ± 0.45	3.00 ± 0.71	2.60 ± 0.55
Atrophy, acinar cell, diffuse	4.00 ± 0.00	3.40 ± 0.89	2.80 ± 1.10

The degree of lesions was graded from one to five depending on severity: 1 = minimal (<1%); 2 = slight (1–25%); 3 = moderate (26–50%); 4 = moderate/severe (51–75%); 5 = severe/high (76–100%).

3.3. HC Altered Insulin and Aldosterone Content in Blood

Insulin levels in the HC (1.32-fold) and SO (1.29-fold) groups increased moderately compared with the control group (Figure 7). Much research has shown that the renin-angiotensin-aldosterone system (RAAS) plays a critical role in diabetes [31–33]. In our previous study, the oral administration of *H. coronarium* aqueous extract (3 g/kg) to Sprague Dawley rats for 90 days, resulted in a decrease of aldosterone levels in the serum. Therefore, we measured the aldosterone level in the present study. Aldosterone was significantly decreased in both HC (0.59-fold) and SO (0.61-fold) groups compared with that in the control group (Figure 8).

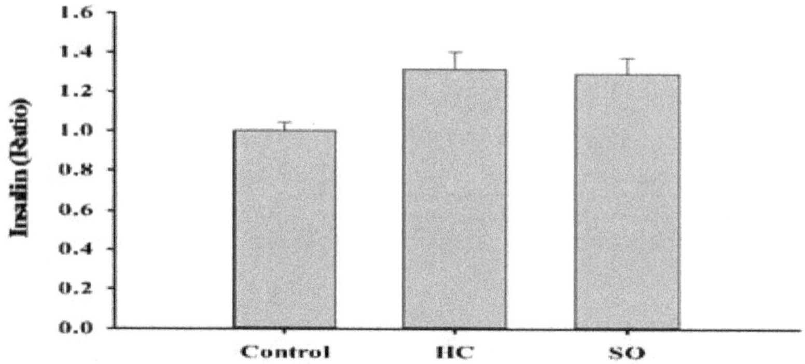

Figure 7. Insulin level in T2DM model rats after 28 days of treatment. No significant difference was found between the control-treated group by one-way ANOVA.

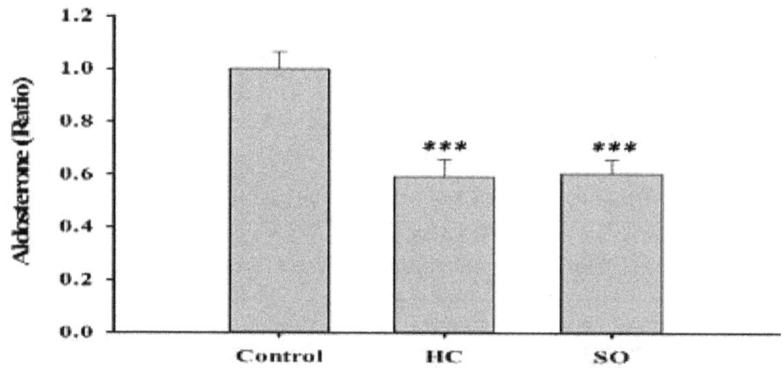

Figure 8. Aldosterone level in T2DM model rats after 28 days of treatment. Significant difference between the control-treated group at *** $p < 0.001$ by one-way ANOVA.

4. Discussion and Conclusions

In this study, we aimed to explore a natural product, *H. coronarium*, and determine if it would benefit people with diabetes. Two types of diabetic rodent models were used to determine the glycemia lowering effect of an aqueous extract of *H. coronarium* leaves. We found that HC significantly increased glucose tolerance in both diabetic models, improved the lipid profile, moderately increased insulin, benefited β-cell structure, and decreased the aldosterone level in an STZ-induced T2DM model. Although HC has been used as a folk medicine worldwide—as a diuretic and for the treatment of inflammation, hypertension, and diabetes—its mechanism of action is yet to be elucidated.

Previous studies have reported that the RAAS has played a major role in diabetes; aldosterone is significantly increased in primary hyperaldosteronism, diabetes, and other metabolic syndromes. An increase in aldosterone causes impaired glucose tolerance, decreased pancreatic β-cell function, and tissue insulin sensitivity [31,34,35]. Aldosterone is a mineralocorticoid hormone that is produced from cholesterol in the cortex of the adrenal gland. It interacts with the mineralocorticoid receptor (MR) to regulate blood pressure, water sodium, and potassium homeostasis [36]. In addition, it has genomic and non-genomic actions. The genomic actions occur through the binding of aldosterone to cytoplasmic MR, and the aldosterone-MR complex translocates to the nucleus and modulates nuclear transcription [37]. As for the rapid non-genomic action, aldosterone increases intracellular Ca^{2+} and protein kinase C (PKC) activation. In addition, aldosterone activates and stimulates Na^+/K^+-ATPase, $Na^+/K^+/2Cl^+$, NHE1, and NBCe1 [38–40], and other pathways, such as the Mitogen-activated protein (MAP) kinases pathway, adenylate cyclase, tyrosine kinase, and cAMP-dependent protein kinase. Therefore, understanding the complete regulation of aldosterone biosynthesis will allow medicinal interventions for the management of hypertension, congestive heart failure, renal disease, and diabetes mellitus [41]. In this study, both HC and SO significantly decreased aldosterone levels and increased glucose tolerance in the STZ-induced T2DM model. These findings suggest that T2DM may be improved by alteration of the aldosterone levels, but more studies are recommended to understand the regulation of this pathway.

Flavonoids may play a role in many metabolic processes involved in T2DM, and Q3GA (also known as miquelianin) is a flavonol glucuronide. Q3GA has been proven to inhibit the production of reactive oxygen species (ROS), low-density lipoprotein (LDL) oxidation [42,43], act as an anti-inflammatory, and improve insulin resistance in skeletal cells [44]. Q3GA also inhibited angiotensin II (Ang II)-induced increases in the DNA binding activity of activator protein (AP)-1, a downstream transcription factor of c-Jun N-terminal kinases (JNK), composed of the c-Jun homo/heterodimer [45]. Angiotensin II interacts with the angiotensin receptor (AT1) membrane receptor that is coupled to cellular second messengers, it is important in the regulation of aldosterone secretion [46]. As Q3GA can reduce the effect of Ang II, it may also contribute to the regulation of aldosterone.

As we would like to develop a new supplement containing HC, we also examined the effect of SO in this study. RYR has been reported to exert anti-inflammatory, hypotensive, cholesterol-lowering, cardioprotective, anticancer, and osteogenic activities [47]. In a previous study, RYR extract (300 mg/kg/day) was reported to decrease the FBG, increase insulin secretion, and protect islet cells in db/db mice [48]. Therefore, we selected RYR for the development of a food supplement containing HC. When the two compounds were combined, we expected an additional effect. In the present study, we also tested the efficacy of SO. SO slightly lowered fasting blood glucose after 28 days of treatment in the STZ -induced T2DM model (Figure 4B). The glucose tolerance (Figure 4C,D) in the SO treatment group was moderately increased compared with that in the HC group after 28 days. However, no differences in insulin, aldosterone, and histopathological findings were observed when the SO group was compared with the HC group. We found that HC exerts beneficial effects in diabetes through modulation of the aldosterone level in the blood to improve glucose tolerance. SO may slightly assist in the improvement of glucose tolerance, although the supplement formula requires improvement. SO also showed effects in two animal models, however, the efficacy of SO in the db/db model was not as strong as HC. The db/db model is known to have as defects in the leptin receptor, leading to increases in insulin and blood glucose, insulin resistance, and obesity [49]. In contrast, STZ is a DNA alkylating agent that targets β-cells [25–28]. As shown by the lipid profile in the STZ model, SO has the ability to ameliorate lipid markers, although not to the same extent as HC (Table 2). This explained how SO lowered the FBG and increased the glucose tolerance after 14 days of treatment, but was not as effective as HC during day 28 in db/db model (Figure 3).

In summary, we treated two types of diabetic rodent models with HC and SO, and found that both HC and SO exerted beneficial effects on T2DM. However, SO treatment did not show a significant difference compared with the HC treatment. The underlying mechanisms of HC, and the interactions of HC and RYR combined, are not wholly investigated yet. Therefore, we suggest that HC could be a suitable candidate for the development of drugs and food supplements for the treatment of T2DM, but more studies should be performed in order to understand the profound mechanism.

Author Contributions: Y.-W.C., C.-H.L. and J.-J.K. planned the experiments; P.-L.L., C.-H.T., and L.-S.T. performed the experiments; L.-S.T. performed data analysis and wrote the manuscript; J.-W.L. is the main pathologist. All authors reviewed the manuscript.

Abbreviations

T2DM	type 2 diabetes;
HDL	high-density lipoproteins cholesterol;
LDL	low-density lipoproteins cholesterol;
OGTT	oral glucose tolerance test’
FBG	fasting blood glucose

Abbreviations

T2DM type 2 diabetes;
HDL high-density lipoproteins cholesterol;
LDL low-density lipoproteins cholesterol;
OGTT oral glucose tolerance test'
FBG fasting blood glucose

References

1. World Health Organization. The Top 10 Causes of Death. Available online: https://www.who.int/news-room/fact-sheets/detail/the-top-10-causes-of-death (accessed on 24 May 2018).
2. Bajaj, H.S.; Zinman, B. Glucose lowering strategies for cardiac benefits: Pathophysiological mechanisms. *Physiology (Bethesda)* **2018**, *33*, 197–210. [CrossRef]
3. Kannel, W.B.; Hjortland, M.; Castelli, W.P. Role of diabetes in congestive heart failure: The Framingham study. *Am. J. Cardiol.* **1974**, *34*, 29–34. [CrossRef]
4. Kannel, W.B.; McGee, D.L. Diabetes and cardiovascular disease. The Framingham study. *JAMA* **1979**, *241*, 2035–2038. [CrossRef] [PubMed]
5. Petropoulos, I.N.; Green, P.; Chan, A.W.; Alam, U.; Fadavi, H.; Marshall, A.; Asghar, O.; Efron, N.; Tavakoli, M.; Malik, R.A. Corneal confocal microscopy detects neuropathy in patients with type 1 diabetes without retinopathy or microalbuminuria. *PLoS ONE* **2015**, *10*, e0123517. [CrossRef] [PubMed]
6. Yorek, M.A. Vascular impairment of epineurial arterioles of the sciatic nerve: Implications for diabetic peripheral neuropathy. *Rev. Diabet. Stud.* **2015**, *12*, 13–28. [CrossRef] [PubMed]
7. Javed, S.; Alam, U.; Malik, R.A. Treating diabetic neuropathy: Present strategies and emerging solutions. *Rev. Diabet. Stud.* **2015**, *12*, 63–83. [CrossRef]
8. Manski-Nankervis, J.A.; Thuraisingam, S.; Sluggett, J.K.; Kilov, G.; Furler, J.; O'Neal, D.; Jenkins, A. Prescribing of diabetes medications to people with type 2 diabetes and chronic kidney disease: A national cross-sectional study. *BMC Fam. Pract.* **2019**, *20*, 29. [CrossRef] [PubMed]
9. Schrijvers, G. Disease management: A proposal for a new definition. *Int. J. Integr. Care* **2009**, *9*, e06. [CrossRef] [PubMed]
10. Raveendran, A.V.; Chacko, E.C.; Pappachan, J.M. Non-pharmacological treatment options in the management of diabetes mellitus. *Eur. Endocrinol.* **2018**, *14*, 31–39. [CrossRef] [PubMed]
11. World Health Organization. *Global Report on Diabetes*; WHO: Geneva, Switzerland, 2016.
12. Perera, P.K.; Li, Y. Functional herbal food ingredients used in type 2 diabetes mellitus. *Pharmacogn. Rev.* **2012**, *6*, 37–45. [PubMed]
13. Van Thanh, B.; Dai, D.N.; Thang, T.D.; Binh, N.Q.; Anh, L.D.; Ogunwande, I.A. Composition of essential oils of four Hedychium species from Vietnam. *Chem. Cent. J.* **2014**, *8*, 54. [CrossRef] [PubMed]
14. Ibrahim, H. *Hedychium*; Backhuys Publisher: Leiden, The Netherlands, 2001; Volume 2, pp. 290–295.
15. Ribeiro Rde, A.; de Barros, F.; de Melo, M.M.; Muniz, C.; Chieia, S.; Wanderley M das, G.; Gomes, C.; Trolin, G. Acute diuretic effects in conscious rats produced by some medicinal plants used in the state of São Paulo, Brasil. *J. Ethnopharmacol.* **1988**, *24*, 19–29. [CrossRef]
16. Ribeiro Rde, A.; Fiuza de Melo, M.M.; De Barros, F.; Gomes, C.; Trolin, G. Acute antihypertensive effect in conscious rats produced by some medicinal plants used in the state of São Paulo. *J. Ethnopharmacol.* **1986**, *15*, 261–269. [CrossRef]
17. Bhandary, M.J.; Chandrashekar, K.R.; Kaveriappa, K.M. Medical ethnobotany of the siddis of Uttara-Kannada District, Karnataka, India. *J. Ethnopharmacol.* **1995**, *47*, 149–158. [CrossRef]
18. Zhan, Z.J.; Wen, Y.T.; Ren, F.Y.; Rao, G.W.; Shan, W.G.; Li, C.P. Diterpenoids and a diarylheptanoid from Hedychium coronarium with significant anti-angiogenic and cytotoxic activities. *Chem. Biodivers.* **2012**, *9*, 2754–2760. [CrossRef] [PubMed]
19. Reuk-ngam, N.; Chimnoi, N.; Khunnawutmanotham, N.; Techasakul, S. Antimicrobial activity of coronarin D and its synergistic potential with antibiotics. *Biomed. Res. Int.* **2014**, *2014*, 581985. [CrossRef] [PubMed]

20. Chen, J.C.; Hsieh, M.C.; Lin, S.H.; Lin, C.C.; Hsi, Y.T.; Lo, Y.S.; Chuang, Y.C.; Hsieh, M.J.; Chen, M.K. Coronarin D induces reactive oxygen species-mediated cell death in human nasopharyngeal cancer cells through inhibition of p38 MAPK and activation of JNK. *Oncotarget* **2017**, *8*, 108006–108019. [CrossRef] [PubMed]
21. Matsuda, H.; Morikawa, T.; Sakamoto, Y.; Toguchida, I.; Yoshikawa, M. Labdane-type diterpenes with inhibitory effects on increase in vascular permeability and nitric oxide production from Hedychium coronarium. *Bioorg. Med. Chem.* **2002**, *10*, 2527–2534. [CrossRef]
22. Li, F.; Sun, X.Y.; Li, X.W.; Yang, T.; Qi, L.W. Enrichment and separation of quercetin-3-*O*-beta-d-glucuronide from lotus leaves (nelumbo nucifera gaertn.) and evaluation of its anti-inflammatory effect. *J. Chromatogr. B Anal. Technol. Biomed. Life Sci.* **2017**, *1040*, 186–191. [CrossRef]
23. Food and Drug Administration. *Guidance for Industry-Estimating the Maximum Safe Starting Dose in Initial Clinical Trials for Therapeutic in Adult Healthy Volunteers*; Center for Drug Evaluation and Research, Ed.; Food and Drug Administration: Rockville, MD, USA, 2005.
24. *BKS.Cg-Dock7m +/+ Leprdb/J*; The Jackson Laboratory: Bar Harbor, ME, USA, 2019.
25. Szkudelski, T. The mechanism of alloxan and streptozotocin action in B cells of the rat pancreas. *Physiol. Res.* **2001**, *50*, 537–546.
26. Szkudelski, T. Streptozotocin-nicotinamide-induced diabetes in the rat. Characteristics of the experimental model. *Exp. Biol. Med. (Maywood)* **2012**, *237*, 481–490. [CrossRef]
27. Islam, M.S.; Wilson, R.D. Experimentally induced rodent models of type 2 diabetes. *Methods Mol. Biol.* **2012**, *933*, 161–174. [PubMed]
28. Ghasemi, A.; Khalifi, S.; Jedi, S. Streptozotocin-nicotinamide-induced rat model of type 2 diabetes. *Acta Physiol. Hung.* **2014**, *101*, 408–420. [CrossRef] [PubMed]
29. Shackelford, C.; Long, G.; Wolf, J.; Okerberg, C.; Herbert, R. Qualitative and quantitative analysis of nonneoplastic lesions in toxicology studies. *Toxicol. Pathol.* **2002**, *30*, 93–96. [CrossRef] [PubMed]
30. Akbarzadeh, A.; Norouzian, D.; Mehrabi, M.R.; Jamshidi, S.; Farhangi, A.; Verdi, A.A.; Mofidian, S.M.; Rad, B.L. Induction of diabetes by Streptozotocin in rats. *Indian J. Clin. Biochem.* **2007**, *22*, 60–64. [CrossRef] [PubMed]
31. Joseph, J.J.; Echouffo-Tcheugui, J.B.; Kalyani, R.R.; Yeh, H.C.; Bertoni, A.G.; Effoe, V.S.; Casanova, R.; Sims, M.; Correa, A.; Wu, W.C.; et al. Aldosterone, renin, and diabetes mellitus in African Americans: The jackson heart study. *J. Clin. Endocrinol. Metab.* **2016**, *101*, 1770–1778. [CrossRef]
32. Lovshin, J.A.; Lytvyn, Y.; Lovblom, L.E.; Katz, A.; Boulet, G.; Bjornstad, P.; Lai, V.; Cham, L.; Tse, J.; Orszag, A.; et al. Retinopathy and RAAS activation: Results from the Canadian study of longevity in type 1 diabetes. *Diabetes Care* **2019**, *42*, 273–280. [CrossRef] [PubMed]
33. Griffin, T.P.; Islam, M.N.; Blake, L.; Bell, M.; Griffin, M.D.; O'Shea, P.M. Effect of sodium glucose co-transporter-2 inhibition on the aldosterone/renin ratio in type 2 diabetes mellitus. *Horm. Metab. Res.* **2018**, *51*, 91–99. [CrossRef] [PubMed]
34. Mosso, L.M.; Carvajal, C.A.; Maiz, A.; Ortiz, E.H.; Castillo, C.R.; Artigas, R.A.; Fardella, C.E. A possible association between primary aldosteronism and a lower beta-cell function. *J. Hypertens.* **2007**, *25*, 2125–2130. [CrossRef] [PubMed]
35. Widimsky, J., Jr.; Sindelka, G.; Haas, T.; Prazny, M.; Hilgertova, J.; Skrha, J. Impaired insulin action in primary hyperaldosteronism. *Physiol. Res.* **2000**, *49*, 241–244. [PubMed]
36. Schmidt, B.M. Rapid non-genomic effects of aldosterone on the renal vasculature. *Steroids* **2008**, *73*, 961–965. [CrossRef] [PubMed]
37. Hermidorff, M.M.; de Assis, L.V.; Isoldi, M.C. Genomic and rapid effects of aldosterone: What we know and do not know thus far. *Heart Fail. Rev.* **2017**, *22*, 65–89. [CrossRef]
38. Alzamora, R.; Brown, L.R.; Harvey, B.J. Direct binding and activation of protein kinase C isoforms by aldosterone and 17beta-estradiol. *Mol. Endocrinol.* **2007**, *21*, 2637–2650. [CrossRef]
39. Mihailidou, A.S.; Mardini, M.; Funder, J.W. Rapid, nongenomic effects of aldosterone in the heart mediated by epsilon protein kinase C. *Endocrinology* **2004**, *145*, 773–780. [CrossRef] [PubMed]
40. Yoshida, T.; Shin-ya, H.; Nakai, S.; Yorimoto, A.; Morimoto, T.; Suyama, T.; Sakurai, M. Genomic and non-genomic effects of aldosterone on the individual variation of the sweat Na^+ concentration during exercise in trained athletes. *Eur. J. Appl. Physiol.* **2006**, *98*, 466–471. [CrossRef]
41. Bollag, W.B. Regulation of aldosterone synthesis and secretion. *Compr. Physiol.* **2014**, *4*, 1017–1055. [PubMed]

42. Terao, J.; Yamaguchi, S.; Shirai, M.; Miyoshi, M.; Moon, J.H.; Oshima, S.; Inakuma, T.; Tsushida, T.; Kato, Y. Protection by quercetin and quercetin 3-*O*-beta-D-glucuronide of peroxynitrite-induced antioxidant consumption in human plasma low-density lipoprotein. *Free Rad. Res.* **2001**, *35*, 925–931. [CrossRef]
43. Moon, J.H.; Tsushida, T.; Nakahara, K.; Terao, J. Identification of quercetin 3-*O*-beta-D-glucuronide as an antioxidative metabolite in rat plasma after oral administration of quercetin. *Free Rad. Biol. Med.* **2001**, *30*, 1274–1285. [CrossRef]
44. Liu, K.; Mei, F.; Wang, Y.; Xiao, N.; Yang, L.; Wang, Y.; Li, J.; Huang, F.; Kou, J.; Liu, B.; et al. Quercetin oppositely regulates insulin-mediated glucose disposal in skeletal muscle under normal and inflammatory conditions: The dual roles of AMPK activation. *Mol. Nutr. Food Res.* **2016**, *60*, 551–565. [CrossRef] [PubMed]
45. Ishizawa, K.; Yoshizumi, M.; Kawai, Y.; Terao, J.; Kihira, Y.; Ikeda, Y.; Tomita, S.; Minakuchi, K.; Tsuchiya, K.; Tamaki, T. Pharmacology in health food: Metabolism of quercetin in vivo and its protective effect against arteriosclerosis. *J. Pharmacol. Sci.* **2011**, *115*, 466–470. [CrossRef]
46. Mulrow, P.J. Angiotensin II and aldosterone regulation. *Regul. Pept.* **1999**, *80*, 27–32. [CrossRef]
47. Patel, S. Functional food red yeast rice (RYR) for metabolic syndrome amelioration: A review on pros and cons. *World J. Microbiol. Biotechnol.* **2016**, *32*, 87. [CrossRef] [PubMed]
48. Wang, J.; Jiang, W.; Zhong, Y.; Lu, B.; Shao, J.; Jiang, S.; Gu, P. Xuezhikang attenuated the functional and morphological impairment of pancreatic islets in diabetic mice via the inhibition of oxidative stress. *J. Cardiovasc. Pharmacol.* **2014**, *63*, 282–289. [CrossRef] [PubMed]
49. Tao, Y.-X. *Glucose Homeostatis and the Pathogenesis of Diabetes Mellitus*, 1st ed.; Academic Press: Cambridge, MA, USA, 2014.

8

Butyrate Reduces HFD-Induced Adipocyte Hypertrophy and Metabolic Risk Factors in Obese LDLr-/-.Leiden Mice

Charlotte E. Pelgrim [1,†], Bart A. A. Franx [1,†], Jessica Snabel [2], Robert Kleemann [2], Ilse A. C. Arnoldussen [1] and Amanda J. Kiliaan [1,*]

1 Donders Institute for Brain, Cognition and Behaviour, Preclinical Imaging Centre, Department of Anatomy, Radboud University Medical Center, 6525 EZ Nijmegen, The Netherlands; charlottepelgrim@gmail.com (C.E.P.); bart.franx@gmail.com (B.A.A.F.); ilse.arnoldussen@radboudumc.nl (I.A.C.A.)

2 Department of Metabolic Health Research, Netherlands Organisation for Applied Scientific Research (TNO), 2301 CE Leiden, The Netherlands; jessica.snabel@tno.nl (J.S.); robert.kleemann@tno.nl (R.K.)

* Correspondence: Amanda.Kiliaan@radboudumc.nl

† Authors contributed equally to this work.

Abstract: Adipose tissue (AT) has a modulating role in obesity-induced metabolic complications like type 2 diabetes mellitus (T2DM) via the production of so-called adipokines such as leptin, adiponectin, and resistin. The adipokines are believed to influence other tissues and to affect insulin resistance, liver function, and to increase the risk of T2DM. In this study, we examined the impact of intervention with the short-chain fatty acid butyrate following a high-fat diet (HFD) on AT function and other metabolic risk factors associated with obesity and T2DM in mice during mid- and late life. In both mid- and late adulthood, butyrate reduced HFD-induced adipocyte hypertrophy and elevations in leptin levels, which were associated with body weight, and cholesterol and triglyceride levels. HFD feeding stimulated macrophage accumulation primarily in epididymal AT in both mid- and late life adult mice, which correlated with liver inflammation in late adulthood. In late-adult mice, butyrate diminished increased insulin levels, which were related to adipocyte size and macrophage content in epididymal AT. These results suggest that dietary butyrate supplementation is able to counteract HFD-induced detrimental changes in AT function and metabolic outcomes in late life. These changes underlie the obesity-induced elevated risk of T2DM, and therefore it is suggested that butyrate has potential to attenuate risk factors associated with obesity and T2DM.

Keywords: obesity; T2DM; high-fat diet; butyrate; adipose tissue; macrophages; adipokines

1. Introduction

In line with the rise of type 2 diabetes mellitus (T2DM) the global prevalence of obesity has more than doubled since 1980 [1]. Moreover, obesity is a major risk factor for T2DM, accounting for 80–85% of the overall risk [2]. Weight or fat loss has the strongest effect on reducing the risk of developing T2DM [3]. It has been suggested that the relationship between obesity and T2DM exists already at a young age [4–6]. In addition, obesity is suggested to exaggerate aging processes [7], and aging is associated with impaired insulin signaling [8], which causes an increase in blood glucose levels. Over time, high blood glucose concentrations combined with high blood pressure and high cholesterol levels affect vascular function, and may evolve into cardiovascular disease, kidney failure, and subsequent cognitive deficits [9,10].

Accumulating evidence suggests that adipose tissue dysfunction—with adipocyte hypertrophy as a first manifestation—may play a role in the development of obesity-induced metabolic conditions that increase the risk for T2DM [11]. Adipocyte hypertrophy results in an elevated recruitment of macrophages surrounding dead or dying adipocytes, which is referred to as crown-like structures (CLS)—an important hallmark of adipose tissue dysfunction— [12]. Macrophages are believed to be major sources of inflammatory cytokines with detrimental effects on insulin signaling in obesity [13]. In addition, adipocyte hypertrophy may lead to the altered production and secretion of adipokines like leptin, resistin, serum amyloid A (SAA), and adiponectin [14–16]. These adipokines play important roles in insulin signaling and the development of a chronic low-grade inflammatory state, which is characteristic for obesity. Overall, amelioration of these obesity-induced and adipose tissue-related changes may provide an important approach to attenuate the risk of developing T2DM.

There is a growing interest in short-chain fatty acids—such as butyrate—as dietary intervention for obesity and related metabolic diseases [17,18]. Butyrate is one of the fatty acids produced during bacterial fermentation in the distal gut of nondigestible carbohydrates like dietary fiber and resistant starch. Both intake of butyrate and dietary fibers have shown positive effects on body weight and insulin sensitivity [17,19–22]. In addition, butyrate has anti-inflammatory properties and affects lipogenesis [17]. A decreased concentration of butyrate-producing bacteria has been observed both in patients with obesity [23] and T2DM [24]. Butyrate may therefore play an essential role in the maintenance of an optimal metabolic state.

It is acknowledged that obesity may differentially affect various organs and tissues, like the brain and cardiovascular system, during midlife as opposed to late life [18,25–27]. Recently, we demonstrated that butyrate is able to restore high-fat diet (HFD)-induced neuroinflammation and changes in brain function in low-density-lipoprotein receptor knockout (LDLr-/-).Leiden mice in mid-adulthood [18]. In addition, mid-adult mice seem to be more susceptible to the development of HFD-induced cardiovascular damage as compared to late-adult mice [18]. However, it has not been elucidated whether diet-induced obesity affects adipose tissue function and its metabolic outcomes differentially during mid- and late adulthood. As follow-up of the previous published study [18], we investigated in the current study the effects of a therapeutic butyrate intervention on adipose tissue function and adipokine levels in the context of manifested HFD-induced obesity in both mid- and late-adult LDLr-/-.Leiden mice.

2. Materials and Methods

2.1. Animals and Diets

The adipose tissues and plasma samples analyzed in this experiment originate from a previously described study [18]. LDLr-/-.Leiden mice were selected because of their high sensitivity to developing HFD-induced obesity and subsequent complications like vascular damage and fatty liver [28–30]. Briefly, male LDLr-/-.Leiden mice (TNO Metabolic Health Research, Leiden, The Netherlands) were housed in individually ventilated cages in a conventional animal room situated in the preclinical imaging center (PRIME) at the central animal laboratory, Radboudumc Nijmegen, the Netherlands. A maximum of five mice were housed per cage with ad libitum access to acidified tap water and food (temperature 21 °C; relative humidity 50–60%; light-dark cycle 7 a.m.–7 p.m.). The experiments were approved by an independent ethical committee on animal care and experimentation (Zeist, The Netherlands), approval project number DEC3682 [18] and carried out in accordance to the ARRIVE guidelines [31].

The intervention regimen of the study [18] is schematically presented in Figure 1. A total group of $n = 60$ LDLr-/-.Leiden mice were divided into a mid- and late-adult cohort ($n = 30$ each). Both cohorts consisted of three diet groups. For the cohort representing mid-adulthood, the first group received a chow diet from birth until the end of the study (Chow). The second group switched to a HFD at three months of age (HFD). The third group switched to a HFD when three months old (m.o.) as well, but this HFD was subsequently enriched with 5% *w/w* butyrate from seven months of age until the end of the study (HDFB) (Figure 1a). The cohort representing late adulthood was subdivided in the same manner, but mice were switched to HFD at six months of age and butyrate intervention started at 10 months of age (Figure 1b).

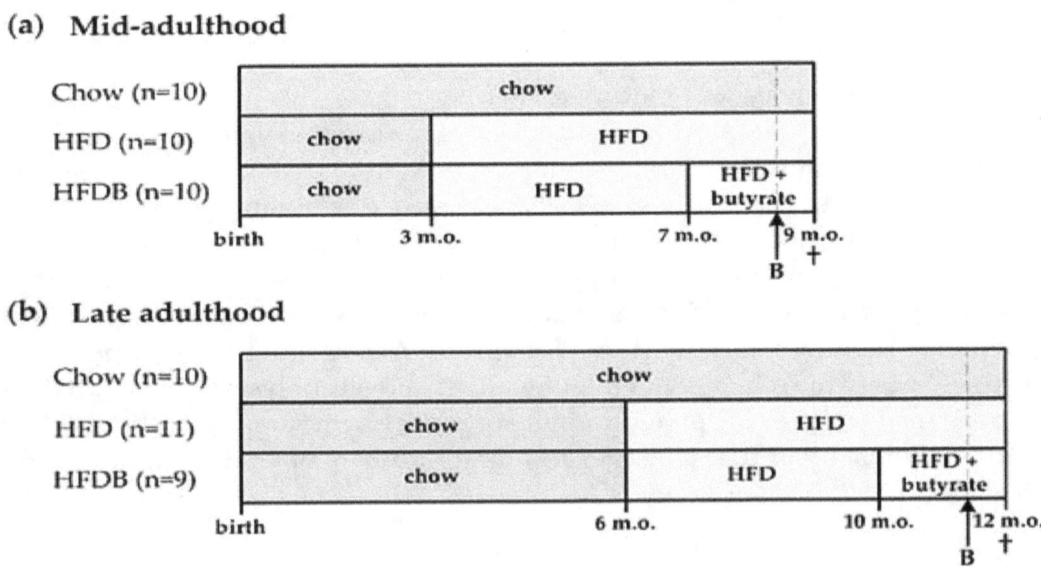

Figure 1. Schematic overview of the study design. (**a**) Mid-adulthood, exposure of the high-fat died HFD started at 3 m.o. in the HFD and HFDB groups. At 7 months of age, the butyrate intervention (HFD supplemented with 5% *w*/*w* butyrate) started in the HFDB group; (**b**) Late adulthood, exposure to the HFD started at 6 months of age in the HFD and HFDB groups, and a butyrate intervention initiated at 10 months of age in the HFDB group. Body weight (individual) and food intake (cage level) were monitored weekly. Blood samples were taken after five hours of fasting. At 9 m.o. and 12 m.o., mice were sacrificed and both liver and adipose tissues were harvested. These tissues were subsequently processed for immunohistochemical staining. B = blood sample collection; HFD = high-fat diet; HFDB = high fat diet enriched with butyrate; m.o. = months old.

2.2. *Plasma Analyses*

Blood was collected after five hours of fasting (8 a.m. to 1 p.m.). Plasma cholesterol, triglyceride and insulin levels were measured using standardized ELISA kits as previously described [18]. Moreover, ELISA kits (Quantikine, R&D systems, Inc., Minneapolis, MN, USA) were used to define plasma leptin (DY498), adiponectin (DY1119), resistin (DY1069) and interleukin-6 (IL-6; M6000B) levels. SAA plasma levels were determined by an ELISA kit as well (KMA0021, Invitrogen, Carlsbad, CA, USA).

2.3. *(Immuno)histochemistry*

Mice were sacrificed by transcardial perfusion with 0.1 M phosphate buffered saline (PBS) after being anesthetized with isoflurane (3.5%, Nicholas Primal (I) limited, London, UK), as described in Arnoldussen et al. [18]. Directly thereafter, the liver and two different adipose tissue depots were harvested and post-fixed in 4% paraformaldehyde for 24 h. Fat depots seem to be differentially active and affected by a HFD and, therefore, we dissected in addition subcutaneous (inguinal) and visceral (epididymal) adipose tissue depots [32,33]. Liver outcomes used for correlation analyses were obtained from a previous experiment [18].

Both epididymal and inguinal adipose tissues were processed for immunohistochemistry on 5 µm paraffin embedded sections. Briefly, paraffin sections were first deparaffinized in xylene and rehydrated in a series of ethanol followed by endogenous peroxidase blocking with 0.3% H_2O_2 in 0.1 M PBS. Antigen retrieval was achieved by treating the tissue in hot 0.05 M sodiumcitrate with a constant temperature of 85 °C. After pre-incubation with 0.1% bovine serum albumin in 0.1 M PBS

(PBS-B), the tissue was incubated overnight at room temperature with primary macrophage (MAC-3) antibodies (1:100; eBioscience, 14-1072) [34]. Next, sections were incubated with secondary donkey anti-rat IgG antibodies (1:200; Jackson ImmunoResearch) in 0.1 M PBS-B at room temperature. Staining was visualized using the ABC method with a Vectastain kit (Vector Laboratories, Burlingame, CA, USA) and diaminobenzidine imidazole solution as chromogen. Finally, sections were dehydrated in a series of ethanol, cleared in xylene, and mounted.

Two entire sections per animal were visualized using a VisionTek live digital microscope (Sakura Finetek, Torrance, CA, USA) at a 10× magnification. Sampling of these sections was carried out with Adobe Illustrator CC 2016 (Adobe, San Jose, CA, USA) using a template with three randomly placed artboards (592.7 × 886.2 mm). Adipocyte cell size (μm^2) and the number of CLS were determined in a total of six samples—three samples per section—per animal. Analyses to determine these measures were performed using CellProfiler [35] version 2.3.0 together with Ilastik version 0.5 [36] for pixel classification. Separate pipelines and classifiers for epididymal and inguinal adipose tissue analyses were used. In order to verify the reliability of these relatively novel analyses, we included an established analysis to determine adipocyte size using ImageJ software as previously described [37]. CLS were determined based on intensity of the cell edge, and total numbers of CLS per animal were calculated per 1000 adipocytes.

2.4. Statistical Analyses

A random and blinded selection procedure was maintained throughout the study. Group means were compared using univariate analysis of variance (ANOVA) with Bonferroni correction for multiple testing with a statistical program, SPSS 24 (IBM SPSS Statistics 24, IBM Corporation, Armonk, NY, USA). Parameter correlation tests were performed using Pearson correlations. Nonparametric tests were used when assumptions of normality and homogeneity of variance were not met. p-values lower than 0.05 were considered significant. Data are presented as mean ± SEM.

3. Results

3.1. Adipocyte Size

Adipocyte size—measured as area (μm^2)—of both epididymal and inguinal adipose tissue depots were determined to assess morphological adaptations. A HFD increased the average epididymal adipocyte size in both mid- and late-adult mice (mid: $p < 0.001$; $F(1,18) = 26.05$, late: $p < 0.02$; $F(1,19) = 7.01$) (Figure 2a). Butyrate intervention significantly reduced adipocyte size in both age cohorts (mid: $p = 0.001$; $F(1,18) = 14.95$, late: $p < 0.02$; $F(1,18) = 7.14$).

Similarly, inguinal adipocyte size was increased by HFD in both mid- and late adulthood ($p = 0.001$; mid: $F(1,18) = 20.49$, late: $F(1,19) = 14.25$) (Figure 2b). After HFD exposure, inguinal adipocyte size was reduced due to butyrate intervention in mid-adult mice ($p < 0.001$; $F(1,18) = 25.69$), but not in late-adult mice. Mean inguinal adipocyte size was significantly larger in late adult as compared to mid-adult high fat diet enriched with butyrate (HFDB) mice ($p < 0.01$; $F(1,18) = 11.28$).

In addition, we compared the number of adipocytes as an additional indication of adipose tissue function. Our analysis indicated that the epididymal adipose tissue contained a lower number of adipocytes than inguinal adipose tissue. The mean adipocyte number in epididymal adipose tissue was higher in mid-adult Chow mice as compared to HFD mice (Table 1). Butyrate intervention increased epididymal adipocyte number solely in mid-adulthood. In both age cohorts, inguinal adipocyte numbers were significantly higher in Chow mice as opposed to HFD mice (Table 1). Only in mid-adulthood did butyrate intervention increase the inguinal adipocyte numbers.

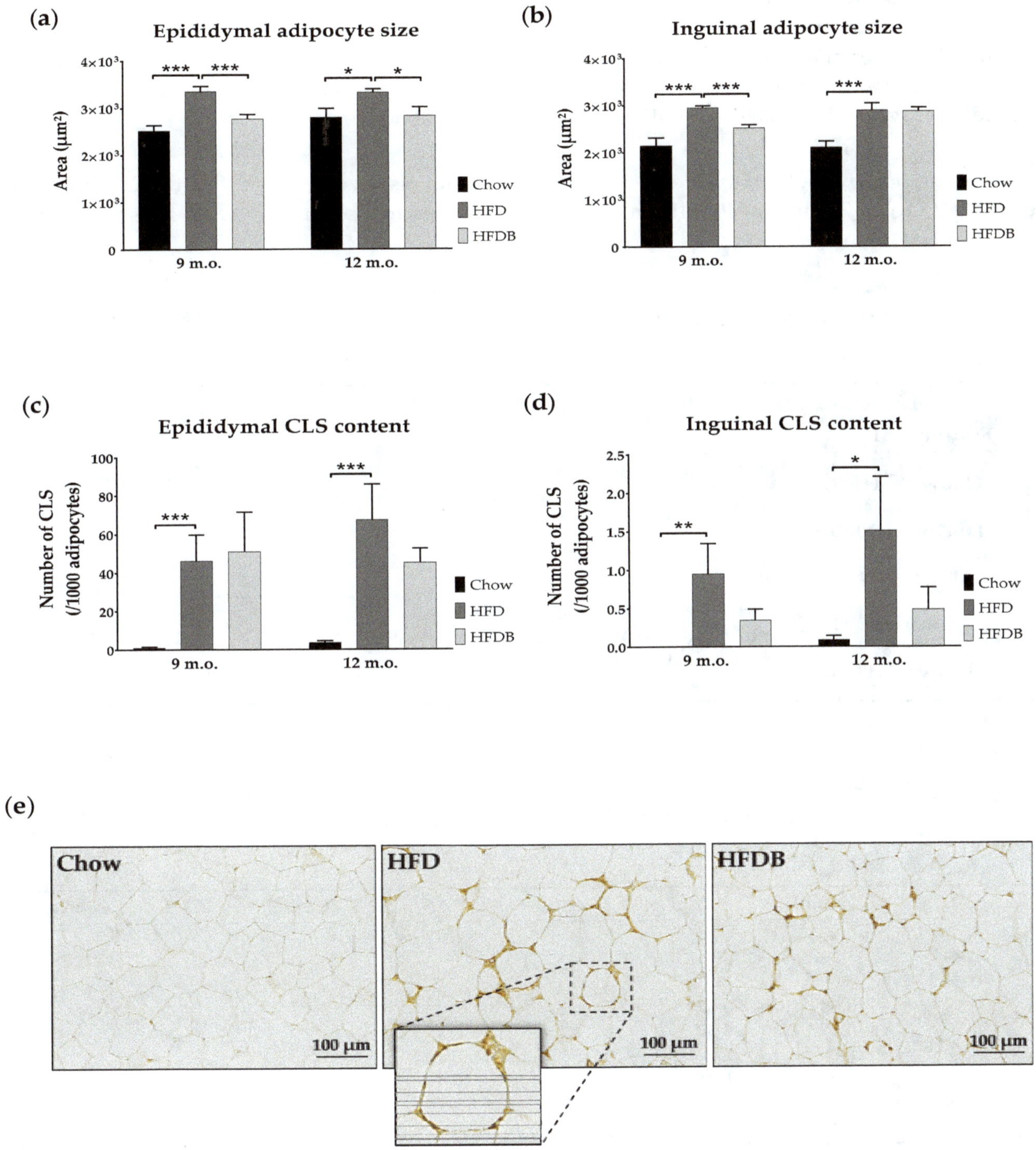

Figure 2. Adipose tissue cell sizes and macrophage infiltration. Mean adipocyte sizes in epididymal (**a**) and inguinal (**b**) adipose tissue depots in both mid- (9 m.o.) and late- (12 m.o.) adult mice. (**c**,**d**) Mean number of crown-like structures (CLS) in epididymal (**c**) and inguinal (**d**) adipose tissue. (**e**) Representative photomicrographs of epididymal adipose tissue stained with antibodies against macrophages (MAC-3) in late-adult mice. In addition, a magnification (40×) of a CLS is represented. These examples are comparable to those observed in mid-adulthood. Data are presented as mean ± standard error of mean (SEM). * $p < 0.05$; ** $p < 0.01$; *** $p \leq 0.001$.

In mid- and late adulthood, both epididymal and inguinal adipocyte size were positively associated with body weight, and cholesterol and triglyceride plasma levels (Tables 2 and 3). In addition, only inguinal adipocyte size was positively correlated with inguinal adipose tissue weight (mid: $p < 0.01$; $R = 0.55$, late: $p < 0.001$; $R = 0.64$). Solely in late adulthood, epididymal adipocyte size correlated positively with plasma insulin levels ($p < 0.01$; Table 3).

Moreover, body weight, cholesterol and triglyceride levels revealed significant and positive inter correlations (Tables 2 and 3). Finally, insulin levels correlated positively with these outcomes in late-adult mice (Table 3).

Table 1. Adipocyte numbers. Represented are the combined mean numbers of two slides.

		Adipocyte Numbers Per 10^6 μm^2 (Mean ± SEM)		
Epididymal				
Chow vs. HFD	mid	468 ± 34 vs. 376 ± 31	$0.05 < p < 0.08$	$F(1,18) = 3.95$
	late	452 ± 40 vs. 410 ± 21	$p = 0.02$	$F(1,18) = 6.54$
HFD vs. HFDB	mid	376 ± 31 vs. 496 ± 35	ns	
	late	410 ± 21 vs. 481 ± 47	ns	
Inguinal				
Chow vs. HFD	mid	665 ± 59 vs. 449 ± 16	$p < 0.01$	$F(1,18) = 12.61$
	late	659 ± 44 vs. 474 ± 41	$p < 0.01$	$F(1,19) = 9.54$
HFD vs. HFDB	mid	449 ± 16 vs. 522 ± 15	$p < 0.01$	$F(1,18) = 11.27$
	late	474 ± 41 vs. 446 ± 18	ns	

ns = not significant.

Table 2. Correlation coefficients among mid-adult mice.

	BW	Chol	Trigl	eAS	iAS	eCLS	iCLS	Leptin	SAA
BW	x								
Chol	0.80^{R} +	x							
Trigl	0.58^{R} +	0.69^{R} +	x						
eAS	0.53^{R} +	0.64^{R} +	0.57^{R} +	x					
iAS	0.55^{R} +	0.57^{R} +	0.37^{R} +	NE	x				
eCLS	$0.53^{\tau b}$ +	$0.49^{\tau b}$ +	$0.15^{\tau b}$ +	$0.24^{\tau b}$ +	NE	x			
iCLS	$0.31^{\tau b}$ +	$0.29^{\tau b}$ +	$0.10^{\tau b}$ +	NE	$0.37^{\tau b}$ +	NE	x		
Leptin	0.78^{R} +	0.87^{R} +	0.62^{R} +	0.76^{R} +	0.67^{R} +	$0.52^{\tau b}$ +	$0.37^{\tau b}$ +	x	
SAA	$0.56^{\tau b}$ +	$0.50^{\tau b}$ +	$0.13^{\tau b}$ +	$0.17^{\tau b}$ +	$0.24^{\tau b}$ +	$0.69^{\tau b}$ +	$0.28^{\tau b}$ +	NE	x

Either the Pearson's (^{R}) or Kendall's tau ($^{\tau b}$) test was used. Not significant. + = positive correlation; Adi = adiponectin; BW = body weight; Chol = cholesterol; eAS = epididymal adipocyte size; eCLS = epididymal CLS; iAS = inguinal adipocyte size; iCLS = inguinal CLS; LI = liver inflammation; NE = not estimated; SAA = serum amyloid A; Trigl = triglycerides.

Table 3. Correlation coefficients among late-adult mice.

	BW	Insulin	Chol	Trigl	eAS	iAS	eCLS	iCLS	LI	Leptin	Adi	SAA
BW	x											
Insulin	0.66 ^{R} +	x										
Chol	0.87 ^{R} +	0.66 ^{R} +	x									
Trigl	0.79 ^{R} +	0.77 ^{R} +	0.81 ^{R} +	x								
eAS	0.52 ^{R} +	0.49 ^{R} +	0.57 ^{R} +	0.53 ^{R} +	x							
iAS	0.47 ^{R} +	0.31 ^{R} +	0.54 ^{R} +	0.50 ^{R} +	NE	x						
eCLS	0.43 $^{\tau b}$ +	0.30 $^{\tau b}$ +	0.55 $^{\tau b}$ +	0.34 $^{\tau b}$ +	0.23 $^{\tau b}$ +	NE	x					
iCLS	0.45 $^{\tau b}$ +	0.21 $^{\tau b}$ +	0.38 $^{\tau b}$ +	0.33 $^{\tau b}$ +	NE	0.37 $^{\tau b}$ +	NE	x				
LI	0.41 $^{\tau b}$ +	0.33 $^{\tau b}$ +	0.45 $^{\tau b}$ +	0.30 $^{\tau b}$ +	0.15 $^{\tau b}$ +	0.22 $^{\tau b}$ +	0.57 $^{\tau b}$ +	0.21 $^{\tau b}$ +	x			
Leptin	0.88 ^{R} +	0.69 ^{R} +	0.91 ^{R} +	0.87 ^{R} +	0.65 ^{R} +	0.64 ^{R} +	0.49 $^{\tau b}$ +	0.41 $^{\tau b}$ +	0.46 $^{\tau b}$ +	x		
Adi	0.56 ^{R} −	0.48 ^{R} −	0.68 ^{R} −	0.47 ^{R} −	0.25 ^{R} −	0.25 ^{R} −	0.19 $^{\tau b}$ −	0.30 $^{\tau b}$ −	0.28 $^{\tau b}$ −	NE	x	
SAA	0.42 $^{\tau b}$ +	0.29 $^{\tau b}$ +	0.57 $^{\tau b}$ +	0.46 $^{\tau b}$ +	0.19 $^{\tau b}$ +	0.53 $^{\tau b}$ +	0.58 $^{\tau b}$ +	0.30 $^{\tau b}$ +	0.44 $^{\tau b}$ +	NE	NE	x

Either the Pearson's (^{R}) or Kendall's tau ($^{\tau b}$) test was used. Not significant. + = positive correlation; − = negative correlation; Adi = adiponectin; BW = Body weight; Chol = cholesterol; eAS = epididymal adipocyte size; eCLS = epididymal CLS; iAS = inguinal adipocyte size; iCLS = inguinal CLS; LI = liver inflammation; NE = not estimated; SAA = serum amyloid A; Trigl = triglycerides.

3.2. *Inflammation in Adipose Tissue and Liver*

To assess the degree of inflammation in adipose tissue, the number of adipocytes infiltrated by macrophages—known as crown-like structures (CLS)—has been determined. Both mid- and late-adult mice on HFD showed higher numbers of CLS in epididymal adipose tissue as opposed to Chow-fed mice (Kruskal Wallis: $p < 0.001$; mid: $\chi^2(1) = 13.50$, late: $\chi^2(1) = 13.02$) (Figure 2c). No effects of butyrate on CLS number in epididymal adipose tissue were observed. In inguinal adipose tissue, the number of CLS was increased after HFD exposure in both mid- (Kruskal-Wallis: $p < 0.01$; $\chi^2(1) = 7.30$) and late- (Kruskal-Wallis: $p < 0.02$; $\chi^2(1) = 6.16$) adult mice (Figure 2d). No significant differences in the number of CLS in inguinal adipose tissue were observed between HFD and HFDB mice (Figure 2d). As scales differ between Figure 2c,d, caution should be taken when interpreting these results. In Figure 2e, examples of epididymal adipose tissue stained for macrophages are shown.

In late adulthood, the number of CLS in epididymal adipose tissue correlated significantly with body weight ($p = 0.001$), and plasma triglyceride ($p < 0.02$), cholesterol ($p < 0.001$) and insulin ($p < 0.05$) levels (Table 3). In mid-adulthood, epididymal adipose tissue CLS content showed only significant correlations with body weight ($p < 0.001$) and plasma cholesterol levels ($p < 0.001$) (Table 2).

In addition to CLS in adipose tissue, data including inflammatory aggregates were used [18] to examine potential relationships to inflammation in the liver, which is another crucial organ regulating insulin sensitivity. Liver inflammation was increased after HFD exposure only in late-adult mice [18]. No significant changes were observed after butyrate intervention. In this age cohort, the number of inflammatory aggregates in the liver was positively correlated with the number of CLS in epididymal adipose tissue ($p < 0.001$) (Table 3).

3.3. *Adipokine Plasma Levels*

Adipokine plasma levels were determined at either nine or 12 months of age. HFD exposure strongly increased leptin plasma levels in both age cohorts ($p < 0.001$; mid: $F(1,18) = 50.10$, late: $F(1,19) = 44.87$) (Figure 3a). Late-adult HFD-fed mice showed higher leptin levels as compared to mid-adult mice fed a HFD ($p < 0.02$; $F(1,19) = 7.71$). Subsequent butyrate intervention resulted in reduced plasma leptin levels, almost reaching control levels in Chow mice ($p < 0.001$; mid: $F(1,18) = 26.49$, late: $F(1,18) = 32.88$). HFD did not affect plasma resistin levels (Figure 3b). Adiponectin plasma levels were reduced after HFD exposure in late-adult mice ($p < 0.001$; $F(1,19) = 17.57$) and were moderately increased after butyrate intervention ($p = 0.053$; $F(1,18) = 4.29$) (Figure 3c). An age effect was observed in both Chow and HFD animals ($p < 0.05$; $F(1,18) = 4.60$ and $F(1,19) = 4.55$, respectively). Serum amyloid A (SAA) plasma levels were increased in mice fed a HFD when compared to Chow-fed mice in both age cohorts (Kruskal-Wallis: $p \leq 0.001$; mid: $\chi^2(1) = 10.14$, late: $\chi^2(1) = 14.46$) (Figure 3d). Plasma levels of interleukin-6 (IL-6) were below detectable levels in all animals in the absence of abnormal positive and negative controls.

In both mid- and late adulthood, plasma leptin levels were positively correlated with body weight ($p < 0.001$), both epididymal and inguinal adipocyte size ($p < 0.001$), and epididymal CLS content ($p < 0.001$) (Tables 2 and 3). Solely in late-adult mice, plasma leptin levels positively correlated with insulin levels ($p < 0.001$) and liver inflammation ($p = 0.001$) (Table 3). Only in late adulthood plasma adiponectin levels showed a negative correlation with body weight ($p < 0.01$), insulin plasma levels ($p < 0.02$), and liver inflammation ($p < 0.05$) (Table 3).

Plasma SAA levels were positively correlated with body weight (mid: $p < 0.001$, late: $p < 0.01$) and the number of CLS in epididymal adipose tissue ($p < 0.001$) in both mid- and late adulthood (Tables 2 and 3). Whereas, SAA plasma levels were positively correlated with insulin levels ($p < 0.05$), inguinal adipocyte size ($p < 0.001$), and liver inflammation ($p < 0.01$) only in late adulthood (Table 3).

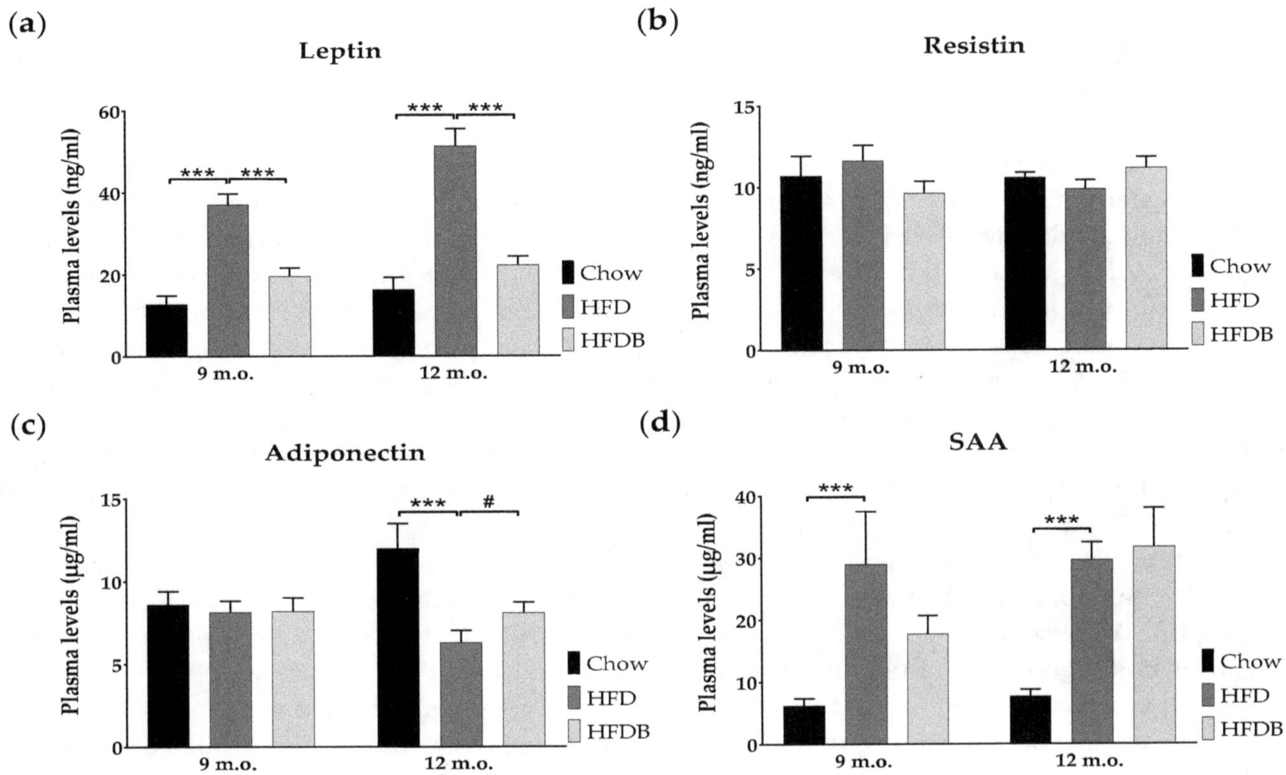

Figure 3. Adipokine plasma levels. Mean plasma levels of leptin (**a**), resistin (**b**), adiponectin (**c**), and serum amyloid A (SAA) (**d**) are represented in both mid- (9 m.o.) and late- (12 m.o.) adult mice as mean ± SEM. *** $p \leq 0.001$; # $p = 0.053$.

4. Discussion

This study describes the detrimental effects of a six-month HFD exposure in mid-adult and late-adult mice, and examined potential health effects of butyrate administered during the last two months of HFD feeding. In this study, HFD exposure caused adipocyte hypertrophy and inflammation, as well as an increase in the plasma levels of proinflammatory adipokines (leptin, SAA) in mid- and late life. Butyrate attenuated HFD-evoked effects, though the effects of butyrate varied in mice that were exposed to HFD in mid-life as compared to late life.

In our study, HFD treatment increased body weight and adiposity, and subsequent butyrate intervention diminished these changes in the LDLr-/-.Leiden mice [18]. Moreover, these changes were observed without significant differences in calorie intake, suggesting that energy intake was similar between the dietary interventions. Other rodent research has shown that a HFD increases body weight and adiposity [38–40], and similar effects of butyrate have been reported in obese mice [38,41]. The LDLr-/-.Leiden mouse model was chosen for this study because of its high sensitivity to develop vascular complications and obesity when fed a HFD even with modest fat content. We found that 12 m.o. LDLr-/-.Leiden mice on standard Chow show a disposition towards pronounced weight gain and are approximately 32% heavier than Chow-fed male C57BL/6 mice of the same age [42], supporting the obesity-prone condition of the model chosen. It is unclear why these mice are susceptible to obesity development, and comparative molecular analysis to C57BL/6 mice have not been made. In our experimental design, a control group of wild-type mice was not included due to restrictions in mice per experiment and time. Therefore, a generalization of the results cannot be made, the more so because the interaction between the LDLr-/- genotype and HFD are still not fully understood. A detailed comparison with wild-type mice and other obesity models would be required to elucidate the role of the LDLr in obesity.

In a previous study, insulin levels were significantly increased in late-adult mice after HFD feeding, whereas no changes in glucose levels were observed [18]. Plasma insulin levels are extremely high due to the experimental conditions employed in this disease model (>20 ng/mL) and much higher than in wild-type mice fed the same diet (<5 ng/mL) [18,30], indicating insulin resistance but no overt T2DM because glucose levels are not elevated and seem to be controlled. Interestingly, butyrate supplementation restored insulin levels to values found in Chow-fed mice, suggesting an improvement in insulin signaling [18]. Previous research described similar effects of butyrate on insulin levels and sensitivity in HFD-fed mice [38,43]. It is not clear whether this effect of butyrate is mediated by improvement of insulin signaling in liver, in peripheral organs, or both. It is possible that both organs are involved, given the time frame in which insulin resistance develops under the conditions employed. For instance, a time resolved clamp study using C57BL/6 mice that were treated with the same HFD as used in the current study showed that the adipose tissue develops insulin resistance after about six to 12 weeks of HFD feeding [44]. Second, the development of insulin resistance in the liver requires longer periods of HFD feeding (about 24 weeks), i.e., a period that is comparable to the duration of HFD exposure herein [44].

Even in the absence of obesity, metabolic dysfunction in adipose tissue induced by adipocyte hypertrophy has consistently been related to insulin resistance and may serve as a predictor for T2DM [45,46]. We observed increased adipocyte size in both epididymal and inguinal adipose tissue depots after HFD feeding. Adipocyte hypertrophy was reduced by butyrate with the exception of inguinal adipose tissue in late-adult mice. Epididymal adipocyte sizes were associated with insulin levels in late adulthood suggesting that epididymal, as opposed to inguinal, adipose tissue may be important in mediating the effects on insulin. Previous studies have demonstrated the significant role of visceral fat in mediating insulin sensitivity in rats [47,48], which may be attributed to the higher degree of metabolic activity of visceral fat as opposed to subcutaneous fat [16,49,50]. The beneficial effects of butyrate on adipocyte size in epididymal adipose tissue have been demonstrated before [51]. Although our knowledge about the exact mechanisms is incomplete, it is likely that butyrate may reverse adipocyte hypertrophy by promoting fatty acid oxidation in adipose tissue [38]. In particular, butyrate may induce a shift from lipid synthesis to utilization resulting in decreased fat storage in white adipose tissue [43]. Our data confirm this hypothesis as adipocyte sizes were significantly associated with both cholesterol and triglyceride levels. Dyslipidemia is a regularly observed condition in T2DM patients [52]. HFD-induced elevations in cholesterol and triglycerides were diminished by butyrate in LDLr-/-.Leiden mice [18], suggesting a mitigation of hyperlipidemia that is not related to enhanced clearance, suggesting effects on very-low-density lipoprotein (VLDL) production. For instance, butyrate may affect hyperlipidemia as it can induce a switch from lipid synthesis to utilization [53]. Unfortunately, our study is limited with respect to functional analyses such as glucose transport, insulin signaling, lipogenesis, and adipogenesis in adipose tissue. Therefore, it would be valuable to investigate these aspects in future studies. The effects of butyrate supplementation on key regulators of adipogenesis in mid-adult versus late-adult mice may provide insight into the pathways by which butyrate may modulate adiposity. It has been shown that butyrate may reduce body weight and improve insulin sensitivity via the modulation of peroxisome proliferator-activated receptor-γ (PPAR-γ) [43], which is a key regulator of adipogenesis [54]. Consistent with this, we recently showed that specific activation of PPAR-γ in adipose tissue attenuates CLS development and, related to this, the development of nonalcoholic fatty liver disease/nonalcoholic steatohepatitis [55]. Anti-inflammatory effects in adipose tissue may attenuate the release of inflammatory mediators and may also affect the development of diseases in other organs such as the liver [56,57]. A notion which is further supported by the coordinated and interactive expression of inflammatory genes in adipose tissue and liver during metabolic overload [58].

It is well established that a correlative and causative relation exists between chronic inflammation and both insulin resistance and T2DM in humans and rodents [13,59]. More specifically, a reduction of macrophage infiltration in adipose tissue can improve insulin sensitivity in diet-induced obese mice by reducing the expression of inflammatory cytokines in adipose tissue [11]. As shown in the present study, HFD feeding results in increased macrophage infiltration mainly in epididymal adipose tissue associated with body weight and insulin levels. Epididymal adipose tissue was characterized by an abundance of CLS, whereas CLS were almost absent in inguinal adipose tissue, which is consistent with previous studies investigating adipose tissue inflammation of various adipose tissue depots in the context of their expandability and maximal storage capacity [30,57]. It is possible that visceral fat may excrete higher amounts of inflammatory proteins and fatty acids affecting insulin signaling, and that macrophages play an important role in this [56,60]. CLS formation in epididymal adipose tissue was not affected by butyrate supplementation in mid-adult mice, whereas a mean reduction of almost 33% was observed in late-adult mice. Consistent with the inflammatory cross-talk between epidydimal adipose tissue and liver, medial lobular inflammation was not affected in mid-adult mice, whereas the number of inflammatory aggregates in the liver was reduced by 44% after dietary butyrate intervention in late-adult mice [18]. Furthermore, liver inflammation in late-adult mice, indicated by inflammatory aggregates in the medial lobe [18], correlated significantly with the number of CLS in epididymal adipose tissue in this study. It is not known via which pathways butyrate can affect inflammation, and future studies may examine the expression of inflammatory mediators at tissue level, in both adipose tissue and the liver. In addition, mechanistic studies examining the expression of transcription factors, such as nuclear factor κB, support the notion that the activation of inflammatory processes in adipose tissue and liver are necessary.

Both the increase in pro-inflammatory and the reduction in anti-inflammatory adipokine secretion by adipose tissue can contribute to systemic and tissue-specific inflammation. In this study, HFD exposure results in increased levels of leptin and serum amyloid A (SAA). These findings are accompanied by a reduction in adiponectin in late adulthood, whereas it remains unclear why adiponectin was not affected by HFD or butyrate treatment in mid-adult mice. An exaggerated metabolic load in adipocytes and inflammatory state may underlie the effects of a HFD on leptin, adiponectin, and SAA levels [16]. Both leptin and SAA are suggested to be pro-inflammatory adipokines, whereas adiponectin has anti-inflammatory properties [61]. Leptin contributes to the inflammatory state in obesity by modulating TNF-α and activating macrophages [62], and butyrate reduced leptin levels in mid-adult and late-adult mice. Leptin can also affect insulin sensitivity by modulating pancreatic β-cells [60]. It thereby contributes to the observed reduction in plasma insulin by butyrate in late-adult mice the more, because butyrate reduced leptin levels nearly to those of Chow-fed mice. Our finding that leptin levels were significantly related to insulin levels in late-adult mice further supports this notion. Although current evidence for the role of SAA in insulin signaling is contradictory [63–65], SAA levels have been correlated with insulin resistance and T2DM [66], which may be related to the pro-inflammatory properties of SAA [14]. Interestingly, adiponectin plasma levels were only affected by HFD feeding in late-adult mice. It is possible that the circulating SAA is mainly released from adipose tissue and that butyrate reduced CLS only in adipose tissue of late-adult mice. Low adiponectin levels may add to an impaired insulin signaling via polarization towards M1 macrophages in adipose tissue [67]. Butyrate intervention reduced changes in both leptin and adiponectin levels, which may in part be attributed to its effect on adipocyte size and its differential effects on CLS, i.e., adipose tissue inflammation, in mid-and late-adult mice.

5. Conclusions

This study provides evidence that dietary supplementation with butyrate constitutes a strategy to counteract features of HFD-induced adipose tissue dysfunction and accompanying metabolic disturbances. These metabolic adaptations often affect insulin signaling and may therefore indicate an increased risk of developing T2DM. Late-adult mice are particularly sensitive to HFD-evoked metabolic risk factors and adaptations. The findings of the current study provide novel insights about the attenuating effects of butyrate on adipose tissue dysfunction and inflammation. Overall, dietary interventions with butyrate may constitute means to ameliorate the risk of developing metabolic disorders such as T2DM in people with obesity.

Acknowledgments: The authors would like to thank Bram Geenen, Jos Dederen, Peter Wielinga and Tim Emmerzaal for their valuable scientific support. In addition, we would like to acknowledge the biotechnicians at TNO Leiden and Preclinical Imaging Centre (PRIME) Radboud university medical center for taking outstanding care of the animals.

Author Contributions: I.A.C.A. and A.J.K. conceived and designed the experiments; C.E.P., B.A.A.F. and J.S. performed the experiments; C.E.P. and B.A.A.F. analyzed the data; J.S. and R.K. contributed reagents/materials/analysis tools; C.E.P., B.A.A.F., I.A.C.A. and A.J.K. wrote the paper.

References

1. World Health Organization. Fact Sheet 311: Obesity and Overweight. 2016. Available online: http://www.who.int/mediacentre/factsheets/fs311/en/ (accessed on 28 February 2017).
2. Diabetes UK. Facts and Stats. 2016. Available online: https://www.diabetes.org.uk/Documents/Position%20statements/DiabetesUK_Facts_Stats_Oct16.pdf (accessed on 27 February 2017).
3. Hamman, R.F.; Wing, R.R.; Edelstein, S.L.; Lachin, J.M.; Bray, G.A.; Delahanty, L.; Hoskin, M.; Kriska, A.M.; Mayer-Davis, E.J.; Pi-Sunyer, X. Effect of weight loss with lifestyle intervention on risk of diabetes. *Diabetes Care* **2006**, *29*, 2102–2107. [CrossRef] [PubMed]
4. Molnar, D. The prevalence of the metabolic syndrome and type 2 diabetes mellitus in children and adolescents. *Int. J. Obes.* **2004**, *28*, S70–S74. [CrossRef] [PubMed]
5. Schwartz, M.S.; Chadha, A. Type 2 diabetes mellitus in childhood: Obesity and insulin resistance. *J. Am. Osteopath. Assoc.* **2008**, *108*, 518–524. [PubMed]
6. Wabitsch, M.; Hauner, H.; Hertrampf, M.; Muche, R.; Hay, B.; Mayer, H.; Kratzer, W.; Debatin, K.; Heinze, E. Type ii diabetes mellitus and impaired glucose regulation in caucasian children and adolescents with obesity living in germany. *Int. J. Obes.* **2004**, *28*, 307–313. [CrossRef] [PubMed]
7. Pérez, L.M.; Pareja-Galeano, H.; Sanchis-Gomar, F.; Emanuele, E.; Lucia, A.; Gálvez, B.G. 'Adipaging': Ageing and obesity share biological hallmarks related to a dysfunctional adipose tissue. *J. Physiol.* **2016**, *594*, 3187–3207. [CrossRef] [PubMed]
8. Fink, R.I.; Kolterman, O.G.; Griffin, J.; Olefsky, J.M. Mechanisms of insulin resistance in aging. *J. Clin. Investig.* **1983**, *71*, 1523. [CrossRef] [PubMed]
9. Inzucchi, S.E.; Bergenstal, R.M.; Buse, J.B.; Diamant, M.; Ferrannini, E.; Nauck, M.; Peters, A.L.; Tsapas, A.; Wender, R.; Matthews, D.R. Management of hyperglycemia in type 2 diabetes: A patient-centered approach. *Diabetes Care* **2012**, *35*, 1364–1379. [CrossRef] [PubMed]
10. Arvanitakis, Z.; Wilson, R.S.; Bienias, J.L.; Evans, D.A.; Bennett, D.A. Diabetes mellitus and risk of alzheimer disease and decline in cognitive function. *Arch. Neurol.* **2004**, *61*, 661–666. [CrossRef] [PubMed]
11. Jung, U.J.; Choi, M.S. Obesity and its metabolic complications: The role of adipokines and the relationship between obesity, inflammation, insulin resistance, dyslipidemia and nonalcoholic fatty liver disease. *Int. J. Mol. Sci.* **2014**, *15*, 6184–6223. [CrossRef] [PubMed]
12. Cinti, S.; Mitchell, G.; Barbatelli, G.; Murano, I.; Ceresi, E.; Faloia, E.; Wang, S.; Fortier, M.; Greenberg, A.S.; Obin, M.S. Adipocyte death defines macrophage localization and function in adipose tissue of obese mice and humans. *J. Lipid Res.* **2005**, *46*, 2347–2355. [CrossRef] [PubMed]
13. Olefsky, J.M.; Glass, C.K. Macrophages, inflammation, and insulin resistance. *Annu. Rev. Physiol.* **2010**, *72*, 219–246. [CrossRef] [PubMed]
14. Poitou, C.; Divoux, A.; Faty, A.; Tordjman, J.; Hugol, D.; Aissat, A.; Keophiphath, M.; Henegar, C.; Commans, S.; Clément, K. Role of serum amyloid a in adipocyte-macrophage cross talk and adipocyte cholesterol efflux. *J. Clin. Endocrinol. Metab.* **2009**, *94*, 1810–1817. [CrossRef] [PubMed]
15. Skurk, T.; Alberti-Huber, C.; Herder, C.; Hauner, H. Relationship between adipocyte size and adipokine expression and secretion. *J. Clin. Endocrinol. Metab.* **2007**, *92*, 1023–1033. [CrossRef] [PubMed]
16. Bays, H.E.; González-Campoy, J.M.; Bray, G.A.; Kitabchi, A.E.; Bergman, D.A.; Schorr, A.B.; Rodbard, H.W.; Henry, R.R. Pathogenic potential of adipose tissue and metabolic consequences of adipocyte hypertrophy and increased visceral adiposity. *Expert Rev. Cardiovasc. Ther.* **2008**, *6*, 343–368. [CrossRef] [PubMed]

17. Canfora, E.E.; Jocken, J.W.; Blaak, E.E. Short-chain fatty acids in control of body weight and insulin sensitivity. *Nat. Rev. Endocrinol.* **2015**, *11*, 577. [CrossRef] [PubMed]
18. Arnoldussen, I.A.; Wiesmann, M.; Pelgrim, C.E.; Wielemaker, E.M.; van Duyvenvoorde, W.; Santos, P.A.; Verschuren, L.; Keijser, B.J.; Heerschap, A.; Kleemann, R.; et al. Butyrate restores hfd induced adaptations in brain function and metabolism in mid-adult obese mice. *Int. J. Obes.* **2017**, *41*, 935–944. [CrossRef] [PubMed]
19. Khan, S.; Jena, G. The role of butyrate, a histone deacetylase inhibitor in diabetes mellitus: Experimental evidence for therapeutic intervention. *Epigenomics* **2015**, *7*, 669–680. [CrossRef] [PubMed]
20. Weickert, M.O.; Möhlig, M.; Schöfl, C.; Arafat, A.M.; Otto, B.; Viehoff, H.; Koebnick, C.; Kohl, A.; Spranger, J.; Pfeiffer, A.F. Cereal fiber improves whole-body insulin sensitivity in overweight and obese women. *Diabetes Care* **2006**, *29*, 775–780. [CrossRef] [PubMed]
21. Weickert, M.O.; Pfeiffer, A.F. Metabolic effects of dietary fiber consumption and prevention of diabetes. *J. Nutr.* **2008**, *138*, 439–442. [PubMed]
22. Marlett, J.A.; McBurney, M.I.; Slavin, J.L. Position of the american dietetic association: Health implications of dietary fiber. *J. Am. Diet. Assoc.* **2002**, *102*, 993–1000. [CrossRef]
23. Elli, M.; Colombo, O.; Tagliabue, A. A common core microbiota between obese individuals and their lean relatives? Evaluation of the predisposition to obesity on the basis of the fecal microflora profile. *Med. Hypotheses* **2010**, *75*, 350–352. [CrossRef] [PubMed]
24. Qin, J.; Li, Y.; Cai, Z.; Li, S.; Zhu, J.; Zhang, F.; Liang, S.; Zhang, W.; Guan, Y.; Shen, D. A metagenome-wide association study of gut microbiota in type 2 diabetes. *Nature* **2012**, *490*, 55–60. [CrossRef] [PubMed]
25. Kivipelto, M.; Ngandu, T.; Fratiglioni, L.; Viitanen, M.; Kåreholt, I.; Winblad, B.; Helkala, E.L.; Tuomilehto, J.; Soininen, H.; Nissinen, A. Obesity and vascular risk factors at midlife and the risk of dementia and alzheimer disease. *Arch. Neurol.* **2005**, *62*, 1556–1560. [CrossRef] [PubMed]
26. Boitard, C.; Etchamendy, N.; Sauvant, J.; Aubert, A.; Tronel, S.; Marighetto, A.; Layé, S.; Ferreira, G. Juvenile, but not adult exposure to high-fat diet impairs relational memory and hippocampal neurogenesis in mice. *Hippocampus* **2012**, *22*, 2095–2100. [CrossRef] [PubMed]
27. Emmerzaal, T.L.; Kiliaan, A.J.; Gustafson, D.R. 2003–2013: A decade of body mass index, alzheimer's disease, and dementia. *J. Alzheimers Dis.* **2015**, *43*, 739–755. [PubMed]
28. Ma, Y.; Wang, W.; Zhang, J.; Lu, Y.; Wu, W.; Yan, H.; Wang, Y. Hyperlipidemia and atherosclerotic lesion development in ldlr-deficient mice on a long-term high-fat diet. *PLoS ONE* **2012**, *7*, e35835. [CrossRef] [PubMed]
29. Radonjic, M.; Wielinga, P.Y.; Wopereis, S.; Kelder, T.; Goelela, V.S.; Verschuren, L.; Toet, K.; van Duyvenvoorde, W.; Stroeve, J.H.; Cnubben, N. Differential effects of drug interventions and dietary lifestyle in developing type 2 diabetes and complications: A systems biology analysis in ldlr−/− mice. *PLoS ONE* **2013**, *8*, e56122. [CrossRef] [PubMed]
30. Morrison, M.C.; Mulder, P.; Salic, K.; Verheij, J.; Liang, W.; Van Duyvenvoorde, W.; Menke, A.; Kooistra, T.; Kleemann, R.; Wielinga, P. Intervention with a caspase-1 inhibitor reduces obesity-associated hyperinsulinemia, non-alcoholic steatohepatitis and hepatic fibrosis in ldlr-/-.Leiden mice. *Int. J. Obes.* **2016**, *40*, 1416–1423. [CrossRef] [PubMed]
31. Kilkenny, C.; Browne, W.J.; Cuthill, I.C.; Emerson, M.; Altman, D.G. Improving bioscience research reporting: The arrive guidelines for reporting animal research. *PLoS Biol.* **2010**, *8*, e1000412. [CrossRef] [PubMed]
32. Gesta, S.; Tseng, Y.-H.; Kahn, C.R. Developmental origin of fat: Tracking obesity to its source. *Cell* **2007**, *131*, 242–256. [CrossRef] [PubMed]
33. Caesar, R.; Manieri, M.; Kelder, T.; Boekschoten, M.; Evelo, C.; Müller, M.; Kooistra, T.; Cinti, S.; Kleemann, R.; Drevon, C.A. A combined transcriptomics and lipidomics analysis of subcutaneous, epididymal and mesenteric adipose tissue reveals marked functional differences. *PLoS ONE* **2010**, *5*, e11525. [CrossRef] [PubMed]
34. Wielinga, P.Y.; Harthoorn, L.F.; Verschuren, L.; Schoemaker, M.H.; Jouni, Z.E.; van Tol, E.A.; Kleemann, R.; Kooistra, T. Arachidonic acid/docosahexaenoic acid-supplemented diet in early life reduces body weight gain, plasma lipids, and adiposity in later life in apoe* 3leiden mice. *Mol. Nutr. Food Res.* **2012**, *56*, 1081–1089. [CrossRef] [PubMed]
35. Carpenter, A.E.; Jones, T.R.; Lamprecht, M.R.; Clarke, C.; Kang, I.H.; Friman, O.; Guertin, D.A.; Chang, J.H.; Lindquist, R.A.; Moffat, J. Cellprofiler: Image analysis software for identifying and quantifying cell phenotypes. *Genome Biol.* **2006**, *7*, R100. [CrossRef] [PubMed]

36. Sommer, C.; Straehle, C.; Koethe, U.; Hamprecht, F.A. Ilastik: Interactive learning and segmentation toolkit. In Proceedings of the 2011 IEEE International Symposium on Biomedical Imaging: From Nano to Macro, Chicago, IL, USA, 30 March–2 April 2011; pp. 230–233.
37. Arnoldussen, I.A.; Zerbi, V.; Wiesmann, M.; Noordman, R.H.; Bolijn, S.; Mutsaers, M.P.; Dederen, P.J.; Kleemann, R.; Kooistra, T.; van Tol, E.A. Early intake of long-chain polyunsaturated fatty acids preserves brain structure and function in diet-induced obesity. *J. Nutr. Biochem.* **2016**, *30*, 177–188. [CrossRef] [PubMed]
38. Gao, Z.; Yin, J.; Zhang, J.; Ward, R.E.; Martin, R.J.; Lefevre, M.; Cefalu, W.T.; Ye, J. Butyrate improves insulin sensitivity and increases energy expenditure in mice. *Diabetes* **2009**, *58*, 1509–1517. [CrossRef] [PubMed]
39. Jakobsdottir, G.; Xu, J.; Molin, G.; Ahrne, S.; Nyman, M. High-fat diet reduces the formation of butyrate, but increases succinate, inflammation, liver fat and cholesterol in rats, while dietary fibre counteracts these effects. *PLoS ONE* **2013**, *8*, e80476. [CrossRef] [PubMed]
40. Bocarsly, M.E.; Fasolino, M.; Kane, G.A.; LaMarca, E.A.; Kirschen, G.W.; Karatsoreos, I.N.; McEwen, B.S.; Gould, E. Obesity diminishes synaptic markers, alters microglial morphology, and impairs cognitive function. *Proc. Natl. Acad. Sci. USA* **2015**, *112*, 15731–15736. [CrossRef] [PubMed]
41. Lin, H.V.; Frassetto, A.; Kowalik, E.J., Jr.; Nawrocki, A.R.; Lu, M.M.; Kosinski, J.R.; Hubert, J.A.; Szeto, D.; Yao, X.; Forrest, G. Butyrate and propionate protect against diet-induced obesity and regulate gut hormones via free fatty acid receptor 3-independent mechanisms. *PLoS ONE* **2012**, *7*, e35240. [CrossRef] [PubMed]
42. Bondolfi, L.; Ermini, F.; Long, J.M.; Ingram, D.K.; Jucker, M. Impact of age and caloric restriction on neurogenesis in the dentate gyrus of c57bl/6 mice. *Neurobiol. Aging* **2004**, *25*, 333–340. [CrossRef]
43. Den Besten, G.; Bleeker, A.; Gerding, A.; van Eunen, K.; Havinga, R.; van Dijk, T.H.; Oosterveer, M.H.; Jonker, J.W.; Groen, A.K.; Reijngoud, D.J. Short-chain fatty acids protect against high-fat diet–induced obesity via a pparγ-dependent switch from lipogenesis to fat oxidation. *Diabetes* **2015**, *64*, 2398–2408. [CrossRef] [PubMed]
44. Mulder, P.; van den Hoek, A.M.; Kleemann, R. The ccr2 inhibitor propagermanium attenuates diet-induced insulin resistance, adipose tissue inflammation and non-alcoholic steatohepatitis. *PLoS ONE* **2017**, *12*, e0169740. [CrossRef] [PubMed]
45. Wang, Y.; Rimm, E.B.; Stampfer, M.J.; Willett, W.C.; Hu, F.B. Comparison of abdominal adiposity and overall obesity in predicting risk of type 2 diabetes among men. *Am. J. Clin. Nutr.* **2005**, *81*, 555–563. [PubMed]
46. Hammarstedt, A.; Graham, T.E.; Kahn, B.B. Adipose tissue dysregulation and reduced insulin sensitivity in non-obese individuals with enlarged abdominal adipose cells. *Diabetol. Metab. Syndr.* **2012**, *4*, 42. [CrossRef] [PubMed]
47. Gabriely, I.; Ma, X.H.; Yang, X.M.; Atzmon, G.; Rajala, M.W.; Berg, A.H.; Scherer, P.; Rossetti, L.; Barzilai, N. Removal of visceral fat prevents insulin resistance and glucose intolerance of aging. *Diabetes* **2002**, *51*, 2951–2958. [CrossRef] [PubMed]
48. Barzilai, N.; She, L.; Liu, B.Q.; Vuguin, P.; Cohen, P.; Wang, J.; Rossetti, L. Surgical removal of visceral fat reverses hepatic insulin resistance. *Diabetes* **1999**, *48*, 94–98. [CrossRef] [PubMed]
49. Arner, P. Obesity and the adipocyte. Regional adipocity in man. *J. Endocrinol.* **1997**, *155*, 191–192. [CrossRef] [PubMed]
50. Tan, G.D.; Goossens, G.H.; Humphreys, S.M.; Vidal, H.; Karpe, F. Upper and lower body adipose tissue function: A direct comparison of fat mobilization in humans. *Obes. Res.* **2004**, *12*, 114–118. [CrossRef] [PubMed]
51. Khan, S.; Jena, G. Sodium butyrate reduces insulin-resistance, fat accumulation and dyslipidemia in type-2 diabetic rat: A comparative study with metformin. *Chem. Biol. Interact.* **2016**, *254*, 124–134. [CrossRef] [PubMed]
52. Mooradian, A.D. Dyslipidemia in type 2 diabetes mellitus. *Nat. Clin. Pract. Endocrinol. Metab.* **2009**, *5*, 150–159. [CrossRef] [PubMed]
53. Den Besten, G.; van Eunen, K.; Groen, A.K.; Venema, K.; Reijngoud, D.J.; Bakker, B.M. The role of short-chain fatty acids in the interplay between diet, gut microbiota, and host energy metabolism. *J. Lipid Res.* **2013**, *54*, 2325–2340. [CrossRef] [PubMed]
54. Camp, H.S.; Ren, D.; Leff, T. Adipogenesis and fat-cell function in obesity and diabetes. *Trends Mol. Med.* **2002**, *8*, 442–447. [CrossRef]

55. Mulder, P.; Morrison, M.C.; Verschuren, L.; Liang, W.; van Bockel, J.H.; Kooistra, T.; Wielinga, P.Y.; Kleemann, R. Reduction of obesity-associated white adipose tissue inflammation by rosiglitazone is associated with reduced non-alcoholic fatty liver disease in ldlr-deficient mice. *Sci. Rep.* **2016**, *6*, 31542. [CrossRef] [PubMed]
56. Morrison, M.C.; Kleemann, R. Role of macrophage migration inhibitory factor in obesity, insulin resistance, type 2 diabetes, and associated hepatic co-morbidities: A comprehensive review of human and rodent studies. *Front. Immunol.* **2015**, *6*, 308. [CrossRef] [PubMed]
57. Mulder, P.; Morrison, M.C.; Wielinga, P.Y.; van Duyvenvoorde, W.; Kooistra, T.; Kleemann, R. Surgical removal of inflamed epididymal white adipose tissue attenuates the development of non-alcoholic steatohepatitis in obesity. *Int. J. Obes.* **2016**, *40*, 675–684. [CrossRef] [PubMed]
58. Liang, W.; Tonini, G.; Mulder, P.; Kelder, T.; van Erk, M.; van den Hoek, A.M.; Mariman, R.; Wielinga, P.Y.; Baccini, M.; Kooistra, T.; et al. Coordinated and interactive expression of genes of lipid metabolism and inflammation in adipose tissue and liver during metabolic overload. *PLoS ONE* **2013**, *8*, e75290. [CrossRef] [PubMed]
59. Xu, H.; Barnes, G.T.; Yang, Q.; Tan, G.; Yang, D.; Chou, C.J.; Sole, J.; Nichols, A.; Ross, J.S.; Tartaglia, L.A. Chronic inflammation in fat plays a crucial role in the development of obesity-related insulin resistance. *J. Clin. Investig.* **2003**, *112*, 1821–1830. [CrossRef] [PubMed]
60. Hajer, G.R.; van Haeften, T.W.; Visseren, F.L. Adipose tissue dysfunction in obesity, diabetes, and vascular diseases. *Eur. Heart J.* **2008**, *29*, 2959–2971. [CrossRef] [PubMed]
61. Antuna-Puente, B.; Feve, B.; Fellahi, S.; Bastard, J.P. Adipokines: The missing link between insulin resistance and obesity. *Diabetes Metab.* **2008**, *34*, 2–11. [CrossRef] [PubMed]
62. Loffreda, S.; Yang, S.; Lin, H.; Karp, C.; Brengman, M.; Wang, D.; Klein, A.; Bulkley, G.; Bao, C.; Noble, P. Leptin regulates proinflammatory immune responses. *FASEB J.* **1998**, *12*, 57–65. [PubMed]
63. De Oliveira, E.M.; Ascar, T.P.; Silva, J.C.; Sandri, S.; Migliorini, S.; Fock, R.A.; Campa, A. Serum amyloid a links endotoxaemia to weight gain and insulin resistance in mice. *Diabetologia* **2016**, *59*, 1760–1768. [CrossRef] [PubMed]
64. Ahlin, S.; Olsson, M.; Olsson, B.; Svensson, P.A.; Sjöholm, K. No evidence for a role of adipose tissue-derived serum amyloid a in the development of insulin resistance or obesity-related inflammation in hsaa1+/− transgenic mice. *PLoS ONE* **2013**, *8*, e72204. [CrossRef] [PubMed]
65. Den Hartigh, L.J.; Wang, S.; Goodspeed, L.; Ding, Y.; Averill, M.; Subramanian, S.; Wietecha, T.; O'Brien, K.D.; Chait, A. Deletion of serum amyloid a3 improves high fat high sucrose diet-induced adipose tissue inflammation and hyperlipidemia in female mice. *PLoS ONE* **2014**, *9*, e108564. [CrossRef] [PubMed]
66. Leinonen, E.; Hurt-Camejo, E.; Wiklund, O.; Hultén, L.M.; Hiukka, A.; Taskinen, M.R. Insulin resistance and adiposity correlate with acute-phase reaction and soluble cell adhesion molecules in type 2 diabetes. *Atherosclerosis* **2003**, *166*, 387–394. [CrossRef]
67. Yamauchi, T.; Kamon, J.; Minokoshi, Y.A.; Ito, Y.; Waki, H.; Uchida, S.; Yamashita, S.; Noda, M.; Kita, S.; Ueki, K. Adiponectin stimulates glucose utilization and fatty-acid oxidation by activating amp-activated protein kinase. *Nat. Med.* **2002**, *8*, 1288–1295. [CrossRef] [PubMed]

9

Glucose and Lipid Dysmetabolism in a Rat Model of Prediabetes Induced by a High-Sucrose Diet

Ana Burgeiro [1,†], Manuela G. Cerqueira [1,†], Bárbara M. Varela-Rodríguez [1], Sara Nunes [1,2], Paula Neto [3], Frederico C. Pereira [1,2], Flávio Reis [1,2,*] and Eugénia Carvalho [1,4,5,6,*]

1 Center of Neuroscience and Cell Biology (CNC) and CNC.IBILI Research Consortium, University of Coimbra, 3004-504 Coimbra, Portugal; burgeiroana@gmail.com (A.B.); manuela.g.cerqueira@gmail.com (M.G.C.); biobvr00@udc.es (B.M.V.-R.); sara_nunes20@hotmail.com (S.N.); fredcp@ci.uc.pt (F.C.P.)

2 Laboratory of Pharmacology and Experimental Therapeutics, Institute for Biomedical Imaging and Life Sciences (IBILI), Faculty of Medicine, University of Coimbra, 3000-548 Coimbra, Portugal

3 Service of Anatomical Pathology, Coimbra University Hospital Centre (CHUC), 3000-075 Coimbra, Portugal; anahepafr@gmail.com

4 The Portuguese Diabetes Association (APDP), 1250-203 Lisbon, Portugal

5 Department of Geriatrics, University of Arkansas for Medical Sciences, Little Rock, AR 72202, USA

6 Arkansas Children's Hospital Research Institute, Little Rock, AR 72202, USA

* Correspondence: freis@fmed.uc.pt (F.R.); ecarvalh@cnc.uc.pt (E.C.);

† These authors contributed equally to this work.

Abstract: Glucotoxicity and lipotoxicity are key features of type 2 diabetes mellitus, but their molecular nature during the early stages of the disease remains to be elucidated. We aimed to characterize glucose and lipid metabolism in insulin-target organs (liver, skeletal muscle, and white adipose tissue) in a rat model treated with a high-sucrose (HSu) diet. Two groups of 16-week-old male Wistar rats underwent a 9-week protocol: HSu diet ($n = 10$)—received 35% of sucrose in drinking water; Control ($n = 12$)—received vehicle (water). Body weight, food, and beverage consumption were monitored and glucose, insulin, and lipid profiles were measured. Serum and liver triglyceride concentrations, as well as the expression of genes and proteins involved in lipid biosynthesis were assessed. The insulin-stimulated glucose uptake and isoproterenol-stimulated lipolysis were also measured in freshly isolated adipocytes. Even in the absence of obesity, this rat model already presented the main features of prediabetes, with fasting normoglycemia but reduced glucose tolerance, postprandial hyperglycemia, compensatory hyperinsulinemia, as well as decreased insulin sensitivity (resistance) and hypertriglyceridemia. In addition, impaired hepatic function, including altered gluconeogenic and lipogenic pathways, as well as increased expression of acetyl-coenzyme A carboxylase 1 and fatty acid synthase in the liver, were observed, suggesting that liver glucose and lipid dysmetabolism may play a major role at this stage of the disease.

Keywords: high-sucrose diet; prediabetes; glucose; lipid; metabolism; hypertriglyceridemia

---

1. Introduction

Type 2 diabetes mellitus (T2DM) has become an epidemic of noncommunicable diseases, with 415 million people worldwide currently living with diabetes [1]. According to the International Diabetes Federation, about 5 million people died from DM in 2015 and the estimates indicate that there will be about 642 million people living with DM by 2040. In addition, there are about 318 million adults with impaired glucose tolerance (IGT), which puts them at high risk for the disease.

Prediabetes (or intermediate hyperglycemia) already displays metabolic alterations and is a high risk state for developing T2DM. According to the American Diabetes Association, prediabetes is distinguished by having impaired fasting glucose (IFG) (100–125 mg/dL glucose), IGT (140–199 mg/dL glucose 2 h after a 75-g oral glucose tolerance test), and glycated hemoglobin (HbA1c) levels between 5.7–6.4%. The prevalence of prediabetes is rapidly increasing with over 470 million people projected with prediabetes by 2030 [2]. This likely anticipates increased morbidity, mortality, and healthcare costs in the near future with DM management. Thus, preventing the progression of IGT and/or IFG to T2DM is the most rational and effective way to combat the DM epidemic and lessen healthcare costs. However, before we can succeed, we need to unravel glucose and lipid metabolism at this stage of the disease.

Diets enriched in sugars including the intake of sugar-sweetened beverages have been consistently linked to the increased risk of hypertriglyceridemia, obesity, T2DM, and cardiovascular disease [3]. A central feature of T2DM is hyperglycemia, as a result of excessive hepatic glucose production, insulin resistance, and deficient secretion of pancreatic insulin. An often overlooked feature is the relationship between glucose and lipids, whose fluxes are indeed closely interlinked through the intersection of metabolic pathways at the acetyl-CoA formation [4]. Impairment of one pathway can indirectly have a major impact on another [4,5]. Molecular and metabolic abnormalities in insulin action, such as peripheral tissues (muscle, liver, and adipose tissues) insulin resistance, together with minor defects in insulin secretion, can be clearly identified before the development of obesity or hyperglycemia. These factors contribute to the increased fatty acid influx into the liver and muscle causing accumulation of toxic lipid metabolites. Particularly, chronically increased levels of plasma nonesterified fatty acids (NEFA) and triglyceride (TG)-rich lipoproteins impair lipid metabolism, a process referred to as lipotoxicity [6]. Furthermore, when the NEFA supply exceeds metabolic capacity, lipids accumulate in peripheral tissues, such as liver and muscle, inducing organ dysfunction [6]. Several recent lines of evidence show that the typical dyslipidemia in T2DM patients, characterized by elevated TGs, low high density lipoprotein cholesterol (HDL-c), and the predominance of small-dense low density lipoprotein (LDL) particles, may not only be the consequence of diabetes but may also cause disturbances of glucose metabolism. In fact, hypertriglyceridemia leads to elevated levels of free fatty acids (FFAs), which contribute to insulin resistance and β-cell dysfunction, putatively by impairing the molecular mechanisms linking insulin receptors with glucose transporters, as well as by directly damaging β-cells. Moreover, hypertriglyceridemia and elevated FFAs can contribute to inflammation, which boosts insulin resistance and β-cell dysfunction [4–7]. In addition, low HDL-c could also influence low-grade inflammation and affect glucose metabolism, thus contributing to diabetes [8]. Collectively, lipotoxicity and glucotoxicity are associated to the progression of DM and its micro- and macrovascular complications [5,9]. However, the nature of glucose and lipid deregulation in the prediabetic state remains to be elucidated.

Therefore, we aim to evaluate glucose and lipid metabolism in a prediabetic rat model, induced by a high-sucrose (HSu) diet [10,11], focusing on the main insulin-target organs: liver, skeletal muscle, and white adipose tissue.

2. Materials and Methods

2.1. Animals and Diets

Male Wistar rats (16 week-old; Charles River Laboratories, Barcelona, Spain) were housed, two per cage, under controlled conditions (12 h light/dark cycle schedule and controlled temperature (22 ± 1 °C) and humidity). After an adaptation period of 1 week, rats were randomly divided into two groups (2 animals per cage) and submitted to a 9-week protocol: (1) control—receiving tap water as vehicle; (2) Hsu—receiving 35% sucrose (S0389; Sigma-Aldrich, St. Louis, MO, USA) in the drinking water. All animals were fed standard rat chow, containing 60% of carbohydrates, 16.1% of protein, 3.1% of lipids, 3.9% of fibers, and 5.1% of minerals (AO4 Panlab, Barcelona, Spain), ad libitum (except during fasting periods). Body weight, food, and beverage consumption were monitored every two days and presented as weekly variation per rat (which is the mean of the two rats per cage). All experiments were conducted in accordance with the European Union (EU) Legislation for the protection of animals used for scientific purposes "Animals (Scientific Procedures) Act", Directive 2010/63/EU, and with the National and Local Authorities, under authorization of the Organ Responsible for Animal Welfare of Faculty of Medicine of Coimbra University (07/2016).

2.2. Chemicals

Collagenase type II was from Roche (Lisbon, Portugal). D-[[^{14}C(U)]-glucose (250 mCi/mmol/L) was from Scopus Research BV (Wageningen, The Netherlands). Human insulin, Actrapid, was kindly supplied by Novo Nordisk A/S (Paço de Arcos, Portugal). N-heptane was from Merck-&-Co., Inc. (Whitehouse Station, NJ, USA). Optiphase Hisafe was from PerkinElmer, Inc. (Waltham, MA, USA). RNeasy® MiniKits were from QIAGEN Sciences (Germantown, MD, USA). High Capacity cDNA Reverse Transcriptase kits were from Applied Biosystems (Forest City, CA, USA). PCR primers were designed using Beacon Designer software and synthesized by IDT-Integrated DNA Technologies, Inc. (BVBA, Leuven, Belgium). SYBRGreen Supermix was from Quanta Biosciences (Gaithersburg, MA, USA). All other reagents were from Sigma (St. Louis, MO, USA). ECF reagent was from GE Healthcare (Little Chalfont, UK).

2.3. Metabolic Characterization

Metabolic characterization was performed as previously described [10] and is detailed in the supplemental material. This included a glucose tolerance test (GTT), an insulin tolerance test (ITT), fasting insulin levels, and insulin resistance (evaluated by the homeostatic model assessment of insulin resistance HOMA-IR index), as well as serum TG to HDL-c ratio (TG/HDL-c), TG-glucose (TyG) index, as well as fed and fasted alanine aminotransferase [6] and aspartate aminotransferase (AST) assessment. Caloric intake was calculated based on the daily food intake, and in HSu-treated animals, the energy related to sucrose consumption was also calculated.

2.4. Blood and Tissues Collection

After a 9-week treatment, blood and tissues (liver, skeletal muscle—from the posterior thigh of the rat leg—and epididymal adipose tissue) were snap frozen and stored at −80 °C. Details are available in the supplemental material.

2.5. Liver Pathology and Triglyceride Content

Liver TG were extracted and quantified as previously reported [12]. Briefly, 50 mg of liver samples were homogenized in 0.5 mL of chlorophorm/methanol (2:1) and incubated for 3 h with agitation at 4 °C. 300 μL of milliQ water were then added to the homogenate and centrifuged (13,000 rpm for 20 min, room temperature). The organic phase was transferred to a clean Eppendorf tube, allowed to evaporate at 4 °C, and finally stored at −20 °C. Liver TG quantification was performed with a specific commercial kit from Spinreact. Colorimetric determination was performed in a spectrophotometer (SPECTRAmax PLUS384, Molecular Devices, Sunnyvale, CA, USA) at a wavelength of 505 nm or 490 nm after TG resuspension in 500 μL of chloroform. Intensity of the formed color was proportional to TG concentration in each sample. Oil red O staining of liver frozen sections was performed to evaluate lipid deposition, according to previously described methodology [13]. Liver pathology was assessed by hematoxylin and eosin (H&E) in paraffin-embedded sections fixed with paraformaldehyde at the moment of sample collection. Data analysis was performed in a blind fashion by a pathologist.

2.6. Cell Size and Weight, Glucose Uptake, and Lipolysis in Isolated Epididymal Adipocytes

Epididymal adipocyte size and weight, insulin-stimulated D-[[^{14}C(U)]-glucose uptake, and isoproterenol-stimulated lipolysis in isolated adipocytes were performed as previously described [14,15]. Briefly, for the insulin-stimulated glucose uptake, the isolated adipocytes were diluted ten times and were stimulated or not with human insulin (1000 μU/mL), for 10 min, at 37 °C, in a shaking water-bath. Subsequently, 0.86 μM D-[[^{14}C(U)]-glucose was added to the medium and the accumulation of glucose followed for 30 min. The cell suspension was then transferred to pre-chilled tubes, containing silicone oil, allowing cells to be separated from the buffer by centrifugation. Cell-associated radioactivity was determined by liquid scintillation counting, which allowed us to calculate the rate of transmembranar glucose transport, according to the formula: cellular clearance of medium glucose = (c.p.m. cells × volume)/(c.p.m. medium × cell number × time).

For isoproterenol-stimulated lipolysis, the isolated adipocytes were diluted ten times and were incubated in the presence or absence of insulin (1000 μU/mL), in a shaking water bath, at 37 °C, for 60 min. The medium was also supplemented or not with isoproterenol (1 μM). Following incubation, cells were separated from the medium by centrifugation and glycerol levels were measured in the medium using an assay kit (Zen Bio, Inc., Research Triangle Park, NC, USA). Further details are available in the supplemental material.

2.7. Liver, Skeletal Muscle, and Adipose Tissue Gene and Protein Expression

Total RNA from liver, skeletal muscle, and epididymal adipose tissue was extracted, and cDNA synthesis and relative mRNA levels for glucose transporter-1(Glut1), -2 (Slc2a2), and -4 (Glut4), phosphoenolpyruvate carboxykinase (Pepck), glucose-6-phosphatase (G6pc), acetyl-CoA carboxylase 1 (Acc1), fatty acid synthase (Fasn), diglyceride acyltransferase (Dgat1), carbohydrate-responsive element-binding protein (Mlxipl/Chrebp), sterol regulatory element-binding transcription factor 1 (Srebf1), and hormone-sensitive lipase (Hsl) were measured (by real time-PCR), as previously described [16]. Protein extraction and Western blot analysis of GLUT1, GLUT2, GLUT4, PEPCK, G6PC, ACC1, FASN, DGAT1, ChREBP, SREBP, and HSL were performed as previously described [14,15]. The supplemental material details the protocols and lists the primer sequences (Table S1) and antibodies (Table S2) used.

2.8. Statistical Analysis

Results were expressed as mean ± standard error of the mean, using GraphPad Prism, version 6 (GraphPad Software, San Diego, CA, USA). Student's *t*-test for normally distributed data or the Mann Whitney test for non-normally distributed data were performed when two groups were considered. One-way or two-way ANOVA, followed by Tukey post hoc test, for multiple comparisons, was used as appropriate. Repeated measures ANOVA, followed by the Tukey post-hoc test, was used to assess the differences between groups and between basal and insulin-stimulated glucose uptake. Differences were considered significant when * $p \leq 0.05$, ** $p \leq 0.01$, *** $p \leq 0.001$, or **** $p \leq 0.0001$.

3. Results

3.1. HSu Diet Increases Beverage Consumption and Caloric Intake, Maintaining Body Weight

During 9 weeks of treatment, the body weight evolution was identical in HSu-treated and control rats (Figure 1A). However, HSu-treated animals had a higher beverage (35% sucrose) consumption but a lower food ingestion (Figure 1B,C). This behavior translated to an increased total caloric intake, mainly from carbohydrates, with a lower calorie consumption from proteins and lipids, when compared with the control animals ((Figure 1D–G).

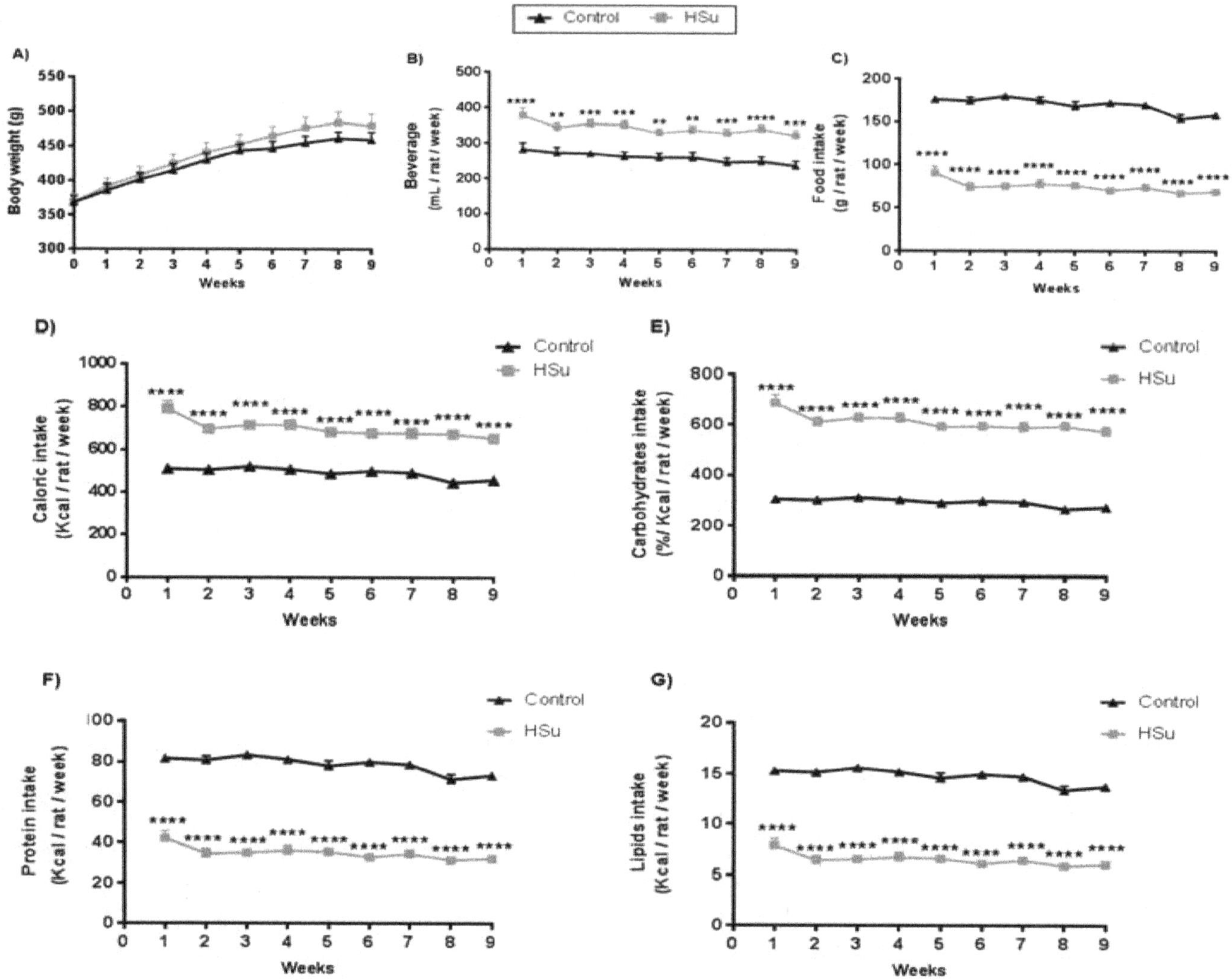

Figure 1. Evolution of body weight (**A**), beverage (**B**) and food (**C**) intake, as well as total caloric consumption (**D**) and caloric intake related with carbohydrates (**E**), protein (**F**), and lipids (**G**), throughout the 9 weeks of treatment. Control (n = 12) and HSu (n = 10). ** $p < 0.01$, *** $p < 0.001$, **** $p < 0.0001$.

3.2. HSu Diet Increases Serum Triglyceride Levels and Impairs Liver Function

The serum TG content in HSu-treated rats was significantly higher than in control animals in the fed state. Also, fed HSu-treated rats presented higher TG concentrations than in fasted HSu animals (Figure 2A). However, no significant differences were found in liver TG levels (Figure 2B). Regardless of the nutritional status (fasted or fed), serum ALT levels were reduced in the HSu-treated rats (Figure 2C); however, no significant differences were found in serum AST levels (Figure 2D). In addition, the liver weight/body weight ratio was increased in HSu-treated animals (Figure 2E).

Despite markers of impaired liver function, no changes in liver structure were found when analyzed by H&E histology (Figure 3(A1,A2)). Oil red O staining showed a slight deposition of lipids in the HSu-treated animals, when compared with the control ones (Figure 3(B1,B2)), respectively).

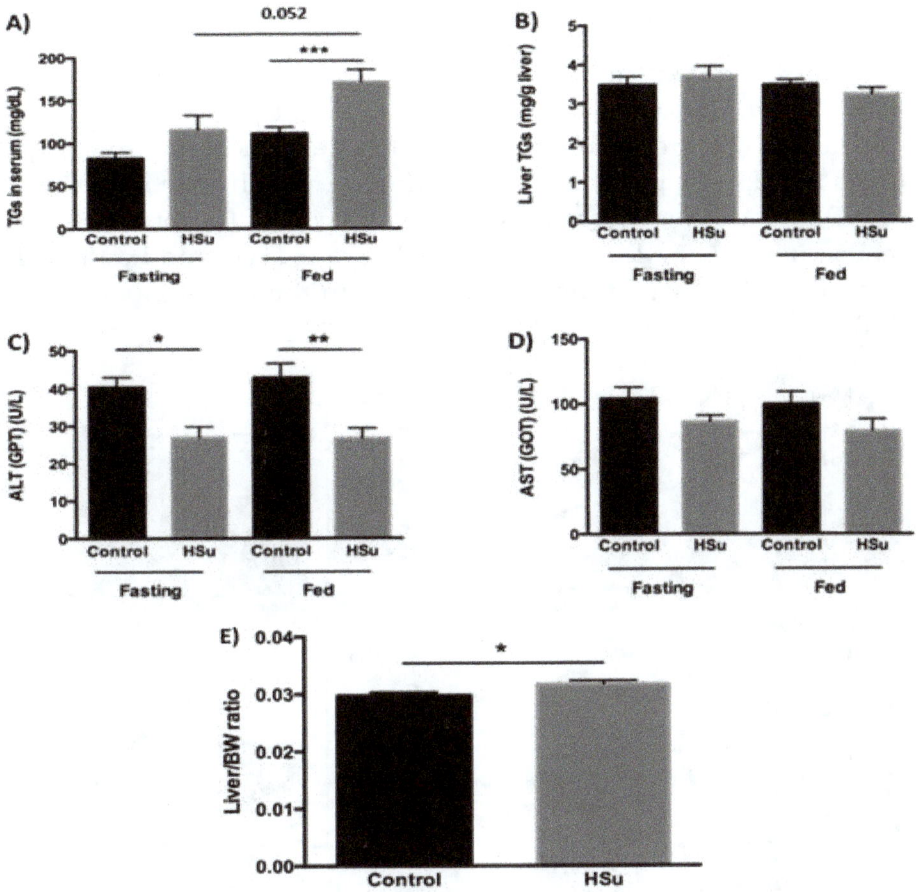

Figure 2. Serum (**A**) and liver (**B**) triglyceride (TG) content, serum alanine aminotransferase (ALT) (**C**) and aspartate aminotransferase (AST) (**D**) levels, as well as liver weight/body weight ratio (**E**) at the end of treatment. Control ($n = 12$) and HSu ($n = 10$). * $p < 0.05$, ** $p < 0.01$, *** $p < 0.001$.

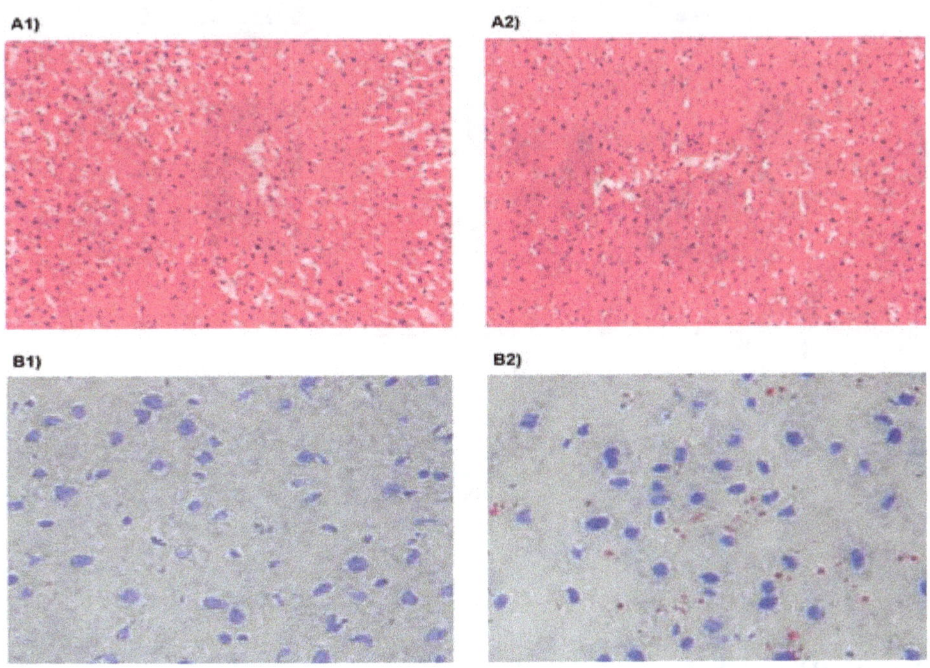

Figure 3. Liver (**A1**,**A2**) Hematoxylin and Eosin (H&E) staining (×200) and (**B1**,**B2**) Oil red O staining (×400) in control (1) and HSu-treated (2) rats. Six sections per group were measured.

3.3. HSu Diet Impairs Glucose Tolerance and Causes Insulin Resistance

Although both groups showed similar fasting glucose levels (Figure 4A,C,E), the HSu-treated rats had significantly slower glucose excursion during a GTT (2 g/kg body weight of glucose), compared to control animals (Figure 4A,B), revealing glucose intolerance. Blood glucose levels were significantly elevated in the HSu-treated rats, 120 min after an insulin injection (0.75 U/kg body weight of insulin) (Figure 4C,D). In addition, serum fasting insulin concentration was significantly elevated in HSu-treated animals (Figure 4F). Moreover, TG/HDL-c ratio, TyG and HOMA-IR indexes, known markers of insulin resistance, were significantly elevated in the HSu-treated rats, compared to the controls (Figure 4G–I).

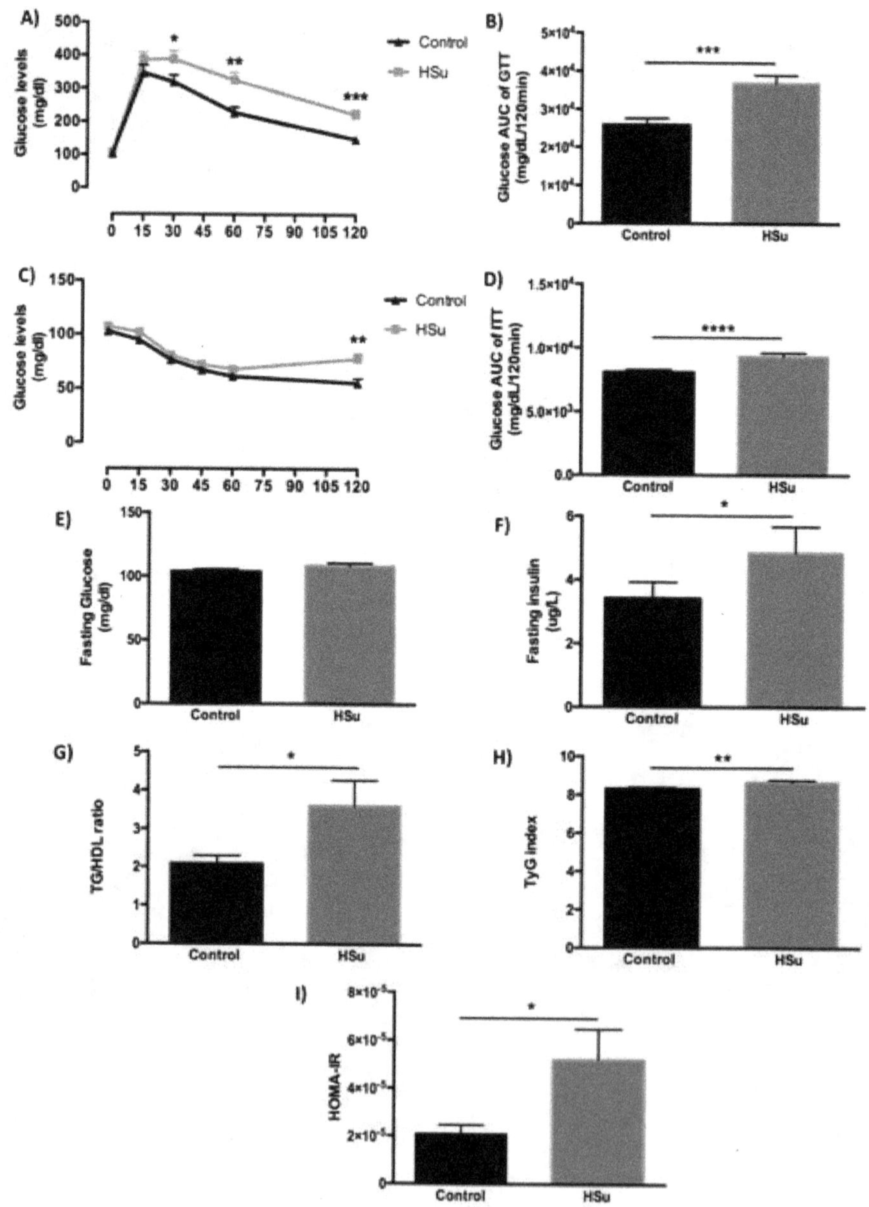

Figure 4. Glucose tolerance test (GTT) and area under the curve (**A**,**B**), insulin tolerance test (ITT) and area under the curve (**C**,**D**), fasting glucose (**E**) and insulin (**F**) levels, as well as insulin resistance markers: triglycerides to high density lipoprotein cholesterol (TG/HDL-c) ratio (**G**), triglyceride glucose (TyG) index (**H**) and homeostatic model assessment of insulin resistance (HOMA-IR) index (**I**) at the end of treatment. Control (n = 12) and HSu (n = 10). * $p < 0.05$, ** $p < 0.01$, *** $p < 0.001$, and **** $p \leq 0.0001$.

3.4. HSu Diet Increases Fat Mass While the Insulin-Stimulated Glucose Uptake in Adipocytes Is Impaired

The epididymal fat pad weight/body weight ratio was significantly higher in the HSu-treated rats when compared to the controls (Figure 5A), while fat cell diameter and weight were unchanged between the groups (Figure 5C,D). Insulin-stimulated glucose uptake was measured in freshly isolated adipocytes. Basal glucose uptake was not significantly different between groups ($p > 0.05$). Adipocytes responded to the stimulatory effect of insulin in the uptake of glucose in both groups (Control − Basal = 20.31 ± 2.59 vs. Insulin = 35.88 ± 4.22, $p < 0.001$; HSu − Basal = 8.55 ± 1.09 vs. Insulin = 17.48 ± 1.16, $p < 0.001$); however, the insulin-stimulated glucose uptake was significantly reduced in adipocytes from HSu-treated rats compared to the controls (17.48 ± 1.16 vs. 35.88 ± 4.22, $p < 0.01$, respectively) (Figure 5B).

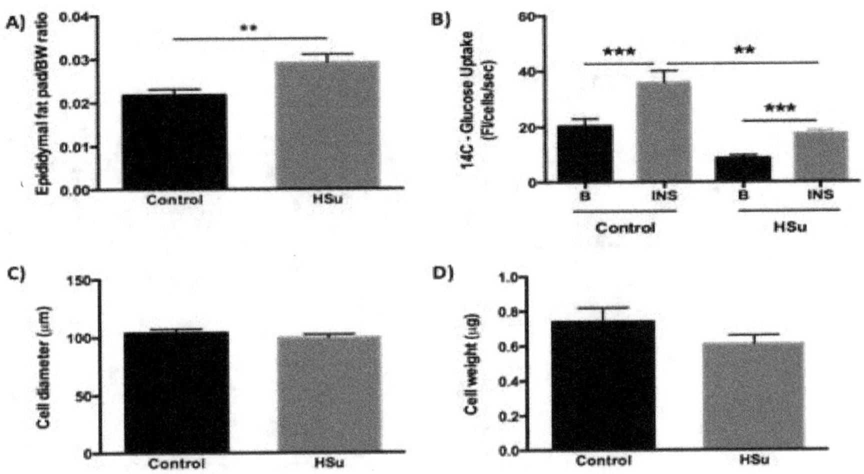

Figure 5. Epididymal fat pad weight/bw ratio (**A**), insulin-stimulated D-[[^{14}C(U)]-glucose uptake in isolated adipocytes (**B**), and adipocyte diameter (**C**) and weight (**D**) at the end of treatment. Control ($n = 12$) and HSu ($n = 10$). ** $p < 0.01$, *** $p < 0.001$.

3.5. HSu Diet Decreased GLUT1 but Increased G6Pase Levels in Liver

The gene and protein levels of mediators of glucose uptake and gluconeogenesis were quantified in liver, skeletal muscle (posterior thigh of the leg), and epididymal adipose tissue. There were no changes in glucose transporter gene levels in all tissues, in the fed state (Figure 6A). Moreover, GLUT1 protein levels were reduced in HSu-treated rats versus controls, with no change in GLUT2 expression, in the liver. In addition, no differences were found in either GLUT1 or GLUT4 protein levels in skeletal muscle or epididymal adipose tissue. To assess hepatic gluconeogenesis, PEPCK and G6Pase gene and protein levels were evaluated. While there was no alteration in gene expression, there was a significant increase in only G6Pase protein levels in the HSu-treated group (Figure 6B).

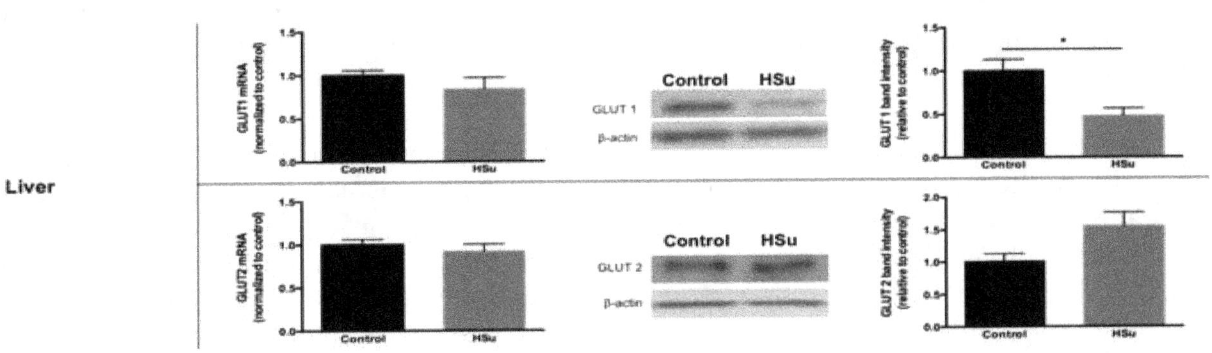

Figure 6. *Cont.*

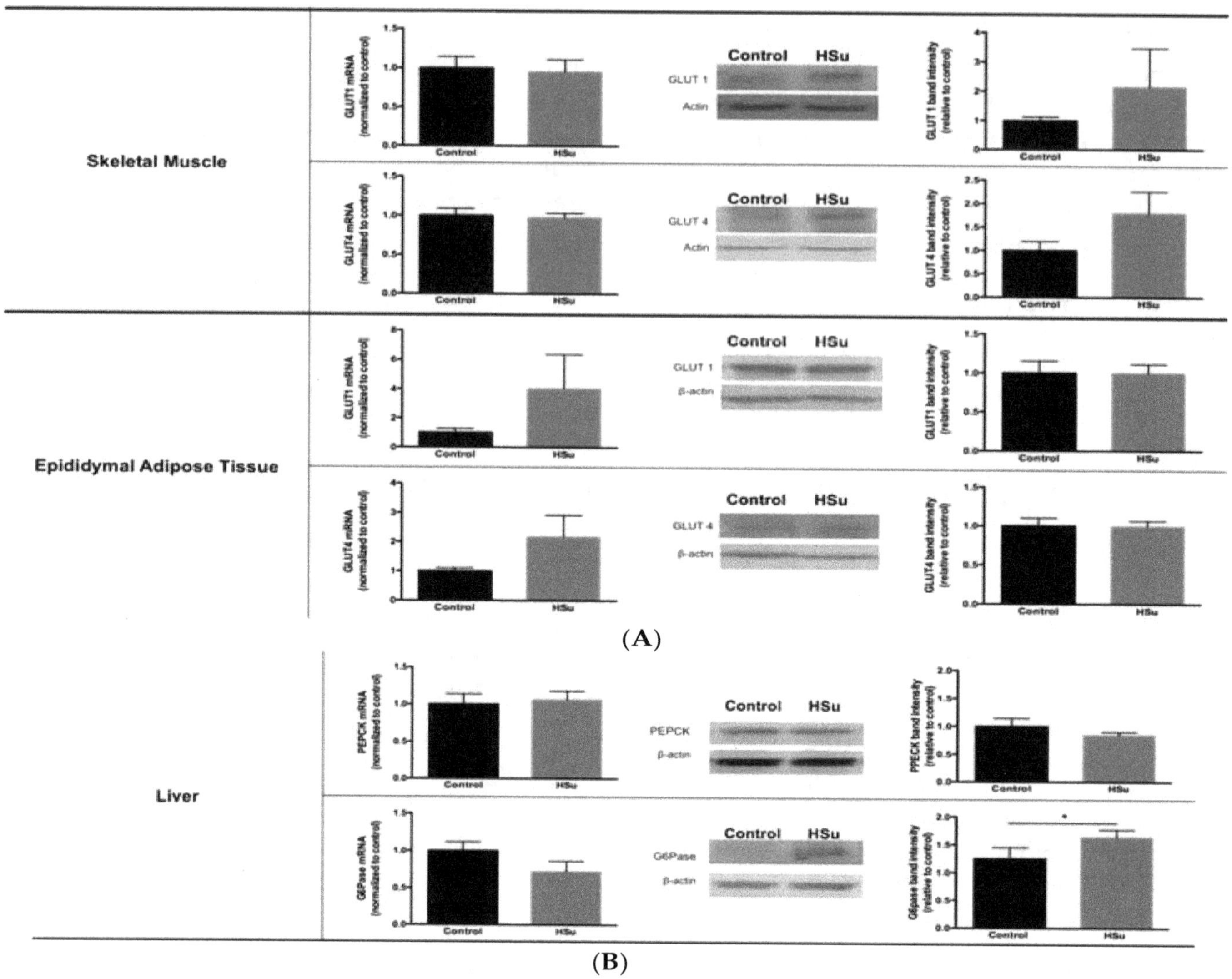

Figure 6. (**A**) Glucose transporters. (**B**) Gluconeogenesis. Gene and protein levels of glucose transporters (**A**) in liver, skeletal muscle (posterior thigh of the leg), and epididymal adipose tissue. Gene and protein levels of mediators of hepatic gluconeogenesis (**B**). Control (n = 12) and HSu (n = 10). * $p \leq 0.05$.

3.6. HSu Diet Increases Hepatic Lipid Biosynthesis, without Alterations in Lipolysis

Gene and protein levels of ACC1, FASN, and DGAT1, that play a major role in lipid biosynthesis in the liver and in fat, were analyzed, together with SREBP and ChREBP. Increased protein levels of ACC1, FASN, and SREBP were observed in the liver of HSu-treated animals, without changes in gene levels (Figure 7A). In addition, in adipose tissue, both gene and protein levels for ChREBP were increased in the HSu-treated rats, without further changes on the other measured mediators (Figure 7A).

Isoproterenol-stimulated lipolysis was performed to measure TG hydrolysis into glycerol and free fatty acids, and to evaluate the antilipolytic effect of insulin in isolated adipocytes (Figure 7(B1)). Both groups responded similarly to the stimulatory effect of isoproterenol (Control: 0.66 ± 0.11; HSu: 0.50 ± 0.08) versus basal (Control: 0.30 ± 0.03; HSu: 0.22 ± 0.03) and insulin levels (Control: 0.34 ± 0.04; HSu: 0.24 ± 0.03). Even though there is a tendency for an antilipolytic effect of insulin after isoproterenol stimulation (Control: 0.50 ± 0.05; HSu: 0.39 ± 0.05), it does not reach significance. Moreover, gene and protein expression levels for HSL were not different between the two groups (Figure 7(B2)).

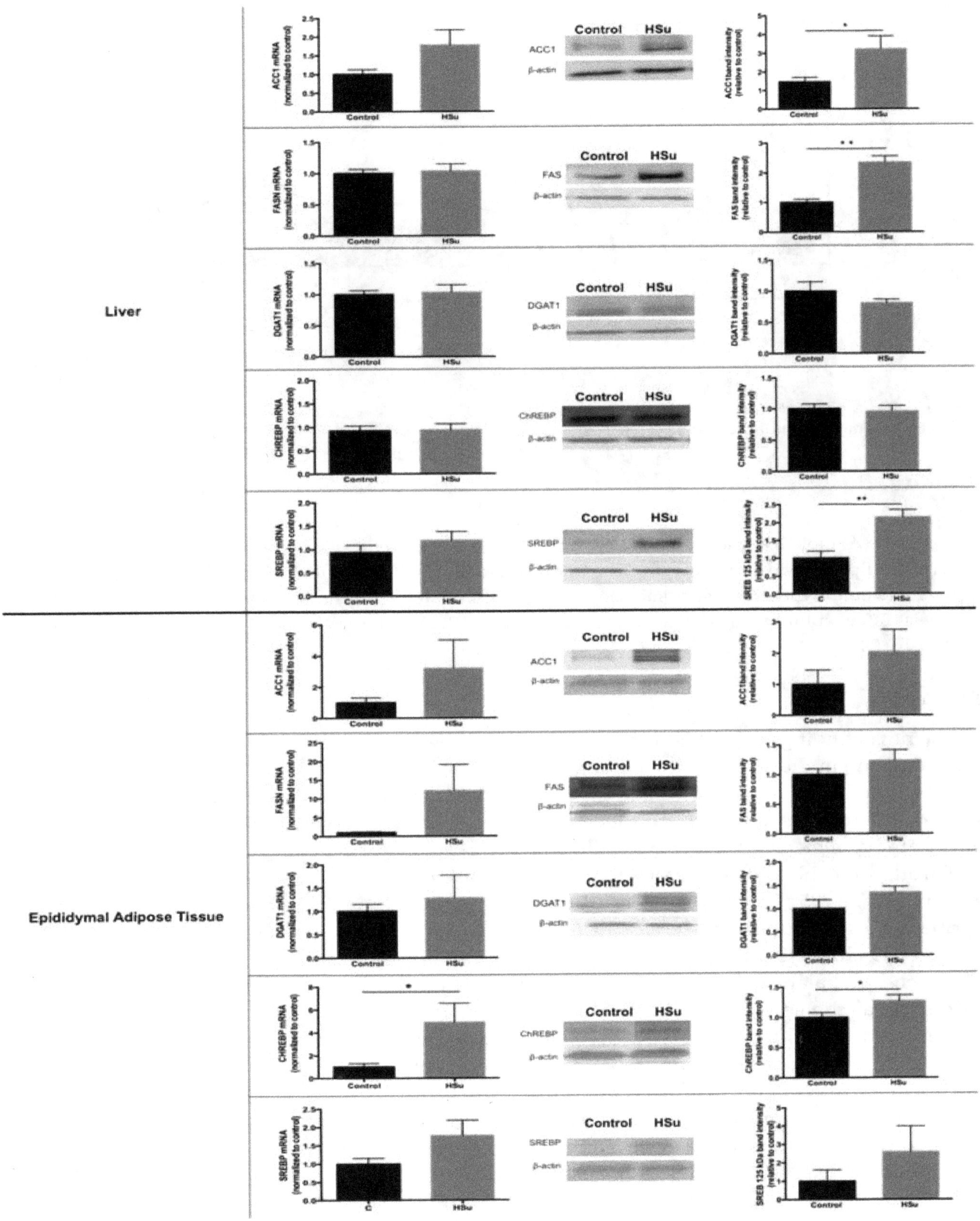

(A)

Figure 7. *Cont.*

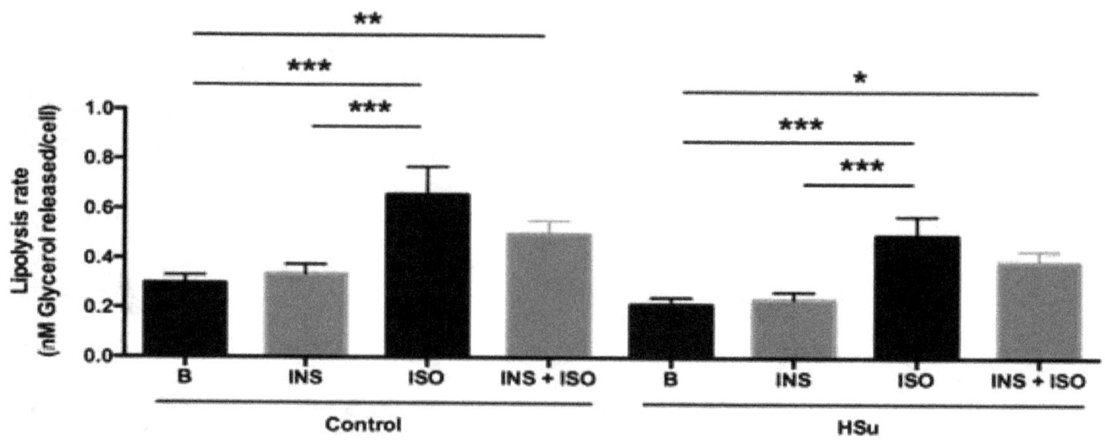

(B1)

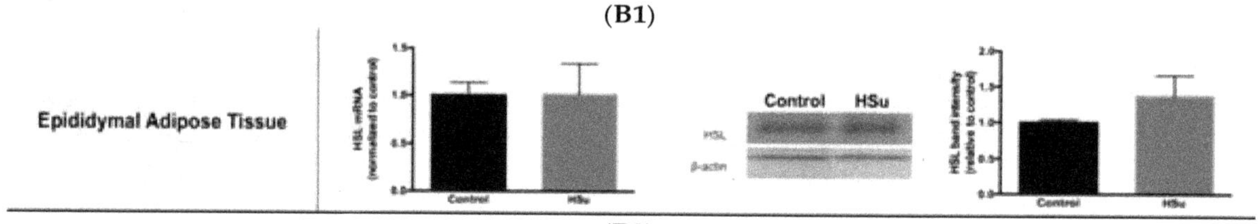

(B2)

Figure 7. (**A**) Lipid biosynthesis. (**B1**,**B2**) Lipolysis. (**B1**) Isoproterenol-stimulated lipolysis. (**B2**) Hormone-sensitive lipase gene and protein. Gene and protein levels of mediators of lipid biosynthesis (**A**) in liver and epididymal adipose tissue. Isoproterenol-stimulated lipolysis (**B1**) and HSL gene and protein levels (**B2**) in epididymal adipose tissue. Control (n = 12) and HSu (n = 10). * $p \leq 0.05$, ** $p < 0.01$, and *** $p < 0.001$.

4. Discussion

The novel findings from this study indicate that a high-sugar diet induces early glucose and lipid dysmetabolism, in the absence of weight gain, only after 9 weeks of treatment. HSu-treated animals developed impaired insulin-stimulated glucose uptake and reduced insulin sensitivity (resistance), together with decreased GLUT1 but increased G6Pase protein levels in the liver. These metabolic changes are paralleled by fed hyperglycemia and hypertriglyceridemia.

Throughout the 9-week treatment, the HSu-treated group had lower food consumption but higher beverage (35% sucrose) and caloric intake, while maintaining body weight, as previously described [17–19]. Similar body weight might have been maintained due to: first, differences in digestion and absorption may have modified the amount of 'bioavailable' energy, affecting the actual positive energy balance; second, the composition of weight gain (fat mass and lean mass) might be different, as the energy cost of protein deposition is higher than that of adipose tissue. In fact, we observed that HSu-treated animals have a greater adiposity translated by an increased epididymal fat pad weight/body weight ratio. Moreover, dietary protein content was suggested to be a critical determinant of weight gain during ad libitum feeding [20].

This prediabetic animal model presented low food intake, which is enriched in 16.1% protein, and increased fluid intake of sucrose-enriched water, in agreement with previous studies [18]. This means that HSu-treated animals ingested a smaller amount of protein and a greater amount of carbohydrates, which can be translated by higher fat mass and smaller lean mass, which allowed the maintenance of body weight. This suggestion might be further confirmed by performing an in vivo non-invasive ecographic magnetic resonance imaging (Echo-MRI) analysis to assess whole body fat, lean, free water, and total water masses.

Indeed, epididymal fat pad weight/body weight ratio was significantly higher in HSu-treated rats. Moreover, high-protein diets are known to reduce adiposity/lipogenesis in the context of high carbohydrate consumption in Western diets [21]. In fact, high-sucrose diets may increase adiposity by stimulating liver lipogenesis [22].

After 9 weeks of treatment, the HSu-treated group had higher serum TG levels, in agreement with previous reports [18,23–25], together with increased lipid deposition in the hepatic tissue, viewed by the Oil Red O staining. In addition, ALT levels were significantly reduced in HSu-treated rats, while a significant increase in the liver weight/body weight ratio was observed, suggesting altered liver function, without liver lesion at this stage of impaired metabolism. The strongest hypothesis to explain the reduced liver function and ALT low levels is malnutrition or an altered nutritional pattern. This prediabetes model had lower food consumption (constituted by 16.1% protein) and increased fluid intake (sucrose-enriched water). Thus, the low serum ALT levels, indicative of liver dysfunction, observed in the HSu-treated rats might be caused by a diet poor in essential nutrients/macromolecules (including proteins and lipids), i.e., malnutrition.

This prediabetes model presented impaired glucose homeostasis. Already at the early stages of the disease, there were initial metabolic deregulations, evidenced by alterations in glucose tolerance during the GTT and ITT, as well as the glucose and insulin levels, indicative of insulin resistance, in agreement with other studies [18,26,27]. At this stage, although fasting glucose levels are maintained within normal values (normoglycemia), due to compensatory hyperinsulinemia, there is already some degree of glucose intolerance and peripheral insulin resistance, in agreement with other reports [18,28–30].

Insulin resistance was demonstrated not only by the increased HOMA-IR index but also by augmented TG/HDL-c ratio and the TyG index, which have previously been used as surrogate measures of impaired insulin sensitivity in obese adolescents with normoglycemia, in prediabetes, as well as in T2DM [31].

In an attempt to explain the glucose, insulin, and lipid dysmetabolism in this model at the prediabetic stage, we assessed possible alterations in glucose and lipid metabolism in fat. Accordingly with previous studies [18], the HSu diet increased fat mass, which is closely linked to the development of severe peripheral IR and prediabetes [32,33]. Moreover, under the fed state, the HSu diet impaired insulin-induced glucose uptake in isolated adipocytes, confirming that visceral adiposity is strongly associated with impaired glucose uptake and IR [34]. Additionally, under IGT, adipocytes are resistant to insulin, and its effectiveness may be impaired, contributing to postprandial hyperglycemia in prediabetic states. Furthermore, the decrease in hepatic GLUT1 in the HSu-treated rats might be mediated by the hyperinsulinemia observed in this animal model [35], although supplementary confirmation of this hypothesis could be achieved by evaluating GLUT1 expression under fasting conditions. On the other hand, both GLUT2 (in the liver) and GLUT4 protein levels (in the adipose tissue and skeletal muscle), were unchanged. The translocation of both GLUT2 and GLUT4 to the plasma membrane is mediated by insulin; however, under IR conditions, this process is impaired [36,37], leading to decreased insulin-stimulated glucose uptake in hepatocytes (mostly by GLUT2), while increasing postprandial blood glucose levels. Even though we did not measure translocation of glucose transporters in this study, it may be possible that these processes are impaired, thus also contributing to the increased postprandial blood glucose levels.

Another factor that may also be contributing to the postprandial hyperglycemia observed in this animal model is that high sucrose consumption increased gluconeogenesis, as previously reported [38]. However, under IGT and/or IR conditions, the derangement of hepatic glucose handling, indicated by changes in GLUT1 and G6Pase may at least in part lead to postprandial hyperglycemia in prediabetic states [39]. Furthermore, in this animal model of IR, insulin may not inhibit the de novo glucose production by the liver, leading therefore to elevated gluconeogenesis, resulting in elevated blood glucose levels in the fed state, as previously reported [35], as well as altered glucose tolerance during a GTT.

Furthermore, the HSu diet increased liver lipid biosynthesis. Our results show that ACC1 and FASN enzymes, as well as the transcription factor SREBP expression levels were increased in the liver of HSu-treated rats, in agreement with previous studies [40–44]. The perturbed liver lipid metabolism that was observed might explain the hypertriglyceridemia present in this prediabetic animal model. In addition, high sucrose consumption may also be contributing to hypertriglyceridemia due to the increased ChREBP gene and protein levels observed in fat [45]. However, the HSu diet did not induce changes in the isoproterenol-stimulated lipolysis in isolated adipocytes, and the HSL protein levels were not different. HSL lipolytic activity is regulated by reversible phosphorylation on five critical residues [46]. Therefore the absence of alterations in lipolysis suggest that HSL phosphorylation was not changed by the HSu diet. Finally, insulin did not show a significant antilipolytic effect at these insulin concentrations. However, it is important to note that we used supra-physiological insulin concentrations (1000 μU/mL), in order to evoke a sustained respond to study the impact of the treatment. Testing physiological insulin concentrations are warranted in both control and HSu animals in future research. In addition, there are other aspects for the forthcoming studies that could consolidate this model, namely lipid profiling of FPLC-separated lipoprotein fractions, quantification of FFA levels, as well as the estimation of VLDL secretion. Furthermore, the impact of the HSu diet on leptin serum levels and on leptin receptor expression would be of interest.

Overall, our study shows that nine week of HSu-diet, which mimics at least in part Western diets [10,11,47], can lead to impaired hepatic glucose and lipid metabolism, typical features of T2DM, already present in this prediabetic model, even in the absence of obesity. This animal model of diet-induced prediabetes shows reduced glucose tolerance, postprandial hyperglycemia, hyperinsulinemia, reduced insulin sensitivity (resistance), and hypertriglyceridemia, together with impaired gluconeogenesis and lipogenesis (Figure 8).

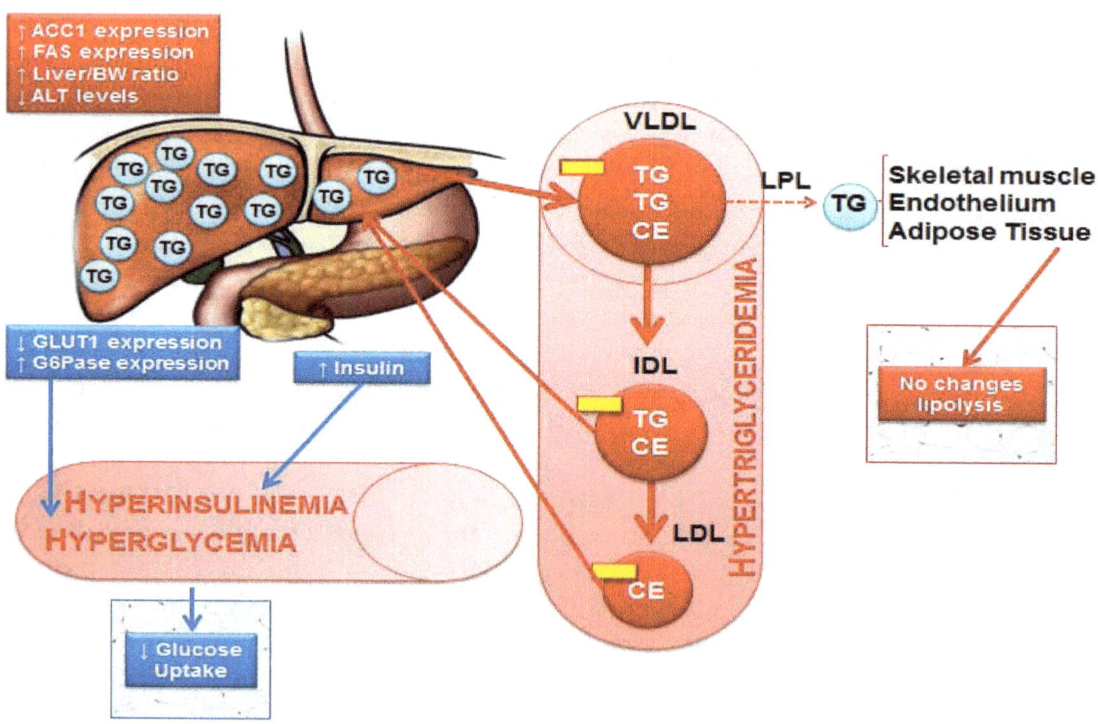

Figure 8. A molecular model describing insulin resistance and prediabetes development after a HSu diet. HSu diet increases serum triglyceride (TG) accumulation and triggers liver lipogenesis, inducing hypertriglyceridemia and interfering with liver function. However, no alterations were observed in lipolysis. The HSu diet alters hepatic proteins involved in basal glucose uptake and gluconeogenesis and impairs the insulin-stimulated glucose uptake in adipocytes, leading to impaired glucose homeostasis and increased IR markers. Legend: ▭ Apolipoprotein; CE—Cholesterol ester; IDL—Intermediate-density protein; LDL—Low-density lipoprotein; LDL—Lipoprotein lipase; TG—Triglycerides; VLDL—Very low-density lipoprotein.

This study should be viewed as an important wake up call for the lifestyle that the general population have been gradually adopting, by consuming large amounts of simple sugars in soft drinks [48]. Importantly, exaggerated consumption of these drinks has been associated with an increased risk for T2DM development by about 26% if the average intake is one/two cans a day, or even more [49]. This feeding behavior is one of the main causes of the uncontrolled increase of IR, T2DM, and associated complications, such as coronary heart disease [50,51].

5. Conclusions

This animal model of prediabetes induced by high-sucrose consumption presents liver glucose and lipid dysmetabolism. It is expected that new insights of impaired metabolism at this early stage of the disease might contribute to disclosing new therapeutic targets and strategies to counteract prediabetes and hinder the natural course of T2DM progression.

Acknowledgments: The authors kindly thank Novo Nordisk A/S for the human insulin (Actrapid), as well as funding support from: SPD/GIFT award, European Foundation for the Study of Diabetes (EFSD), EXCL/DTP-PIC/0069/2012, CNC.IBILI Strategic Project 2015-UID/NEU/04539/2013 funded by the Portuguese Foundation for Science and Technology (FCT) and by FEDER through Operational Programme Competitiveness Factors (COMPETE): FCOMP-01-0124-FEDER-028417 and POCI-01-0145-FEDER-007440,, SFRH/BD/109017/2015 (Sara Nunes PhD scholarship by FCT) as well as Centro 2020 Regional Operational Programmes (CENTRO-01-0145-FEDER-000012: HealthyAging2020 and CENTRO-01-0145-FEDER-000008: BrainHealth 2020). E.C. is partly supported by NIH P30AG028718 and NIH RO1 AG033761.

Author Contributions: A.B., F.C.P., F.R. and E.C. designed the study. All authors participated in rat housing/feeding and/or in the analytical assays. P.N. performed the histopathological analysis. A.B., M.C., B.M.V.-R. and S.N. performed statistical analyses. A.B. and M.C. prepared figures and drafted the manuscript. A.B., F.C.P., F.R. and E.C. edited and revised the manuscript. All authors read and approved the final version.

References

1. Lau, D.C.; Teoh, H. Current and emerging pharmacotherapies for weight management in prediabetes and diabetes. *Can. J. Diabetes* **2015**, *39* (Suppl. S5), S134–S141. [CrossRef] [PubMed]
2. Tabak, A.G.; Herder, C.; Rathmann, W.; Brunner, E.J.; Kivimaki, M. Prediabetes: A high-risk state for diabetes development. *Lancet* **2012**, *379*, 2279–2290. [CrossRef]
3. Malik, V.S.; Hu, F.B. Fructose and Cardiometabolic Health: What the Evidence from Sugar-Sweetened Beverages Tells Us. *J. Am. Coll. Cardiol.* **2015**, *66*, 1615–1624. [CrossRef] [PubMed]
4. Parhofer, K.G. Interaction between glucose and lipid metabolism: More than diabetic dyslipidemia. *Diabetes Metab. J.* **2015**, *39*, 353–362. [CrossRef] [PubMed]
5. Erion, D.M.; Park, H.J.; Lee, H.Y. The role of lipids in the pathogenesis and treatment of type 2 diabetes and associated co-morbidities. *BMB Rep.* **2016**, *49*, 139–148. [CrossRef] [PubMed]
6. Van Raalte, D.H.; van der Zijl, N.J.; Diamant, M. Pancreatic steatosis in humans: Cause or marker of lipotoxicity? *Curr. Opin. Clin. Nutr. Metab. Care* **2010**, *13*, 478–485. [CrossRef] [PubMed]
7. Rachek, L.I. Free fatty acids and skeletal muscle insulin resistance. *Prog. Mol. Biol. Transl. Sci.* **2014**, *121*, 267–292. [PubMed]
8. Drew, B.G.; Rye, K.A.; Duffy, S.J.; Barter, P.; Kingwell, B.A. The emerging role of HDL in glucose metabolism. *Nat. Rev. Endocrinol.* **2012**, *8*, 237–245. [CrossRef] [PubMed]
9. Cusi, K. The role of adipose tissue and lipotoxicity in the pathogenesis of type 2 diabetes. *Curr. Diabetes Rep.* **2010**, *10*, 306–315. [CrossRef] [PubMed]
10. Nunes, S.; Soares, E.; Fernandes, J.; Viana, S.; Carvalho, E.; Pereira, F.C.; Reis, F. Early cardiac changes in a rat model of prediabetes: Brain natriuretic peptide overexpression seems to be the best marker. *Cardiovasc. Diabetol.* **2013**, *12*, 44. [CrossRef] [PubMed]
11. Soares, E.; Prediger, R.D.; Nunes, S.; Castro, A.A.; Viana, S.D.; Lemos, C.; De Souza, C.M.; Agostinho, P.; Cunha, R.A.; Carvalho, E.; et al. Spatial memory impairments in a prediabetic rat model. *Neuroscience* **2013**, *250*, 565–577. [CrossRef] [PubMed]
12. Silva, A.M.; Martins, F.; Jones, J.G.; Carvalho, R. 2H2O incorporation into hepatic acetyl-CoA and de novo lipogenesis as measured by Krebs cycle-mediated 2H-enrichment of glutamate and glutamine. *Magn. Reson. Med.* **2011**, *66*, 1526–1530. [CrossRef] [PubMed]

13. Kho, M.C.; Lee, Y.J.; Park, J.H.; Kim, H.Y.; Yoon, J.J.; Ahn, Y.M.; Tan, R.; Park, M.C.; Cha, J.D.; Choi, K.M.; et al. Fermented red ginseng potentiates improvement of metabolic dysfunction in metabolic syndrome rat models. *Nutrients* **2016**, *8*, E369. [CrossRef] [PubMed]
14. Pereira, M.J.; Palming, J.; Rizell, M.; Aureliano, M.; Carvalho, E.; Svensson, M.K.; Eriksson, J.W. mTOR inhibition with rapamycin causes impaired insulin signalling and glucose uptake in human subcutaneous and omental adipocytes. *Mol. Cell. Endocrinol.* **2012**, *355*, 96–105. [CrossRef] [PubMed]
15. Pereira, M.J.; Palming, J.; Rizell, M.; Aureliano, M.; Carvalho, E.; Svensson, M.K.; Eriksson, J.W. The immunosuppressive agents rapamycin, cyclosporin A and tacrolimus increase lipolysis, inhibit lipid storage and alter expression of genes involved in lipid metabolism in human adipose tissue. *Mol. Cell. Endocrinol.* **2013**, *365*, 260–269. [CrossRef] [PubMed]
16. Burgeiro, A.; Fuhrmann, A.; Cherian, S.; Espinoza, D.; Jarak, I.; Carvalho, R.A.; Loureiro, M.; Patrício, M.; Antunes, M.; Carvalho, E. Glucose uptake and lipid metabolism are impaired in epicardial adipose tissue from heart failure patients with or without diabetes. *Am. J. Physiol. Endocrinol. Metab.* **2016**, *310*, E550–E564. [CrossRef] [PubMed]
17. Ritze, Y.M.; Bardos, G.; D'Haese, J.G.; Ernst, B.; Thurnheer, M.; Schultes, B.; Bischoff, S.C. Effect of high sugar intake on glucose transporter and weight regulating hormones in mice and humans. *PLoS ONE* **2014**, *9*, e101702. [CrossRef] [PubMed]
18. Lirio, L.M.; Forechi, L.; Zanardo, T.C.; Batista, H.M.; Meira, E.F.; Nogueira, B.V.; Mill, J.G.; Baldo, M.P. Chronic fructose intake accelerates non-alcoholic fatty liver disease in the presence of essential hypertension. *J. Diabetes Complicat.* **2016**, *30*, 85–92. [CrossRef] [PubMed]
19. Glendinning, J.I.; Breinager, L.; Kyrillou, E.; Lacuna, K.; Rocha, R.; Sclafani, A. Differential effects of sucrose and fructose on dietary obesity in four mouse strains. *Physiol. Behav.* **2010**, *101*, 331–343. [CrossRef] [PubMed]
20. Galgani, J.; Ravussin, E. Energy metabolism, fuel selection and body weight regulation. *Int. J. Obes.* **2008**, *32* (Suppl. S7), S109–S119. [CrossRef] [PubMed]
21. Chaumontet, C.; Even, P.C.; Schwarz, J.; Simonin-Foucault, A.; Piedcoq, J.; Fromentin, G.; Azzout-Marniche, D.; Tomé, D. High dietary protein decreases fat deposition induced by high-fat and high-sucrose diet in rats. *Br. J. Nutr.* **2015**, *114*, 1132–1142. [CrossRef] [PubMed]
22. Borsheim, E.; Bui, Q.U.; Tissier, S.; Cree, M.G.; Rønsen, O.; Morio, B.; Ferrando, A.A.; Kobayashi, H.; Newcomer, B.R.; Wolfe, R.R. Amino acid supplementation decreases plasma and liver triacylglycerols in elderly. *Nutrition* **2009**, *25*, 281–288. [CrossRef] [PubMed]
23. Simental-Mendia, L.E.; Rodriguez-Moran, M.; Guerrero-Romero, F. The hypertriglyceridemia is associated with isolated impaired glucose tolerance in subjects without insulin resistance. *Endocr. Res.* **2015**, *40*, 70–73. [CrossRef] [PubMed]
24. Ram, J.; Snehalatha, C.; Nanditha, A.; Selvam, S.; Shetty, S.A.; Godsland, I.F.; Johnston, D.G.; Ramachandran, A. Hypertriglyceridaemic waist phenotype as a simple predictive marker of incident diabetes in Asian-Indian men with prediabetes. *Diabet. Med.* **2014**, *31*, 1542–1549. [CrossRef] [PubMed]
25. Daly, M.E.; Vale, C.; Walker, M.; Alberti, K.G.; Mathers, J.C. Dietary carbohydrates and insulin sensitivity: A review of the evidence and clinical implications. *Am. J. Clin. Nutr.* **1997**, *66*, 1072–1085. [PubMed]
26. Giorelli Gde, V.; Matos, L.N.; Saado, A.; Soibelman, V.L.; Dias, C.B. No association between 25-hydroxyvitamin D levels and prediabetes in Brazilian patients. A cross-sectional study. *Sao Paulo Med. J.* **2015**, *133*, 73–77. [CrossRef] [PubMed]
27. Jenkins, N.T.; Hagberg, J.M. Aerobic training effects on glucose tolerance in prediabetic and normoglycemic humans. *Med. Sci. Sports Exerc.* **2011**, *43*, 2231–2240. [CrossRef] [PubMed]
28. Fiorini, F.; Raffa, M.; Patrone, E.; Castelluccio, A. Glucose metabolism and chronic renal insufficiency. *Arch. Ital. Urol. Androl.* **1994**, *66*, 51–56. [PubMed]
29. Pagliassotti, M.J.; Prach, P.A.; Koppenhafer, T.A.; Pan, D.A. Changes in insulin action, triglycerides, and lipid composition during sucrose feeding in rats. *Am. J. Physiol.* **1996**, *271*, R1319–R1326. [PubMed]
30. Dutta, K.; Podolin, D.A.; Davidson, M.B.; Davidoff, A.J. Cardiomyocyte dysfunction in sucrose-fed rats is associated with insulin resistance. *Diabetes* **2001**, *50*, 1186–1192. [CrossRef] [PubMed]
31. Mohd Nor, N.S.; Lee, S.; Bacha, F.; Tfayli, H.; Arslanian, S. Triglyceride glucose index as a surrogate measure of insulin sensitivity in obese adolescents with normoglycemia, prediabetes, and type 2 diabetes mellitus: Comparison with the hyperinsulinemic-euglycemic clamp. *Pediatr. Diabetes* **2016**, *17*, 458–465. [CrossRef] [PubMed]

32. Weiss, R.; Dufour, S.; Taksali, S.E.; Tamborlane, W.V.; Petersen, K.F.; Bonadonna, R.C.; Boselli, L.; Barbetta, G.; Allen, K.; Rife, F.; et al. Prediabetes in obese youth: A syndrome of impaired glucose tolerance, severe insulin resistance, and altered myocellular and abdominal fat partitioning. *Lancet* **2003**, *362*, 951–957. [CrossRef]
33. Neeland, I.J.; Turer, A.T.; Ayers, C.R.; Powell-Wiley, T.M.; Vega, G.L.; Farzaneh-Far, R.; Grundy, S.M.; Khera, A.; McGuire, D.K.; de Lemos, J.A. Dysfunctional adiposity and the risk of prediabetes and type 2 diabetes in obese adults. *JAMA* **2012**, *308*, 1150–1159. [CrossRef] [PubMed]
34. Kim, G.; Jo, K.; Kim, K.J.; Lee, Y.H.; Han, E.; Yoon, H.J.; Wang, H.J.; Kang, E.S.; Yun, M. Visceral adiposity is associated with altered myocardial glucose uptake measured by (18)FDG-PET in 346 subjects with normal glucose tolerance, prediabetes, and type 2 diabetes. *Cardiovasc. Diabetol.* **2015**, *14*, 148. [CrossRef] [PubMed]
35. Tal, M.; Kahn, B.B.; Lodish, H.F. Expression of the low Km GLUT-1 glucose transporter is turned on in perivenous hepatocytes of insulin-deficient diabetic rats. *Endocrinology* **1991**, *129*, 1933–1941. [CrossRef] [PubMed]
36. Tobin, V.; Le Gall, M.; Fioramonti, X.; Stolarczyk, E.; Blazquez, A.G.; Klein, C.; Prigent, M.; Serradas, P.; Cuif, M.H.; Magnan, C.; et al. Insulin internalizes GLUT2 in the enterocytes of healthy but not insulin-resistant mice. *Diabetes* **2008**, *57*, 555–562. [CrossRef] [PubMed]
37. Carvalho, E.; Rondinone, C.; Smith, U. Insulin resistance in fat cells from obese Zucker rats—Evidence for an impaired activation and translocation of protein kinase B and glucose transporter 4. *Mol. Cell. Biochem.* **2000**, *206*, 7–16. [CrossRef] [PubMed]
38. Basu, R.; Barosa, C.; Jones, J.; Dube, S.; Carter, R.; Basu, A.; Rizza, R.A. Pathogenesis of prediabetes: Role of the liver in isolated fasting hyperglycemia and combined fasting and postprandial hyperglycemia. *J. Clin. Endocrinol. Metab.* **2013**, *98*, E409–E417. [CrossRef] [PubMed]
39. Dinneen, S.F. The postprandial state: Mechanisms of glucose intolerance. *Diabet. Med.* **1997**, *14* (Suppl. S3), S19–S24. [CrossRef]
40. Ryu, M.H.; Cha, Y.S. The effects of a high-fat or high-sucrose diet on serum lipid profiles, hepatic acyl-CoA synthetase, carnitine palmitoyltransferase-I, and the acetyl-CoA carboxylase mRNA levels in rats. *J. Biochem. Mol. Biol.* **2003**, *36*, 312–318. [CrossRef] [PubMed]
41. Bruckdorfer, K.R.; Khan, I.H.; Yudkin, J. Fatty acid synthetase activity in the liver and adipose tissue of rats fed with various carbohydrates. *Biochem. J.* **1972**, *129*, 439–446. [CrossRef] [PubMed]
42. Agheli, N.; Kabir, M.; Berni-Canani, S.; Petitjean, E.; Boussairi, A.; Luo, J.; Bornet, F.; Slama, G.; Rizkalla, S.W. Plasma lipids and fatty acid synthase activity are regulated by short-chain fructo-oligosaccharides in sucrose-fed insulin-resistant rats. *J. Nutr.* **1998**, *128*, 1283–1288. [PubMed]
43. Im, S.S.; Kang, S.Y.; Kim, S.Y.; Kim, H.I.; Kim, J.W.; Kim, K.S.; Ahn, Y.H. Glucose-stimulated upregulation of GLUT2 gene is mediated by sterol response element-binding protein-1c in the hepatocytes. *Diabetes* **2005**, *54*, 1684–1691. [CrossRef] [PubMed]
44. Ducluzeau, P.H.; Perretti, N.; Laville, M.; Andreelli, F.; Vega, N.; Riou, J.P.; Vidal, H. Regulation by insulin of gene expression in human skeletal muscle and adipose tissue. Evidence for specific defects in type 2 diabetes. *Diabetes* **2001**, *50*, 1134–1142. [CrossRef] [PubMed]
45. Herman, M.A.; Peroni, O.D.; Villoria, J.; Schön, M.R.; Abumrad, N.A.; Blüher, M.; Klein, S.; Kahn, B.B. A novel ChREBP isoform in adipose tissue regulates systemic glucose metabolism. *Nature* **2012**, *484*, 333–338. [CrossRef] [PubMed]
46. Lampidonis, A.D.; Rogdakis, E.; Voutsinas, G.E.; Stravopodis, D.J. The resurgence of Hormone-Sensitive Lipase (HSL) in mammalian lipolysis. *Gene* **2011**, *477*, 1–11. [CrossRef] [PubMed]
47. Bouchard-Mercier, A.; Rudkowska, I.; Lemieux, S.; Couture, P.; Vohl, M.C. The metabolic signature associated with the Western dietary pattern: A cross-sectional study. *Nutr. J.* **2013**, *12*, 158. [CrossRef] [PubMed]
48. Hu, F.B. Resolved: There is sufficient scientific evidence that decreasing sugar-sweetened beverage consumption will reduce the prevalence of obesity and obesity-related diseases. *Obes. Rev.* **2013**, *14*, 606–619. [CrossRef] [PubMed]
49. Malik, V.S.; Popkin, B.M.; Bray, G.A.; Despres, J.P.; Willett, W.C.; Hu, F.B. Sugar-sweetened beverages and risk of metabolic syndrome and type 2 diabetes: A meta-analysis. *Diabetes Care* **2010**, *33*, 2477–2483. [CrossRef] [PubMed]
50. Fung, T.T.; Malik, V.; Rexrode, K.M.; Manson, J.E.; Willett, W.C.; Hu, F.B. Sweetened beverage consumption and risk of coronary heart disease in women. *Am. J. Clin. Nutr.* **2009**, *89*, 1037–1042. [CrossRef] [PubMed]

10

Integrated Assessment of Pharmacological and Nutritional Cardiovascular Risk Management: Blood Pressure Control in the DIAbetes and LifEstyle Cohort Twente (DIALECT)

Christina M. Gant [1,2,†], S. Heleen Binnenmars [1,2,†], Else van den Berg [2], Stephan J. L. Bakker [2], Gerjan Navis [2] and Gozewijn D. Laverman [1,2,*]

1 Department of Internal Medicine/Nephrology, Ziekenhuisgroep Twente, Zilvermeeuw 1, 7609 PP Almelo, The Netherlands; c.gant@zgt.nl (C.M.G.); s.h.binnenmars@umcg.nl (S.H.B.)

2 Department of Internal Medicine, Division of Nephrology, University of Groningen, University Medical Center Groningen, Hanzeplein 1, 9713 GZ Groningen, The Netherlands; e.van.den.berg@umcg.nl (E.v.d.B.); s.j.l.bakker@umcg.nl (S.J.L.B.); G.j.navis@umcg.nl (G.N.)

* Correspondence: g.laverman@zgt.nl

† These authors contributed equally.

Abstract: Cardiovascular risk management is an integral part of treatment in Type 2 Diabetes Mellitus (T2DM), and requires pharmacological as well as nutritional management. We hypothesize that a systematic assessment of both pharmacological and nutritional management can identify targets for the improvement of treatment quality. Therefore, we analysed blood pressure (BP) management in the DIAbetes and LifEstyle Cohort Twente (DIALECT). DIALECT is an observational cohort from routine diabetes care, performed at the ZGT Hospital (Almelo and Hengelo, The Netherlands). BP was measured for 15 min with one minute intervals. Sodium and potassium intake was derived from 24-hour urinary excretion. We determined the adherence to pharmacological and non-pharmacological guidelines in patients with BP on target (BP-OT) and BP not on target (BP-NOT). In total, 450 patients were included from August 2009 until January 2016. The mean age was 63 ± 9 years, and the majority was male (58%). In total, 53% had BP-OT. In those with BP-NOT, pharmacological management was suboptimal (zero to two antihypertensive drugs) in 62% of patients, and nutritional guideline adherence was suboptimal in 100% of patients (only 8% had a sodium intake on target, 66% had a potassium intake on target, 3% had a sodium-to-potassium ratio on target, and body mass index was <30 kg/m^2 in 35%). These data show pharmacological undertreatment and a low adherence to nutritional guidelines. Uncontrolled BP is common in T2DM, and our data show a window of opportunity for improving BP control, especially in nutritional management. To improve treatment quality, we advocate to incorporate the integrated monitoring of nutritional management in quality improvement cycles in routine care.

Keywords: Type 2 diabetes mellitus; blood pressure; pharmacological management; nutrition; dietary sodium intake

1. Introduction

Type 2 Diabetes Mellitus (T2DM), with an estimated number of 422 million patients worldwide, is one of the major conditions associated with cardiovascular events and cardiovascular death [1]. Therefore, the prevention of the development and progression of such complications is a main goal in the treatment of T2DM, and evidence-based recommendations to reach this goal are incorporated in treatment guidelines. Treatment consists of pharmacological and non-pharmacological management, the latter consisting in large part of nutritional guidance. Still, cardiovascular complications develop in the majority of T2DM patients, demonstrating the large challenge of adequate treatment [2,3]. One explanation for this could be a failure to reach guideline treatment targets. Indeed, several studies have shown that targets for blood pressure, glycemic control, and Low Density Lipoprotein (LDL) cholesterol are not reached in a large number of patients [4–8].

Pharmacological and nutritional management are often studied as separate entities, despite the fact that both are crucial elements of treatment. We hypothesize that a systematic assessment of both pharmacological and nutritional management can identify targets for the improvement of treatment quality. The DIAbetes and LifEstyle Cohort Twente (DIALECT) cohort study was specifically designed for this purpose. DIALECT is an observational study in T2DM patients in a well-defined region in The Netherlands, and uses validated and detailed real-world data on nutritional habits, pharmacological treatment, and current clinical condition. To obtain non-biased data on individual nutrient intake, 24-hour urine collections were used and stored in a biobank to allow for future analyses [9].

We aim to address how well the targets for blood pressure management are reached, and how this is related to (1) pharmacological management; and (2) nutritional management (i.e., the dietary intake of salt [10,11], potassium [12,13], body mass index (BMI), and alcohol). Moreover, we assessed additional nutritional parameters for which no specific counselling was given, but have been shown to be relevant to cardiovascular risk in diabetic kidney disease (magnesium [14–16] and phosphate [17,18]). Because the presence of diabetic kidney disease implicates different blood pressure targets, we analysed patients without and with renal involvement separately.

2. Materials and Methods

2.1. Study Design and Participants

DIALECT is a prospective cohort study in patients with T2DM, performed in the ZGT Hospital, which is located in Almelo and Hengelo, The Netherlands. It is designed to study pharmacological and non-pharmacological management in a regional T2DM population treated in a secondary health care center. All patients with T2DM and aged 18+ years treated in the outpatient clinic of our hospital were eligible, with the only exclusion criteria being an inability to understand the informed consent procedure, insufficient knowledge of the Dutch language, or a dependency on renal replacement therapy.

This paper reports on the DIALECT-1 population, consisting of the first 450 patients, recruited between September 2009 and January 2016. The inclusion of new patients in DIALECT-2 will be performed until December 2019, or until the number of 850 is reached. The study is performed according to the guidelines of good clinical practice and the Declaration of Helsinki. It has been approved by the local institutional review boards (METC-registration numbers NL57219.044.16 and 1009.68020), and is registered in the Netherlands Trial Register (NTR trial code 5855).

2.2. Study Procedures

Patients were screened for eligibility in the electronic patient file, and subsequently invited for a study visit. At the clinic, all of the information relevant to the medical condition was recorded in a database (Figure 1, Supplementary Table S1). Height, weight, and waist and hip circumference were measured. Body mass index was calculated as weight divided by height squared (kg/m^2), and body surface area was estimated by applying the universally adopted formula of DuBois [19]. Blood pressure was measured in a supine position by an automated device (Dinamap®; GE Medical systems, Milwaukee, WI, USA) for 15 min with a one-minute interval. The mean systolic and diastolic pressure of the last three measurements was used for further analysis.

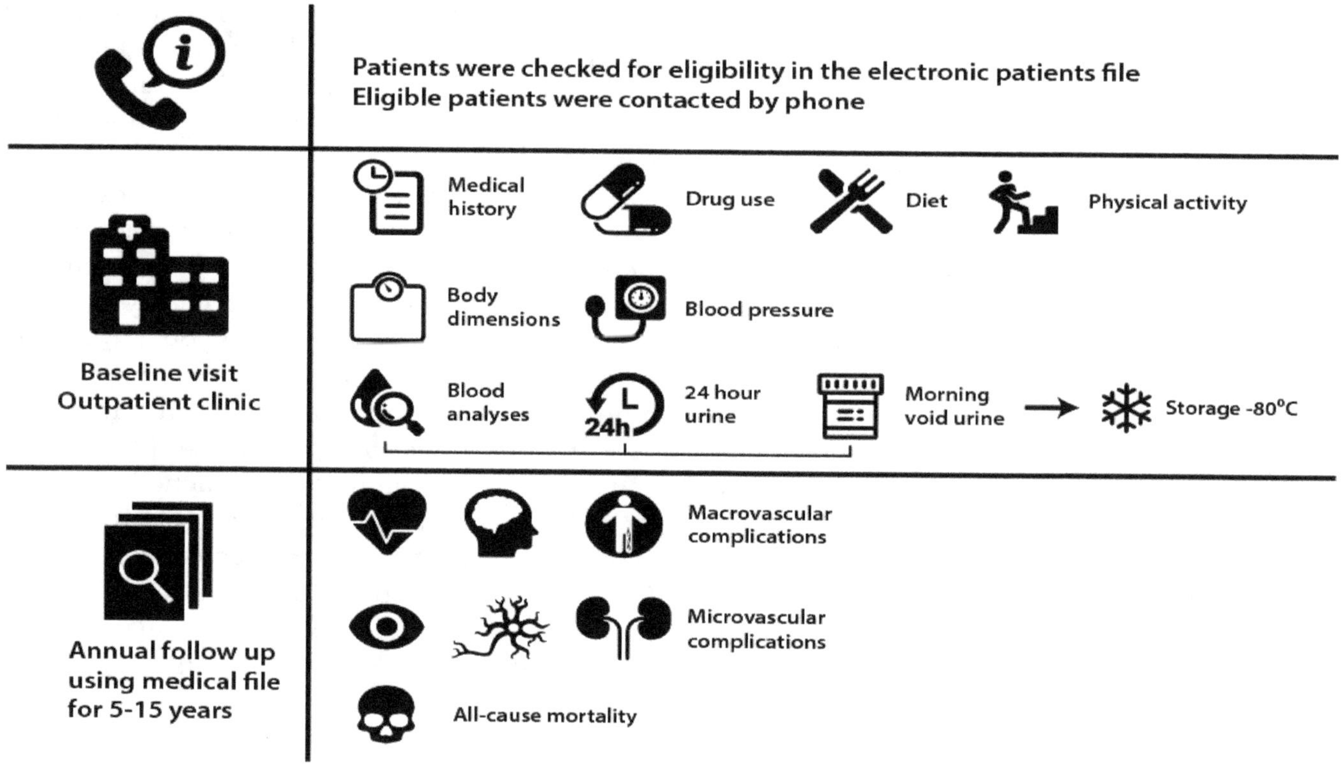

Figure 1. Patient inclusion and data collection.

Physical activity was assessed using the Short Questionnaire to Asses Health enhancing physical activity (SQUASH) questionnaire, which was previously validated in [20]. The 24-hour urinary content of specific substances was measured where possible and appropriate.

Routine laboratory tests were performed in venous blood, including blood count tests, liver function tests, renal function tests, HbA1c, and cholesterol. The estimated glomerular filtration rate (eGFR) was calculated using the Chronic Kidney Disease Epidemiology Collaboration (CKD-EPI) formula [21]. From samples of a 24-hour urine collection, the following parameters were measured: sodium, potassium, creatinine, calcium, phosphate, chloride, albumin, protein, urea, and uric acid excretion. Twenty-four-hour urinary excretion was calculated by multiplying these concentrations with the volume of the 24-hour urine collection. Creatinine clearance was calculated from the 24-hour urine creatinine excretion and the plasma creatinine concentration. For the proper collection of the 24-hour urine sample, patients were instructed to dispose of the first morning void urine, and thereafter collect all urine in the provided canister until the first morning void urine of the next day. In between voids, they were instructed to store the canister in a dark cool place, preferably in a refrigerator. A separate single morning void urine was used to assess the urinary albumin-to-creatinine ratio.

The samples of blood, 24-hour urine collection, and morning void urine were stored in a biobank at −80 degrees Celsius for additional analyses, as specified in Supplementary Table S1.

2.3. Routine Clinical Care

Diabetes care in the Netherlands is standardised, both in the outpatient clinic and at the general practitioner. It consists of three to four outpatient clinic visits per year. The development of albuminuria is assessed yearly using the albumin–creatinine ratio in a single morning void urine. Retinopathy is assessed at one to two year intervals. Neuropathy is assessed yearly using monofilament and vibration tests with a tuning fork.

Lifestyle management in T2DM consists of guidance regarding weight loss, increasing physical activity, and smoking cessation, and of referral to a dietician for dietary guidance on weight loss and the adherence to dietary guidelines, including sodium restriction and stimulating an intake of fruit and vegetables. The frequency of dietary follow-up visits is targeted at the individual goals and needs of patients depending on personal preferences as well as comorbidity. At each doctor visit, target HbA1c and blood pressure are monitored, and pharmacological intervention is adjusted accordingly. Cholesterol levels are monitored yearly. Targets for HbA1c and LDL cholesterol are often individualized; the general targets are <53 mmol/L and <2.5 mmol/L, respectively.

2.4. Definitions

The blood pressure (BP) targets in our analyses were derived from the international guidelines for diabetes management, which have been adopted for use in The Netherlands [22,23]. In patients with diabetic kidney disease, the BP target was set according to the Kidney Diseases Improving Global Outcomes (KDIGO) guidelines, which are internationally acclaimed guidelines for chronic kidney disease, and are also applied in The Netherlands [23]. Patients with diabetic kidney disease without albuminuria (eGFR <60, no albuminuria) had a BP target of $\leq$140/90 mmHg, while patients with albuminuria and either an eGFR $\geq$60 mL/min or an eGFR <60 mL/min had a BP target of $\leq$130/80 mmHg. For patients with T2DM without diabetic kidney disease, the European Association for the Study of Diabetes (EASD) guidelines are used, which stipulate a blood pressure (BP) target of <140/85 mmHg [22]. Accordingly, the patients were grouped by eGFR above or below 60 mL/min and by the presence of albuminuria. Albuminuria was defined as a 24-hour urinary albumin excretion >30 mg/day. As the EASD and KDIGO guidelines for those without albuminuria differ slightly, we performed all of the analyses using the EASD guidelines for those with eGFR <60 and no albuminuria as well. The results were virtually similar, and for the sake of conciseness, the data is not shown.

The targets for nutritional management were set according to the Dutch guidelines when available. The target dietary salt intake was $\leq$6 g/day [24], and the target dietary potassium intake was set at $\geq$3.5 g/day, according to best evidence [13]. The target alcohol intake was $\leq$2 units per day for women, and $\leq$3 units per day for men. It should be noted that in 2015, the Health Council of The Netherlands changed the guidelines for alcohol consumption to zero units per day; however, our patients were included in the study before the introduction of these new guidelines [25]. The target BMI was <30 kg/m^2. The target for smoking was either no smoking history, or having previously stopped smoking.

The data on dietary intake of salt, potassium, and proteins were derived from 24-hour urinary excretion. For this, it is important to realise that the patients in our cohort were assessed under steady state conditions, in which the net renal excretion of sodium is almost equal to the dietary intake of sodium, with only approximately 5–10% being excreted by other routes (e.g., sweat or feces) [9]. Therefore, 24-hour urinary sodium excretion is considered the gold standard for the assessment of sodium intake [9,26], and dietary salt intake was calculated by multiplying the net 24-hour sodium excretion (in mol/day) with the molar weight of salt (NaCl, 58.44 g/mol). Dietary potassium intake was calculated from urinary potassium excretion under the assumption of a renal excretion rate of 77% [13,27]. Dietary protein intake was calculated from urinary urea nitrogen excretion using the Maroni formula [28]. As the renal excretion of magnesium is lower in patients with a low eGFR, dietary magnesium intake could not be calculated from urinary magnesium excretion with the same formula (using the assumption of an intestinal absorption of 30%) [16]. Therefore, we present the urinary daily excretion of magnesium. Also, while no consensus exists to calculate dietary phosphate intake from the urinary excretion, urinary phosphate excretion does reflect variability in intestinal phosphate uptake [29,30], so we present the urinary excretion values.

2.5. Statistical Analyses

All of the statistical analyses were performed using Statistical Package for the Social Sciences (SPSS), version 23.0. Normally distributed data are presented as mean $\pm$ standard deviation. Skewed variables are expressed as median [interquartile range]. Dichotomous variables are presented in number and percentage. First, we divided the population according to the presence of albuminuria and/or a reduced eGFR (<60 mL/min), as in these groups the target BP is different (<140/85 for those without diabetic kidney disease, ≤140/90 mmHg for patients without albuminuria and an eGFR <60 mL/min, and ≤130/80 mmHg for those with albuminuria). Second, we divided the population into two groups, according to the reached blood pressure. These groups are denoted as "Blood pressure on target" (BP-OT) and "Blood pressure not on target" (BP-NOT), respectively. The differences between the groups were analysed using the student *t*-test, one-way ANOVA, the Mann–Whitney U test, the Kruskall–Wallis test, and the Chi Square test when appropriate. To perform a multivariate analysis of the determinants of not on target BP, multivariate logistic regression was used. In order to adjust for age and gender, the differences in nutritional data among the groups were also determined using mixed model analyses with Sidak post-hoc tests.

3. Results

Between September 2009 and January 2016, 1082 eligible patients were identified and invited to participate in the study, of whom 470 were enrolled in the study and performed the baseline visit. The most common causes for not participating in the study were: No interest in research, and inability due to co-morbidity (Figure 2). Twenty patients were excluded after the baseline visit, as in closer analysis their correct diagnosis was Type 1 Diabetes Mellitus instead of Type 2. All of the remaining 450 patients were included in our data analysis.

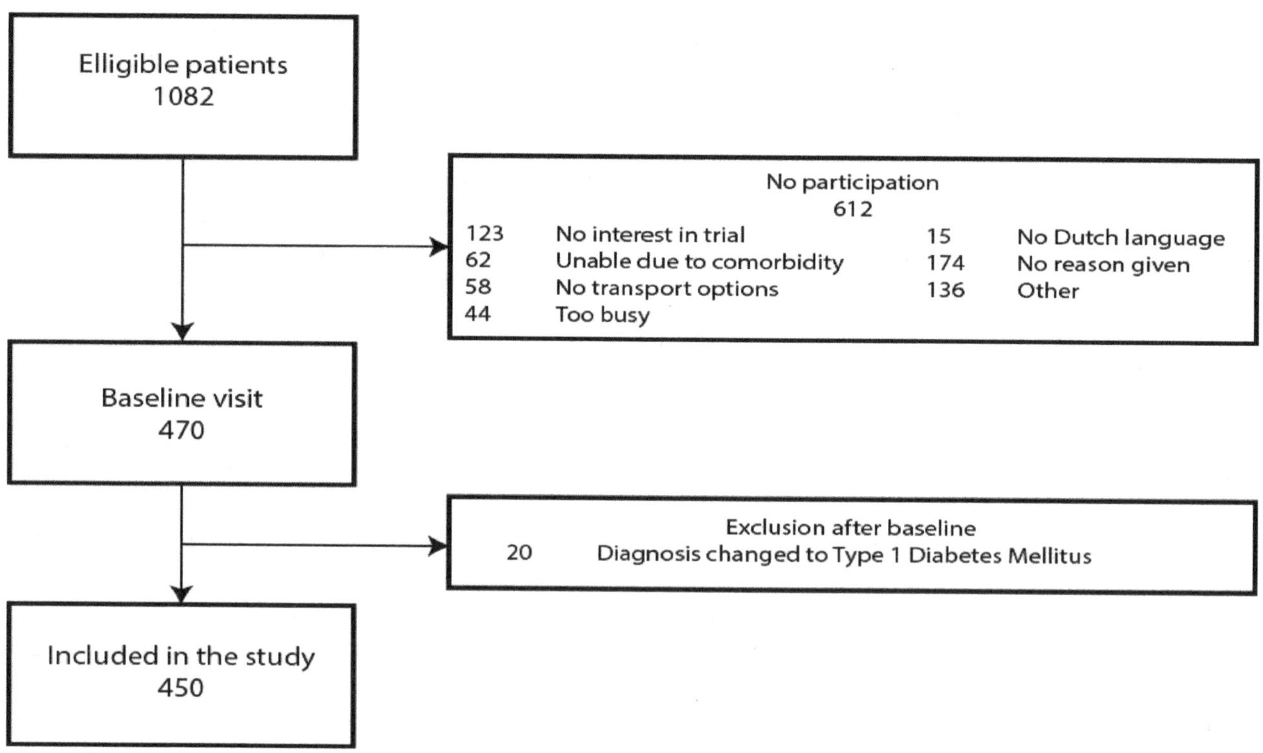

Figure 2. Patient recruitment flowchart.

3.1. *Baseline Pharmacological and Nutritional Characteristics*

The baseline data are presented in Table 1, by a break-up according to reduced eGFR (<60 mL/min) and the presence of albuminuria. The mean age of the participants was 63 $\pm$ 9 years, and was higher in the groups with eGFR <60 (Table 1). There were more men (58%) than women, and men were over-represented in the albuminuria groups (74% and 77% respectively for eGFR ≥60 and <60). The mean BMI was 32.9 $\pm$ 6.2 kg/m^2, reflecting a predominantly obese T2DM population, and BMI did not differ among the groups (Table 1).

Table 1. DIALECT-1 Baseline, nutritional, and pharmacological characteristics.

Variable	Total Population	eGFR ≥60 Albuminuria No	eGFR ≥60 Albuminuria Yes	eGFR <60 Albuminuria No	eGFR <60 Albuminuria Yes	*p*-Value
Number of patients (% of population)	450	257 (57)	85 (19)	52 (12)	51 (11)	
Patient characteristics						
Age (years)	63 ± 9	61 ± 9	62 ± 8	67 ± 8 *,†	69 ± 7 *,†	<0.001
Male, *n* (%)	259 (58)	139 (54)	63 (74)	19 (37)	39 (77)	<0.001
Years T2DM (years)	11 (7–18)	11 (7–18)	14 (8–19)	12 (6–17)	10 (6–15)	0.45
Serum HbA1C (mmol/mol)	57 ± 12	58 ± 11	59 ± 13	54 ± 11	57 ± 13	0.15
Insulin use, *n* (%)	284 (63)	160 (62)	64 (75)	31 (60)	28 (55)	0.07
Systolic blood pressure (mmHg)	139 ± 16	136 ± 15	140 ± 19	131 ± 13 †	139 ± 17	0.009
Diastolic blood pressure (mmHg)	76 ± 9	75 ± 9	76 ± 10	70 ± 9 *,†	75 ± 10 ‡	0.004
BP on target, *n* (%)	236 (53)	155 (60)	28 (33)	41 (79)	12 (24)	<0.001
Macrovascular disease, *n* (%)	158 (35)	68 (27)	36 (42)	25 (48)	31 (61)	<0.001
eGFR (mL/min)	84 (62–97)	92 (78–100)	88 (74–99)	47 (36–54)	39 (33–45)	<0.001
Albumin excretion (mg/day)	11 (3–66)	5 (2–11)	94 (62–202)	4 (1–12)	332 (93–661)	<0.001
Pharmacological management						
RAASi, *n* (%)	296 (67)	152 (59)	63 (74)	39 (75)	42 (82)	0.001
β-blockers, *n* (%)	207 (46)	100 (39)	37 (44)	36 (69)	33 (65)	<0.001
Thiazide diuretics, *n* (%)	137 (31)	81 (32)	15 (18)	21 (40)	18 (35)	0.02
Calcium antagonists, *n* (%)	101 (23)	43 (17)	26 (31)	13 (25)	19 (37)	0.002
Loop diuretics, *n* (%)	81 (18)	26 (10)	18 (21)	17 (33)	20 (39)	<0.001
Potassium sparing diuretics, *n* (%)	43 (10)	11 (4)	8 (9)	12 (23)	12 (24)	<0.001
Number of antihypertensives	2 (1–3)	2 (0–3)	2 (1–3)	3 (2–3)	3 (2–4)	<0.001
No antihypertensive therapy, *n* (%)	83 (19)	65 (25)	12 (14)	1 (2)	2 (4)	<0.001
1 drug, *n* (%)	101 (23)	61 (24)	17 (20)	6 (12)	6 (12)	
2 drugs, *n* (%)	106 (24)	57 (22)	28 (33)	13 (25)	11 (22)	
3 drugs, *n* (%)	91 (20)	44 (17)	15 (18)	21 (40)	12 (24)	
4 drugs, *n* (%)	56 (13)	24 (9)	10 (12)	8 (15)	13 (26)	
5+ drugs, *n* (%)	11 (3)	6 (2)	3 (4)	3 (6)	7 (14)	
Hypertension requiring 4+ drugs, *n* (%)	117 (26)	48 (19)	23 (27)	16 (31)	30 (59)	<0.001
Total number of drugs	7 ± 3	6 ± 3	7 ± 2	8 ± 3 *	9 ± 3 *,†	<0.001

Table 1. *Cont.*

Variable	Total Population	eGFR ≥60 Albuminuria No	eGFR ≥60 Albuminuria Yes	eGFR <60 Albuminuria No	eGFR <60 Albuminuria Yes	*p*-Value
Non-pharmacological management						
BMI (kg/m^2)	32.9 ± 6.2	32.9 ± 6.5	32.9 ± 5.4	33.3 ± 6.2	32.3 ± 6.1	0.89
Current smoker, *n* (%)	74 (17)	41 (16)	15 (18)	10 (19)	8 (16)	0.93
Alcohol intake (units per month)	5 (0–30)	5 (0–28)	10 (0–47)	3 (0–24)	12 (0–40)	0.22
25(OH) Vitamin D (nmol/L)	42 ± 20	43 ± 18	37 ± 19	42 ± 26	44 ± 22	0.09
Urinary excretion						
Urinary creatinine excretion (mmol/day)	13.8 ± 4.8	13.9 ± 4.9	14.8 ± 5.4	12.8 ± 4.2	12.8 ± 3.6	0.03
Urinary magnesium excretion (mmol/day)	4.0 ± 2.1	4.1 ± 2.1	4.4 ± 2.3	3.3 ± 1.7 *,†	3.2 ± 1.4 *,†	0.001
Urinary phosphate excretion (mmol/day)	27.5 ± 11.6	28.2 ± 12.2	30.3 ± 12.6	22.7 ± 7.7 *,†	25.0 ± 7.9	0.001
Sodium-to-potassium ratio (mmol/mmol)	2.5 ± 1.0	2.5 ± 1.0	2.8 ± 1.2	2.2 ± 0.7 †	2.3 ± 0.8	0.004
Calculated intake						
Dietary salt intake (g/day)	10.9 ± 4.7	11.0 ± 4.3	12.7 ± 5.6 *	8.7 ± 4.0 *,†	9.7 ± 3.9 †	<0.001
Salt intake ≤6 g/day	53 (12)	26 (10)	5 (6)	15 (29)	7 (14)	<0.001
Dietary potassium intake (g/day)	3.9 ± 1.3	4.0 ± 1.4	4.1 ± 1.1	3.5 ± 1.3	3.6 ± 0.9	0.01
Potassium intake ≥3.5 g/day	290 (66)	173 (69)	62 (73)	27 (53)	29 (59)	0.06
Dietary protein intake (g/day)	92 ± 27	94 ± 28	98 ± 29	80 ± 23 *,†	84 ± 21 †	0.001

* $p < 0.05$ vs. eGFR ≥60/Albuminuria (Alb)−; † $p < 0.05$ vs. eGFR ≥60/Alb+. ‡ $p < 0.05$ vs. eGFR <60/Alb−. Abbreviations: T2DM, Type 2 Diabetes Mellitus; BP, blood pressure.

There was no renal involvement in 57% of the patients (eGFR ≥60/Alb−; Table 1). Of all of the patients, 30% (n = 136) had albuminuria, either with a preserved (n = 85, eGFR ≥60/Alb+) or reduced renal function (n = 51, eGFR <60/Alb+). Fifty-two patients (12%) had a reduced renal function without albuminuria (eGFR <60/Alb−). The mean systolic blood pressure was 139 ± 16 mmHg, and the mean diastolic BP was 76 ± 9 mmHg. Most of the patients (81%) used one or more antihypertensive drugs. The target BP was reached in 53% of all patients, while 47% had BP not on target. In patients with albuminuria, 33% and 24% reached the target blood pressure in eGFR ≥60 and in eGFR <60, respectively (Table 1). Additionally, a blood pressure of ≤140/90 mmHg was reached in 48% and 41% of albuminuria patients with an eGFR ≥60 and eGFR <60, respectively. The group with albuminuria and eGFR <60 received the largest number of antihypertensive drugs (3 (2–4) drugs, Table 1). Additionally, the number of patients with hypertension requiring 4+ drugs was highest in this group (59%, $p < 0.001$). In contrast, the antihypertensive drug use in the eGFR ≥60/Alb+ group is not higher than in the other groups (2 (1–3) drugs). Patients without chronic kidney disease (CKD) (Table 1, group eGFR ≥60/Alb−) most commonly used renin-angiotensin-aldosterone-system inhibition (RAASi) (59%), followed by β-blockers (39%), and thiazide diuretics (32%). This was different in those with CKD (groups eGFR ≥60/Alb+, eGFR <60/Alb−, and eGFR <60/Alb+): RAASi (77%), β-blockers (62%), and Calcium antagonists (31%). There were two patients with an eGFR <60 that used a phosphate binder, one in the Alb− group, and one in the Alb+ group.

The mean dietary salt intake was high, namely, 10.9 g of salt per day, and was considerably higher in the groups with preserved eGFR. When adjusting for age and gender, these differences remained virtually similar (data not shown). In the overall population, only 53 patients (12%) adhered to the dietary guidelines for dietary salt intake, ≤6 g/day, and in the eGFR ≥60/Alb+ group this percentage was even lower, i.e., 6%. In total, 8% of patients had a salt intake of ≤5 g/day as recommended by the WHO. The mean potassium intake was 3.9 ± 1.3 g/day, and 66% of patients had an intake, as recommended, above 3.5 g/day (Table 1). The mean urinary magnesium excretion was 4.0 ± 2.1 mmol/day, and as expected was lower in patients with an eGFR <60 mL/min than in those with an eGFR ≥ 60mL/min. The mean urinary phosphate excretion was 27.5 ± 11.6 mmol/day, and the mean calculated dietary protein intake was 92 ± 27 g/day.

3.2. Pharmacological and Nutritional Management in BP-On Target (BP-OT) and BP-Not On Target (BP-NOT) Groups

Table 2 shows the patients' characteristics by a break-up of BT-OT and BP-NOT. Patients with BP-NOT were more often men (64% vs. 53%, P = 0.018), and had a higher HbA1C (59 ± 12 vs. 56 ± 11 mmol/L, P = 0.031). While the presence of albuminuria was a strong predictor of uncontrolled BP (46% vs. 17%, $p < 0.001$), poor BP control was not associated with an eGFR <60 mL/min (24% vs. 22%).

Patients with BP-OT used loop diuretics more often than those with BP-NOT (Table 2). There were no other differences in the pharmacological treatment between the BP groups; neither in the types of prescribed drugs, nor in the total number of prescribed antihypertensive drugs. Surprisingly, of the patients with BP-NOT, 21% did not use any antihypertensive drug, while 20% used only one, and 21% used two antihypertensive drugs.

Adherence to the recommended nutritional guidelines by a breakup of BP-OT and BP-NOT is shown in Figure 3. In both groups, adherence to the recommended lifestyle guidelines was poor, and the total number of lifestyle targets adhered to did not differ between the groups (3 (2–3) in BP-OT vs. 3 (2–3) in BP-NOT, p = 0.22). In patients with BP-NOT, 8% had a dietary salt intake below the recommended 6 g/day, which was lower than those with BP-OT (15%, p = 0.025). Adherence to the potassium guideline (66% of patients) did not differ among the groups. Only 3% of patients had a sodium-to-potassium ratio ≤1.0 in both BP groups. There were only three patients (1%) who adhered to both the recommended intakes of salt and potassium. BMI was ≤30 kg/m^2 in 35% of patients, and this proportion did not differ among the BP groups. The smoking and alcohol guidelines were adhered to by 83% and 86% of all patients, and these proportions were not different among the BP groups. We found no differences in the other nutritional factors between the BP-OT and BP-NOT groups (Table 2). In the total population, there was only one patient (with BP-OT) who adhered to all of the lifestyle guidelines simultaneously. There were no differences in lifestyle guidelines adherence between those with zero to two antihypertensives and those with three-plus antihypertensives.

Table 2. DIALECT-1 pharmacological and nutritional management by a breakup of BP on target/not on target.

Variable	BP On Target	BP Not On Target	*p*-Value
Patient characteristics	*n* = 239	*n* = 210	
Age (years)	63 ± 9	63 ± 9	0.36
Male, *n* (%)	126 (53)	134 (64)	0.02
Years T2DM (years)	11 (7–17)	12 (7–18)	0.26
Serum HbA1C (mmol/mol)	56 ± 11	59 ± 12	0.03
Insulin use, *n* (%)	149 (62)	136 (65)	0.60
Systolic blood pressure (mmHg)	125 ± 10	149 ± 13	<0.001
Diastolic blood pressure (mmHg)	70 ± 8	80 ± 9	<0.001
eGFR <60, *n* (%)	53 (22)	51 (24)	0.60
Albuminuria, *n* (%)	40 (17)	95 (46)	<0.001
Pharmacological management			
RAASi, *n* (%)	163 (68)	134 (64)	0.33
β-blockers, *n* (%)	115 (48)	93 (44)	0.42
Thiazide diuretics, *n* (%)	71 (30)	66 (31)	0.69
Calcium antagonists, *n* (%)	50 (21)	52 (25)	0.33
Loop diuretics, *n* (%)	52 (22)	29 (14)	0.03
Potassium sparing diuretics, *n* (%)	22 (9)	21 (10)	0.78
Number of antihypertensives	2 (1–3)	2 (1–3)	0.51
No antihypertensive therapy, *n* (%)	39 (16)	44 (21)	0.85
1 drug, *n* (%)	47 (20)	42 (20)	
2 drugs, *n* (%)	64 (27)	45 (21)	
3 drugs, *n* (%)	50 (21)	43 (21)	
4 drugs, *n* (%)	29 (12)	27 (13)	
5+ drugs, *n* (%)	10 (4)	9 (4)	
Hypertension requiring 4+ drugs, *n* (%)	39 (16)	79 (38)	<0.001
Total number of drugs	7.0 ± 2.6	6.7 ± 2.8	0.30
Non-pharmacological management			
BMI (kg/m^2)	32.8 ± 5.8	32.9 ± 6.7	0.89
Serum 25 (OH) Vitamin D (nmol/L)	43 ± 20	41 ± 20	0.22
Urinary excretion			
Urinary creatinine excretion (mmol/day)	13.6 ± 4.9	14.1 ± 4.7	0.22
Urinary magnesium excretion (mmol/day)	3.9 ± 2.1	4.0 ± 1.9	0.43
Urinary phosphate excretion (mmol/day)	26.9 ± 12.3	28.2 ± 10.7	0.26
Sodium-to-potassium ratio (mmol/mmol)	2.5 ± 1.0	2.5 ± 0.9	0.49
Calculated intake			
Dietary salt intake (g/day)	10.7 ± 4.8	11.1 ± 4.4	0.47
Dietary potassium intake (g/day)	3.8 ± 1.3	4.0 ± 1.2	0.15
Dietary protein intake (g/day)	90 ± 29	93 ± 26	0.29

In the multivariate logistic regression analysis, albuminuria and the use of loop diuretics remained the only significant predictors of BP-NOT (data not shown).

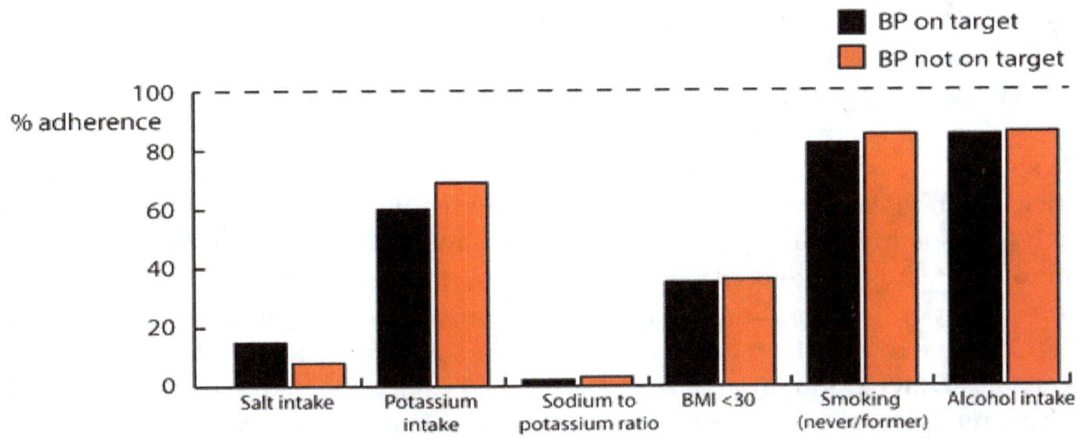

Figure 3. % Adherence to nutritional guidelines, by a breakup of blood pressure on target/not on target. Alcohol intake is self-reported, and the target intake was ≤2 units per day for women and ≤3 units per day for men.

4. Discussion

In this paper, we present the blood pressure management of Type 2 diabetes patients (T2DM), using combined data on pharmacological and nutritional management in a real-life secondary health care setting. As anticipated, the prevalence of hypertension was high, and 81% of patients were on antihypertensives. However, BP control was poor, as the target BP was not reached in 47% of patients. An integrated assessment of pharmacological and nutritional management demonstrated a large window of opportunity for improving BP control in T2DM, both by intensifying antihypertensive drug treatment, and increasing nutritional guideline adherence.

The proportion of patients with their blood pressure on target (BP-OT) in our cohort is in line with findings in other T2DM cohorts [31], as well as diabetic kidney disease cohorts [5,32]. The proportion was lower than found in T2DM patients treated in the primary care setting, in whom adequate blood pressure control was found in 85% of patients [33,34], which may well reflect the referral policy, with more difficult patients being referred to secondary care. In the baseline data of the LEADER-4 trial (a randomized clinical trial in T2DM patients) [31], where 51% of patients had BP-NOT, the antihypertensive use was lower than we report, as about 80% of all patients used zero to two antihypertensive drugs. In diabetic kidney disease studies (i.e., studies with T2DM and either albuminuria and/or eGFR <60), the antihypertensive drug use is mostly in line with our findings, with >90% of patients using antihypertensive drugs, and RAASi being the most frequently used drug [5,32]. In line with our findings, Smits et al. found that RAASi was the most commonly used class of antihypertensive drugs in a Dutch T2DM cohort in primary care, followed by betablockers and diuretics [33]. The number of used antihypertensive drugs they report is largely comparable to our findings, albeit that the use of four to five drugs seems more common in our secondary care cohort. It should be noted that in these studies regarding BP control in a real world setting, data regarding nutrient intake is not available.

An important issue when evaluating the pharmacological management of blood pressure is treatment non-adherence, which reportedly ranges from 31 to 40% in patients with poorly controlled blood pressure [35,36]. Thus, establishing an infrastructure that allows the monitoring of adherence would be of great value. Yet, even assuming a drug-treatment non-adherence rate of 40% in our patients, the non-adherence to lifestyle measures seems to stand out as an additional important target for intervention.

What can be done to improve BP control in T2DM? Our data, and data from other trials, clearly show that true therapy-resistant hypertension, defined as hypertension persisting despite three antihypertensive drugs at maximum tolerable dosage of which one is a diuretic, is not the issue in most patients with BP-NOT. The majority of BP-NOT patients (62%) do not use more than two antihypertensive drugs, illustrating the opportunity for intensifying pharmacological treatment. One promising option in this regard is the removal of excess extracellular fluid with diuretics, especially in those patients with a high salt intake.

Our data show that, especially for nutritional management, there is a large window of opportunity for improvement, as in the total population only one patient adhered to all of the nutritional guidelines simultaneously. This is highly relevant, since lifestyle interventions have the potential to not only reduce BP, but to also reduce the overall cardiovascular risk [11,37–40]. Even though dietary counselling has already been part of their routine care, the mean daily salt intake in our population was almost 11 g/day, roughly twice that of the recommended 6 g/day, and considerably higher than the mean salt intake in the general Dutch population of 8.5 g/day [41]. Previously, Mente et al demonstrated that for each 1-gram increment in estimated sodium excretion, blood pressure was 2/1 mmHg higher, where this slope was more pronounced and steeper in those with hypertension, high-sodium diets (>5g/day), and older persons [42]. Therefore, the most obvious step to improve non-pharmacological management would be to reduce dietary salt intake. This is underscored by a previous study, performed in T2DM patients in the same region, which has shown that, although the aim to reduce dietary salt intake to <6 g/day was not reached, even a relatively modest reduction in salt intake from 12 to 9 g/day can reduce blood pressure by 6/3 mmHg and albuminuria by 42% while under RAASi [43]. Furthermore, reducing salt intake is associated with potentiating the antihypertensive effects of RAASi [44–46].

There is evidence that a combined dietary approach aimed at reducing salt while increasing potassium intake has the potential to improve cardiovascular risk management [12,47]. However, the potassium intake in our patients was generally already above the recommended intake of 3.5 g/day. Therefore, the finding that the sodium-to-potassium ratio was higher than the deemed optimal ratio of 1 mmol/mmol in 97% of patients is primarily determined by high salt intake.

To improve blood pressure control, dietary intervention could also be aimed at reducing body weight. The mean BMI in our cohort was above 30 kg/m^2. While a relationship between obesity and blood pressure has previously been demonstrated [7,48], we did not find such an association here. This might be due to the fact that we had few participants with a BMI < 25 kg/m^2, and therefore did not have a large enough dispersion to differentiate between the BP groups. Intentional weight loss has been associated with beneficial effects, both on BP and on other cardiovascular risk factors such as LDL cholesterol and glycemic control [49]. Therefore, even though weight loss is notoriously difficult to achieve, especially in patients on insulin treatment, it should remain a priority in the non-pharmacological treatment of T2DM, and also in secondary health care centres.

Finally, an association between the intake of magnesium and phosphate and blood pressure has been reported previously [14,17,18,50,51]. Here, we did not find differences in urinary magnesium excretion or in urinary phosphate excretion between those with BP-OT and BP-NOT. As the urinary excretion of magnesium and phosphate is lower in those with a low eGFR, these results might be misleading. However, the proportion of patients with a low eGFR was similar in both the BP-OT and BP-NOT groups, making it less likely that differences in the urinary excretion of magnesium and phosphate between the BP groups were masked by differences in urinary excretion due to a low eGFR. In the general population, a continuous relationship between lower magnesium excretion and the risk for hypertension was reported [16]; moreover, patients with a low magnesium intake had a greater risk of developing ischemic heart disease [52]. While no nutritional recommendations are currently available for magnesium to stratify adequate/inadequate intake, in our population approximately 28% of patients had a magnesium excretion below the values associated with ischemic heart disease in the general population. Regarding phosphate intake, population-based studies as well as studies in CKD have shown associations with outcome, albeit not equivocal [53,54], and it has been proposed that excess phosphate intake is a risk factor that is generally overlooked in patients with early stages of CKD by lack of measurements [55]. While more research is needed on the relation between magnesium and phosphate excretion and adverse outcomes, our data illustrate that 24-hour urine, collected to assess the intake of established nutritional targets such as salt and potassium, can simply be used to establish a more complete nutritional profile, which could be useful for future improvements in nutritional studies and counselling.

It should be noted that the adherence to nutritional guidelines was equally poor in the BP-OT and BP-NOT groups. While in the BP-NOT group there is more urgency to adhere to these guidelines, namely to correct BP, the adherence to the guidelines in the BP-OT group should not be overlooked. In regard to salt intake, previously it has been shown that a higher salt intake while under RAASi is associated with worse cardiovascular outcomes, even independent of BP [46]. Furthermore, as stated above, intentional weight loss has many benefits that surpass BP management [49], and therefore can also greatly improve outcomes if BP is already on target. Lastly, in a population-based cohort, low potassium intake has been associated with the occurrence of chronic kidney disease [56].

The DIALECT study has several strengths, including the use of real-world data from a cohort representative of secondary health care in T2DM, at least in the context of the Dutch referral health care setting. Second, we study the integrated role of non-biased data on both pharmacological and non-pharmacological parameters on BP, which is an important approach, as in cardiovascular risk management pharmacological and non-pharmacological interventions go hand in hand. Third, through the use of 24-hour urine collections, we provide objective measurements of dietary intake and several relevant nutrients.

There are also some limitations. An observational study cannot prove causal relationships. Also, there is some risk of response bias, although patient characteristics were similar between those who did and did not participate.

What are the implications of our study? Adequate management equals the sum of measures taken in combination with compliance. Our data on poor nutritional management do not distinguish between a lack of adequate nutritional counselling and a lack of compliance. However, it is well established that sustained lifestyle change is difficult to achieve, demonstrating that currently no modus of adequate counselling and therefore adequate management exists. The question, therefore, is how to establish this. Previous well-designed studies, using interventions of intensive nurse practitioner support and self-management, both did not lead to neither long-standing changes in nutritional habits, nor a reduction of cardiovascular outcomes [57,58]. As alternative approach, improvement strategies as tested for pharmacological management could be considered. In particular, it has been shown that the systematic evaluation of prescription quality as assessed by prescription quality indicators not only improved pharmacological compliance with guidelines, but also patient outcomes [59]. To the best of our knowledge, such approaches have never been developed and tested for nutritional management. As several objective parameters are available, such as the urinary excretion of sodium and potassium, this would be feasible in routine clinical care. Therefore, to improve blood pressure control, in our opinion, the use of nutritional quality indicators may have the potential to improve treatment quality as a whole.

5. Conclusions

Uncontrolled BP is common in T2DM, especially in those with microalbuminuria. An integrated assessment of pharmacological and nutritional management demonstrated a window of opportunity for improving BP treatment, especially in nutritional management. We advocate that incorporating the integrated monitoring of pharmacological and nutritional management in quality control cycles has the potential to improve treatment quality in T2DM.

Acknowledgments: We thank Willeke van Kampen, Sanne van Huizen, Anne Davina, Jolien Jaspers, and Manon Harmelink for their contribution to patient inclusion. Furthermore, we would like to thank Bettine Haandrikman for her help with setting up the biobank. Lastly, we would like to thank Job van der Palen and Marloes Vermeer for their support in statistical analyses.

Author Contributions: E.v.d.B., S.J.L.B., G.J.N. and G.D.L. conceived and designed the study. C.M.G., H.B. and E.v.d.B. included patients and performed the measurements. C.M.G. and H.B. analysed the data. S.J.L.B., G.J.N. and G.D.L. contributed materials. C.M.G., H.B., S.J.L.B., G.J.N. and G.D.L. wrote the paper.

References

1. World Health Organization. *Global Report on Diabetes*; WHO Press: Geneva, Switzerland, 2016.
2. Tancredi, M.; Rosengren, A.; Svensson, A.M.; Kosiborod, M.; Pivodic, A.; Gudbjornsdottir, S.; Wedel, H.; Clements, M.; Dahlqvist, S.; Lind, M. Excess Mortality among Persons with Type 2 Diabetes. *N. Engl. J. Med.* **2015**, *373*, 1720–1732. [CrossRef] [PubMed]
3. Fox, C.S.; Coady, S.; Sorlie, P.D.; Levy, D.; Meigs, J.B.; D'Agostino, R.B., Sr.; Wilson, P.W.; Savage, P.J. Trends in Cardiovascular Complications of Diabetes. *JAMA* **2004**, *292*, 2495–2499. [CrossRef] [PubMed]
4. Langsted, A.; Freiberg, J.J.; Nordestgaard, B.G. Extent of Undertreatment and Overtreatment with Cholesterol-Lowering Therapy According to European Guidelines in 92,348 Danes without Ischemic Cardiovascular Disease and Diabetes in 2004–2014. *Atherosclerosis* **2016**, *257*, 9–15. [CrossRef] [PubMed]
5. De Cosmo, S.; Viazzi, F.; Piscitelli, P.; Giorda, C.; Ceriello, A.; Genovese, S.; Russo, G.; Guida, P.; Fioretto, P.; Pontremoli, R.; et al. Blood Pressure Status and the Incidence of Diabetic Kidney Disease in Patients with Hypertension and Type 2 Diabetes. *J. Hypertens.* **2016**, *34*, 2090–2098. [CrossRef] [PubMed]
6. Gorter, K.; van Bruggen, R.; Stolk, R.; Zuithoff, P.; Verhoeven, R.; Rutten, G. Overall Quality of Diabetes Care in a Defined Geographic Region: Different Sides of the Same Story. *Br. J. Gen. Pract.* **2008**, *58*, 339–345. [CrossRef] [PubMed]
7. Baptista, D.R.; Thieme, R.D.; Reis, W.C.; Pontarolo, R.; Correr, C.J. Proportion of Brazilian Diabetes Patients that Achieve Treatment Goals: Implications for Better Quality of Care. *Diabetol. Metab. Syndr.* **2015**, *7*, 113. [CrossRef] [PubMed]
8. Laxy, M.; Knoll, G.; Schunk, M.; Meisinger, C.; Huth, C.; Holle, R. Quality of Diabetes Care in Germany Improved from 2000 to 2007 to 2014, but Improvements Diminished since 2007. Evidence from the Population-Based KORA Studies. *PLoS ONE* **2016**, *11*, e0164704. [CrossRef] [PubMed]
9. McLean, R.M. Measuring Population Sodium Intake: A Review of Methods. *Nutrients* **2014**, *6*, 4651–4662. [CrossRef] [PubMed]
10. WHO. *Guideline: Sodium Intake for Adults and Children*; WHO Press: Geneva, Switzerland, 2012.
11. Fox, C.S.; Golden, S.H.; Anderson, C.; Bray, G.A.; Burke, L.E.; de Boer, I.H.; Deedwania, P.; Eckel, R.H.; Ershow, A.G.; Fradkin, J.; et al. Update on Prevention of Cardiovascular Disease in Adults with Type 2 Diabetes Mellitus in Light of Recent Evidence: A Scientific Statement from the American Heart Association and the American Diabetes Association. *Diabetes Care* **2015**, *38*, 1777–1803. [CrossRef] [PubMed]
12. Filippini, T.; Violi, F.; D'Amico, R.; Vinceti, M. The Effect of Potassium Supplementation on Blood Pressure in Hypertensive Subjects: A Systematic Review and Meta-Analysis. *Int. J. Cardiol.* **2017**, *230*, 127–135. [CrossRef] [PubMed]
13. WHO. *Guideline: Potassium Intake for Adults and Children*; WHO Press: Geneva, Switzerland, 2012.
14. Zhang, X.; Li, Y.; Del Gobbo, L.C.; Rosanoff, A.; Wang, J.; Zhang, W.; Song, Y. Effects of Magnesium Supplementation on Blood Pressure: A Meta-Analysis of Randomized Double-Blind Placebo-Controlled Trials. *Hypertension* **2016**, *68*, 324–333. [CrossRef] [PubMed]
15. Bain, L.K.; Myint, P.K.; Jennings, A.; Lentjes, M.A.; Luben, R.N.; Khaw, K.T.; Wareham, N.J.; Welch, A.A. The Relationship between Dietary Magnesium Intake, Stroke and its Major Risk Factors, Blood Pressure and Cholesterol, in the EPIC-Norfolk Cohort. *Int. J. Cardiol.* **2015**, *196*, 108–114. [CrossRef] [PubMed]
16. Joosten, M.M.; Gansevoort, R.T.; Mukamal, K.J.; Kootstra-Ros, J.E.; Feskens, E.J.; Geleijnse, J.M.; Navis, G.; Bakker, S.J. PREVEND Study Group. Urinary Magnesium Excretion and Risk of Hypertension: The Prevention of Renal and Vascular End-Stage Disease Study. *Hypertension* **2013**, *61*, 1161–1167. [CrossRef] [PubMed]
17. Bozic, M.; Panizo, S.; Sevilla, M.A.; Riera, M.; Soler, M.J.; Pascual, J.; Lopez, I.; Freixenet, M.; Fernandez, E.; Valdivielso, J.M. High Phosphate Diet Increases Arterial Blood Pressure Via a Parathyroid Hormone Mediated Increase of Renin. *J. Hypertens.* **2014**, *32*, 1822–1832. [CrossRef] [PubMed]

18. Mizuno, M.; Mitchell, J.H.; Crawford, S.; Huang, C.L.; Maalouf, N.; Hu, M.C.; Moe, O.W.; Smith, S.A.; Vongpatanasin, W. High Dietary Phosphate Intake Induces Hypertension and Augments Exercise Pressor Reflex Function in Rats. *Am. J. Physiol. Regul. Integr. Comp. Physiol.* **2016**, *311*, R39–R48. [CrossRef] [PubMed]
19. Du Bois, D.; Du Bois, E.F. A Formula to Estimate the Approximate Surface Area if Height and Weight be Known. 1916. *Nutrition* **1989**, *5*, 303–311. [PubMed]
20. Wendel-Vos, G.C.; Schuit, A.J.; Saris, W.H.; Kromhout, D. Reproducibility and Relative Validity of the Short Questionnaire to Assess Health-Enhancing Physical Activity. *J. Clin. Epidemiol.* **2003**, *56*, 1163–1169. [CrossRef]
21. Levey, A.S.; Stevens, L.A.; Schmid, C.H.; Zhang, Y.L.; Castro, A.F., 3rd; Feldman, H.I.; Kusek, J.W.; Eggers, P.; Van Lente, F.; Greene, T.; et al. A New Equation to Estimate Glomerular Filtration Rate. *Ann. Intern. Med.* **2009**, *150*, 604–612. [CrossRef] [PubMed]
22. Authors/Task Force Members; Ryden, L.; Grant, P.J.; Anker, S.D.; Berne, C.; Cosentino, F.; Danchin, N.; Deaton, C.; Escaned, J.; Hammes, H.P.; et al. ESC Guidelines on Diabetes, Pre-Diabetes, and Cardiovascular Diseases Developed in Collaboration with the EASD: The Task Force on Diabetes, Pre-Diabetes, and Cardiovascular Diseases of the European Society of Cardiology (ESC) and Developed in Collaboration with the European Association for the Study of Diabetes (EASD). *Eur. Heart J.* **2013**, *34*, 3035–3087. [PubMed]
23. Kidney Disease: Improving Global Outcomes (KDIGO) Blood Pressure Work Group. KDIGO Clinical Practice Guideline for the Management of Blood Pressure in Chronic Kidney Disease. *Kidney Int. Suppl.* **2012**, *2*, 337–414.
24. Kromhout, D.; Spaaij, C.J.; de Goede, J.; Weggemans, R.M. The 2015 Dutch Food-Based Dietary Guidelines. *Eur. J. Clin. Nutr.* **2016**, *70*, 869–878. [CrossRef] [PubMed]
25. Gezondheidsraad. *Richtlijnen Goede Voeding 2015*; Gezondheidsraad: The Hague, The Netherlands, 2015.
26. Bock, H.A.; Stein, J.H. Diuretics and the Control of Extracellular Fluid Volume: Role of Counterregulation. *Semin. Nephrol.* **1988**, *8*, 264–272. [PubMed]
27. Holbrook, J.T.; Patterson, K.Y.; Bodner, J.E.; Douglas, L.W.; Veillon, C.; Kelsay, J.L.; Mertz, W.; Smith, J.C., Jr. Sodium and Potassium Intake and Balance in Adults Consuming Self-Selected Diets. *Am. J. Clin. Nutr.* **1984**, *40*, 786–793. [PubMed]
28. Maroni, B.J.; Steinman, T.I.; Mitch, W.E. A Method for Estimating Nitrogen Intake of Patients with Chronic Renal Failure. *Kidney Int.* **1985**, *27*, 58–65. [CrossRef] [PubMed]
29. Newsome, B.; Ix, J.H.; Tighiouart, H.; Sarnak, M.J.; Levey, A.S.; Beck, G.J.; Block, G. Effect of Protein Restriction on Serum and Urine Phosphate in the Modification of Diet in Renal Disease (MDRD) Study. *Am. J. Kidney Dis.* **2013**, *61*, 1045–1046. [CrossRef] [PubMed]
30. Block, G.A.; Wheeler, D.C.; Persky, M.S.; Kestenbaum, B.; Ketteler, M.; Spiegel, D.M.; Allison, M.A.; Asplin, J.; Smits, G.; Hoofnagle, A.N.; et al. Effects of Phosphate Binders in Moderate CKD. *J. Am. Soc. Nephrol.* **2012**, *23*, 1407–1415. [CrossRef] [PubMed]
31. Petrie, J.R.; Marso, S.P.; Bain, S.C.; Franek, E.; Jacob, S.; Masmiquel, L.; Leiter, L.A.; Haluzik, M.; Satman, I.; Omar, M.; et al. LEADER-4: Blood Pressure Control in Patients with Type 2 Diabetes and High Cardiovascular Risk: Baseline Data from the LEADER Randomized Trial. *J. Hypertens.* **2016**, *34*, 1140–1150. [CrossRef] [PubMed]
32. Halimi, J.M.; Joly, D.; Combe, C.; Choukroun, G.; Dussol, B.; Fauvel, J.P.; Quere, S.; Fiquet, B. Blood Pressure and Proteinuria Control Remains a Challenge in Patients with Type 2 Diabetes Mellitus and Chronic Kidney Disease: Experience from the Prospective Observational ALICE-PROTECT Study. *BMC Nephrol.* **2016**, *17*, 135. [CrossRef] [PubMed]
33. Smits, K.P.; Sidorenkov, G.; Kleefstra, N.; Bouma, M.; Meulepas, M.; Voorham, J.; Navis, G.; Bilo, H.J.; Denig, P. Development and Validation of Prescribing Quality Indicators for Patients with Type 2 Diabetes. *Int. J. Clin. Pract.* **2017**, *71*. [CrossRef] [PubMed]
34. Walraven, I.; Mast, M.R.; Hoekstra, T.; Jansen, A.P.; Rauh, S.P.; Rutters, F.R.; van der Heijden, A.A.; Elders, P.J.; Moll, A.C.; Polak, B.C.; et al. Real-World Evidence of Suboptimal Blood Pressure Control in Patients with Type 2 Diabetes. *J. Hypertens.* **2015**, *33*, 2091–2098. [CrossRef] [PubMed]
35. Vrijens, B.; Antoniou, S.; Burnier, M.; de la Sierra, A.; Volpe, M. Current Situation of Medication Adherence in Hypertension. *Front. Pharmacol.* **2017**, *8*, 100. [CrossRef] [PubMed]

36. De Jager, R.L.; de Beus, E.; Beeftink, M.M.; Sanders, M.F.; Vonken, E.J.; Voskuil, M.; van Maarseveen, E.M.; Bots, M.L.; Blankestijn, P.J. SYMPATHY Investigators. Impact of Medication Adherence on the Effect of Renal Denervation: The SYMPATHY Trial. *Hypertension* **2017**, *69*, 678–684. [CrossRef] [PubMed]
37. Dunkler, D.; Kohl, M.; Heinze, G.; Teo, K.K.; Rosengren, A.; Pogue, J.; Gao, P.; Gerstein, H.; Yusuf, S.; Oberbauer, R.; et al. Modifiable Lifestyle and Social Factors Affect Chronic Kidney Disease in High-Risk Individuals with Type 2 Diabetes Mellitus. *Kidney Int.* **2015**, *87*, 784–791. [CrossRef] [PubMed]
38. Knowler, W.C.; Barrett-Connor, E.; Fowler, S.E.; Hamman, R.F.; Lachin, J.M.; Walker, E.A.; Nathan, D.M. Diabetes Prevention Program Research Group. Reduction in the Incidence of Type 2 Diabetes with Lifestyle Intervention Or Metformin. *N. Engl. J. Med.* **2002**, *346*, 393–403. [PubMed]
39. Bibbins-Domingo, K.; Chertow, G.M.; Coxson, P.G.; Moran, A.; Lightwood, J.M.; Pletcher, M.J.; Goldman, L. Projected Effect of Dietary Salt Reductions on Future Cardiovascular Disease. *N. Engl. J. Med.* **2010**, *362*, 590–599. [CrossRef] [PubMed]
40. Wong, M.M.; Arcand, J.; Leung, A.A.; Thout, S.R.; Campbell, N.R.; Webster, J. The Science of Salt: A Regularly Updated Systematic Review of Salt and Health Outcomes (December 2015–March 2016). *J. Clin. Hypertens. (Greenwich)* **2017**, *19*, 322–332. [CrossRef] [PubMed]
41. Hendriksen, M.; Etemad, Z.; van den Bogaard, C.H.; van der A, D.L. *Salt, Iodine and Potassium Intake among Adults in Doetinchem in 2015*; RIVM Report 2016–0081; Rijksinstituut voor Volksgezondheid en Milieu: Bilthoven, The Netherlands, 2016.
42. Mente, A.; O'Donnell, M.J.; Rangarajan, S.; McQueen, M.J.; Poirier, P.; Wielgosz, A.; Morrison, H.; Li, W.; Wang, X.; Di, C.; et al. Association of Urinary Sodium and Potassium Excretion with Blood Pressure. *N. Engl. J. Med.* **2014**, *371*, 601–611. [CrossRef] [PubMed]
43. Kwakernaak, A.J.; Krikken, J.A.; Binnenmars, S.H.; Visser, F.W.; Hemmelder, M.H.; Woittiez, A.J.; Groen, H.; Laverman, G.D.; Navis, G. Holland Nephrology Study (HONEST) Group. Effects of Sodium Restriction and Hydrochlorothiazide on RAAS Blockade Efficacy in Diabetic Nephropathy: A Randomised Clinical Trial. *Lancet Diabetes Endocrinol.* **2014**, *2*, 385–395. [CrossRef]
44. Lambers Heerspink, H.J.; de Borst, M.H.; Bakker, S.J.; Navis, G.J. Improving the Efficacy of RAAS Blockade in Patients with Chronic Kidney Disease. *Nat. Rev. Nephrol.* **2013**, *9*, 112–121. [CrossRef] [PubMed]
45. Vogt, L.; Waanders, F.; Boomsma, F.; de Zeeuw, D.; Navis, G. Effects of Dietary Sodium and Hydrochlorothiazide on the Antiproteinuric Efficacy of Losartan. *J. Am. Soc. Nephrol.* **2008**, *19*, 999–1007. [CrossRef] [PubMed]
46. Lambers Heerspink, H.J.; Holtkamp, F.A.; Parving, H.H.; Navis, G.J.; Lewis, J.B.; Ritz, E.; de Graeff, P.A.; de Zeeuw, D. Moderation of Dietary Sodium Potentiates the Renal and Cardiovascular Protective Effects of Angiotensin Receptor Blockers. *Kidney Int.* **2012**, *82*, 330–337. [CrossRef] [PubMed]
47. Kieneker, L.M.; Gansevoort, R.T.; Mukamal, K.J.; de Boer, R.A.; Navis, G.; Bakker, S.J.; Joosten, M.M. Urinary Potassium Excretion and Risk of Developing Hypertension: The Prevention of Renal and Vascular End-Stage Disease Study. *Hypertension* **2014**, *64*, 769–776. [CrossRef] [PubMed]
48. Adeniyi, O.V.; Yogeswaran, P.; Longo-Mbenza, B.; Ter Goon, D. Uncontrolled Hypertension and its Determinants in Patients with Concomitant Type 2 Diabetes Mellitus (T2DM) in Rural South Africa. *PLoS ONE* **2016**, *11*, e0150033. [CrossRef] [PubMed]
49. Zomer, E.; Gurusamy, K.; Leach, R.; Trimmer, C.; Lobstein, T.; Morris, S.; James, W.P.; Finer, N. Interventions that Cause Weight Loss and the Impact on Cardiovascular Risk Factors: A Systematic Review and Meta-Analysis. *Obes. Rev.* **2016**, *17*, 1001–1011. [CrossRef] [PubMed]
50. Verma, H.; Garg, R. Effect of Magnesium Supplementation on Type 2 Diabetes Associated Cardiovascular Risk Factors: A Systematic Review and Meta-Analysis. *J. Hum. Nutr. Diet.* **2017**. [CrossRef] [PubMed]
51. Humalda, J.K.; Keyzer, C.A.; Binnenmars, S.H.; Kwakernaak, A.J.; Slagman, M.C.; Laverman, G.D.; Bakker, S.J.; de Borst, M.H.; Navis, G.J. Concordance of Dietary Sodium Intake and Concomitant Phosphate Load: Implications for Sodium Interventions. *Nutr. Metab. Cardiovasc. Dis.* **2016**, *26*, 689–696. [CrossRef] [PubMed]
52. Joosten, M.M.; Gansevoort, R.T.; Mukamal, K.J.; van der Harst, P.; Geleijnse, J.M.; Feskens, E.J.; Navis, G.; Bakker, S.J.; PREVEND Study Group. Urinary and Plasma Magnesium and Risk of Ischemic Heart Disease. *Am. J. Clin. Nutr.* **2013**, *97*, 1299–1306. [CrossRef] [PubMed]

53. Chang, A.R.; Grams, M.E. Serum Phosphorus and Mortality in the Third National Health and Nutrition Examination Survey (NHANES III): Effect Modification by Fasting. *Am. J. Kidney Dis.* **2014**, *64*, 567–573. [CrossRef] [PubMed]
54. Palomino, H.L.; Rifkin, D.E.; Anderson, C.; Criqui, M.H.; Whooley, M.A.; Ix, J.H. 24-Hour Urine Phosphorus Excretion and Mortality and Cardiovascular Events. *Clin. J. Am. Soc. Nephrol.* **2013**, *8*, 1202–1210. [CrossRef] [PubMed]
55. Ritz, E.; Hahn, K.; Ketteler, M.; Kuhlmann, M.K.; Mann, J. Phosphate Additives in Food—A Health Risk. *Dtsch. Arzteblatt Int.* **2012**, *109*, 49–55.
56. Kieneker, L.M.; Bakker, S.J.; de Boer, R.A.; Navis, G.J.; Gansevoort, R.T.; Joosten, M.M. Low Potassium Excretion but Not High Sodium Excretion is Associated with Increased Risk of Developing Chronic Kidney Disease. *Kidney Int.* **2016**, *90*, 888–896. [CrossRef] [PubMed]
57. Meuleman, Y.; Hoekstra, T.; Dekker, F.W.; Navis, G.; Vogt, L.; van der Boog, P.J.M.; Bos, W.J.W.; van Montfrans, G.A.; van Dijk, S.; ESMO Study Group. Sodium Restriction in Patients with CKD: A Randomized Controlled Trial of Self-Management Support. *Am. J. Kidney Dis.* **2017**, *69*, 576–586. [CrossRef] [PubMed]
58. Van Zuilen, A.D.; Bots, M.L.; Dulger, A.; van der Tweel, I.; van Buren, M.; Ten Dam, M.A.; Kaasjager, K.A.; Ligtenberg, G.; Sijpkens, Y.W.; Sluiter, H.E.; et al. Multifactorial Intervention with Nurse Practitioners does Not Change Cardiovascular Outcomes in Patients with Chronic Kidney Disease. *Kidney Int.* **2012**, *82*, 710–717. [CrossRef] [PubMed]
59. Smits, K.P.J.; Sidorenkov, G.; Navis, G.; Bouma, M.; Meulepas, M.A.; Bilo, H.J.G.; Denig, P. Prescribing Quality and Prediction of Clinical Outcomes in Patients with Type 2 Diabetes: A Prospective Cohort Study. *Diabetes Care* **2017**, *40*, e83–e84. [CrossRef] [PubMed]

11

Carbohydrates from Sources with a Higher Glycemic Index during Adolescence: Is Evening Rather than Morning Intake Relevant for Risk Markers of Type 2 Diabetes in Young Adulthood?

Tanja Diederichs [1], Christian Herder [2,3], Sarah Roßbach [1], Michael Roden [2,3,4], Stefan A. Wudy [5], Ute Nöthlings [1], Ute Alexy [1,*] and Anette E. Buyken [1,6]

1 IEL-Nutritional Epidemiology, DONALD Study, Rheinische Friedrich-Wilhelms-University Bonn, Heinstueck 11, 44225 Dortmund, Germany; tdiederi@uni-bonn.de (T.D.); srossbac@uni-bonn.de (S.R.); noethlings@uni-bonn.de (U.N.); anette.buyken@uni-paderborn.de (A.E.B.)

2 Institute for Clinical Diabetology, German Diabetes Center, Leibniz Center for Diabetes Research at Heinrich Heine University Düsseldorf, Düsseldorf, Auf'm Hennekamp 65, 40225 Düsseldorf, Germany; christian.herder@ddz.uni-duesseldorf.de (C.H.); michael.roden@ddz.uni-duesseldorf.de (M.R.)

3 German Center for Diabetes Research (DZD), Ingolstädter Landstr. 1, 85764 München-Neuherberg, Germany

4 Department of Endocrinology and Diabetology, Medical Faculty, Heinrich Heine University Düsseldorf, Moorenstraße 5, 40225 Düsseldorf, Germany

5 Pediatric Endocrinology and Diabetology, Laboratory for Translational Hormone Analytics, Peptide Hormone Research Unit, Center of Child and Adolescent Medicine, Justus Liebig University Giessen, Feulgenstraße 10-12, 35392 Gießen, Germany; Stefan.Wudy@paediat.med.uni-giessen.de

6 Institute of Nutrition, Consumption and Health, Faculty of Natural Sciences, University Paderborn, Warburger Straße 100, 33098 Paderborn, Germany

* Correspondence: alexy@uni-bonn.de

Abstract: Background: This study investigated whether glycemic index (GI) or glycemic load (GL) of morning or evening intake and morning or evening carbohydrate intake from low- or higher-GI food sources (low-GI-CHO, higher-GI-CHO) during adolescence are relevant for risk markers of type 2 diabetes in young adulthood. **Methods:** Analyses included DOrtmund Nutritional and Anthropometric Longitudinally Designed (DONALD) study participants who had provided at least two 3-day weighed dietary records (median: 7 records) during adolescence and one blood sample in young adulthood. Using multivariable linear regression analyses, estimated morning and evening GI, GL, low-GI-CHO (GI < 55) and higher-GI-CHO (GI $\geq$ 55) were related to insulin sensitivity ($N = 252$), hepatic steatosis index (HSI), fatty liver index (FLI) (both $N = 253$), and a pro-inflammatory-score ($N = 249$). **Results:** Morning intakes during adolescence were not associated with any of the adult risk markers. A higher evening GI during adolescence was related to an increased HSI in young adulthood ($p = 0.003$). A higher consumption of higher-GI-CHO in the evening was associated with lower insulin sensitivity ($p = 0.046$) and an increased HSI ($p = 0.006$), while a higher evening intake of low-GI-CHO was related to a lower HSI ($p = 0.009$). Evening intakes were not related to FLI or the pro-inflammatory-score (all $p > 0.1$). **Conclusion:** Avoidance of large amounts of carbohydrates from higher-GI sources in the evening should be considered in preventive strategies to reduce the risk of type 2 diabetes in adulthood.

Keywords: glycaemic index; glycaemic load; daytime; adolescence; type 2 diabetes mellitus

1. Introduction

Diets low in glycemic index (GI) or glycemic load (GL) are related to a lower risk of developing type 2 diabetes mellitus [1,2]. Their preferred use has hence been advocated particularly during periods of physiological insulin resistance, such as puberty [3]. This is supported by our recent observations linking a higher dietary GI/GL during puberty to a lower insulin sensitivity and increased liver enzyme activities [4] as well as increased levels of interleukin-(IL)-6 [5] in young adulthood, i.e., metabolic markers indicating an increased risk of developing type 2 diabetes in later life [6].

Recent discussions on preventive procedures also account for chronobiological aspects of metabolism [7]. This originates from the observation that extreme circadian (circa dies (lat.) = about 24 h) misalignment—as experienced during shiftwork—enhances the risk of type 2 diabetes among adults [8]. In a subsample from a Finnish population-based study, behavioral traits towards eveningness (based on a questionnaire assessing morningness-eveningness) were linked to notably higher odds for type 2 diabetes [9]. Persons with a late chronotype (i.e., those with a preference for a delayed timing of sleep on free days, i.e., without social obligations) are at particular risk of experiencing mild, but chronic misalignment resulting from the discrepancy between their circadian clock and socially determined, fixed schedules [10]. Misalignment may extend to their dietary behavior if it does not match metabolic processes, most of which follow a circadian rhythm [7]. Hence, dietary misalignment can emerge due to a discrepancy between the biological and the social timing or result from a general mismatch of dietary intake to metabolic circadian rhythmicity, e.g., to the decrease in insulin sensitivity over the day [11,12]. It is conceivable that adolescents are vulnerable to dietary misalignment since adolescence is characterized by a pronounced "lateness" in chronotype, i.e., a preference for a delayed timing of sleep on free days [13], which may be exacerbated by the physiological insulin resistance occurring during adolescence [14]. We hence hypothesize that recurring postprandial glycemic excursions elicited by carbohydrate-containing foods with a higher GI are particularly detrimental in evening hours and will have longer-term downstream adverse effects on adult metabolic health. It is possible that these are specific to either the *relative* glycemic response to the carbohydrate-containing foods consumed in evening hours, i.e., their GI [15], to their estimated postprandial glucose and insulin responses (i.e., their GL) and/or the intake of carbohydrates from low-GI (GI < 55) or higher-GI (GI ≥ 55, thus including sources with moderate- as well as high-GI) sources (low-GI-CHO, higher-GI-CHO).

Therefore, the aim of our current analysis was to separately examine the habitual dietary GI and GL of morning and evening intake during adolescence as well as morning and evening low-GI-CHO and higher-GI-CHO intake for prospective associations with risk markers of type 2 diabetes in young adulthood. Primary outcome measures comprised established risk parameters (insulin sensitivity, hepatic steatosis index (HSI), fatty liver index (FLI) and a pro-inflammatory score). Newly emerging risk markers of type 2 diabetes (fetuin A, fibroblast growth factor 21 (FGF-21) [16], interleukin-1 receptor antagonist (IL-1ra) and omentin [17]) were considered as secondary outcomes.

2. Methods

2.1. DONALD Study

The DONALD (DOrtmund Nutritional and Anthropometric Longitudinally Designed) study is an ongoing, open cohort study conducted in Dortmund, Germany, that was previously described [18]. In brief, since 1985, detailed data on diet, growth, development, and metabolism between infancy and early adulthood have been collected from approximately 1550 healthy children. Each year, 30–35 infants are newly recruited and first examined at the ages of three or six months. Participants regularly return to the study center thereafter; assessment during adolescence is scheduled annually. Since 2005, participants aged 18+ years are requested to provide a fasting blood sample in addition to the regular examination. The study was approved by the Ethics Committee of the University of Bonn (project identification code: 098/06, date of approval 21 June 2006); all examinations are performed with written consent from the parents and/or the participants.

2.2. Dietary Assessment

Nutritional data are assessed by 3-day weighed dietary records on three consecutive days. Participants are free to choose the days of recording. Dietary records include information on the timing of meal consumption. Parents and/or participants are instructed by dietitians to weigh all consumed foods and beverages, including leftovers, to the nearest 1 g. To this end, they receive regularly calibrated electronic food scales (initially Soehnle Digita 8000 (Leifheit AG, Nassau, Germany), now WEDO digi 2000 (Werner Dorsch GmbH, Muenster/Dieburg, Germany)). When exact weighing is not possible, semi-quantitative measures (e.g., number of spoons) are allowed. Moreover, information on recipes and on the types and brands of food items consumed is requested. The dietary records are collected as well as reviewed by the dietitians and analyzed using the continuously updated in-house nutrient database LEBTAB [19]. It includes information from standard nutrient tables, product labels, or recipe simulations based on the listed ingredients and nutrients.

2.3. Blood Analysis

Venous blood samples are drawn after an overnight fast, centrifuged at 4 °C and frozen at −80 °C in the DONALD Study Center. Fasting plasma glucose was determined on a Roche/Hitachi Cobas c 311 analyzer (Basel, Switzerland). Plasma insulin concentration was measured at the Laboratory for Translational Hormone Analytics of the University of Giessen using an immunoradiometric assay (IRMA, DRG Diagnostics, Marburg, Germany). All other measurements were performed at the German Diabetes Center with assay characteristics as described [5,20–22]: plasma activities of alanine-aminotransferase (ALT), aspartate-aminotransferase (AST), gamma-glutamyltransferase (GGT), plasma triglycerides (TG) and plasma high-sensitivity C-reactive protein (hsCRP) with the Roche/Hitachi Cobas c311 analyzer (Roche diagnostics, Mannheim, Germany), plasma high-sensitivity interleukin-(IL)-6 using the Human IL-6 Quantikine HS, plasma adiponectin with the Human Total Adiponectin/Acrp30 Quantikine ELISA, serum leptin with the Leptin Quantikine ELISA, serum interleukin-1 receptor antagonist (IL-1ra) with the Human IL-1ra/IL-1F3 ELISA, plasma fibroblast growth factor (FGF-21) with the Human FGF-21 kits all from R & D Systems (Wiesbaden, Germany), serum IL-18 using the Human IL-18 ELISA kit from MBL (Nagoya, Japan), and plasma chemerin with the Human Chemerin ELISA, plasma omentin-1 with the Human Omentin-1 ELISA, plasma chemerin with the Human Chemerin ELISA and plasma fetuin-A with the Human Fetuin-A ELISA kits from BioVendor (Brno, Czech Republic).

Insulin sensitivity was assessed using the updated HOMA2 sensitivity (in %) based on fasting insulin and blood glucose [23]. Indices of hepatic steatosis were calculated as follows:

Hepatic steatosis index (HSI):

- $\text{HSI} = 8 \times \text{ALT}/\text{AST} + \text{BMI}$

  (+2, if female; +2, if diabetes mellitus, but not applied, as the DONALD study excludes participants with chronic disease) [24],
- Fatty liver index (FLI):

  $\text{FLI} = e^x/(1 + e^x) \times 100$

  with $x = 0.953 \times \ln(\text{TG}) + 0.139 \times \text{BMI} + 0.718 \times \ln(\text{GGT}) + 0.053 \times \text{waist circumference} - 15.745$ [25].

To estimate associations with chronic low-grade inflammation a pro-inflammatory score of established inflammation markers—assumed to be more predictive of inflammation than single markers [26]—was obtained by averaging inflammation markers, that were standardized (z) by sex (mean = 0, SD = 1) beforehand. To align anti-inflammatory adiponectin in the pro-inflammatory score it was multiplied by −1:

$$\text{Pro-inflammatory score} = (z\text{-hsCRP} + z\text{-IL-6} + z\text{-IL18} + z\text{-chemerin} + z\text{-adiponectin} \times (-1) + z\text{-leptin})/6.$$

2.4. Anthropometric Data

Anthropometric measurements are performed by trained nurses according to standard procedures, with the participants dressed only in underwear and barefoot. Standing height is measured to the nearest 0.1 cm (digital stadiometer: Harpenden Ltd., Crymych, UK) and body weight to the nearest 0.1 kg (electronic scale: model 753 E; Seca, Hamburg, Germany). Waist circumference is measured at the midpoint between the lower rib and the iliac crest to the nearest 0.1 cm. Measurements of skinfold thicknesses are taken on the right side of the body at the biceps, triceps, subscapular and suprailiac sites to the nearest 0.1 mm (Holtain caliper: Holtain Ltd., Crymych, UK).

From these measures, adolescent body mass index (BMI, kg/m^2) and its sex- and age-specific SD-scores (SDS) were calculated using current German BMI standards [27]. The prevalence of overweight in adolescence was calculated using standards of the International Obesity TaskForce (IOTF) [28]. Percent body fat (%BF) in adolescence and adulthood was estimated using the Slaughter [29] and the Durnin-Womersley equations [30], respectively. From these, body fat mass (kg) was calculated [(%BF $\times$ body mass)/100] and related to the square of height to obtain fat mass index (FMI, kg/m^2).

2.5. Family Characteristics

On a child's admission to the study, information on gestational characteristics and birth anthropometrics are abstracted from a standardized document (Mutterpass), given to all pregnant women in Germany. Moreover, parents are interviewed concerning the child's early life data as well as family and socio-economic characteristics at regular intervals. Additionally, parents are regularly weighed and measured using the same equipment used for participants.

2.6. Definition of Morning and Evening Intake

The definition of morning and evening was described in earlier analyses [31,32]. Briefly, for each age (year), the time between the end of the night and 11 a.m. and the time between 6 p.m. and the start of the night, respectively, was used to define morning and evening.

For estimation of morning and evening GI and GL as well as morning and evening carbohydrate intake from low- or higher-GI food sources, each carbohydrate containing food recorded in the corresponding day-time window was assigned a published GI value [33,34], based on glucose as reference food and according to a standardized procedure [35]. Carbohydrate content of each food consumed in the morning or in the evening was then multiplied by the food's GI to obtain the GL of the corresponding day-time window. Subsequently, overall morning/evening GI was obtained by dividing morning/evening GL by morning/evening carbohydrate intake. To distinguish carbohydrates from low- and higher-GI food sources, a value of 55 (cutoff proposed for low-GI foods [34]) was chosen for categorization. Accordingly, morning and evening carbohydrate intake from low-GI sources (low-GI-CHO (GI < 55) in g) and from moderate- or high-GI sources (higher-GI-CHO (GI ≥ 55) in g) was calculated.

2.7. Study Sample

Due to the open-cohort design of the study, many subjects have not yet reached young adulthood, when blood samples are taken. At the time of this analysis $N = 414$ young adults had provided at least one fasting blood sample, in which risk markers of type 2 diabetes were quantified. As only term (gestational age 37–42 weeks) singletons with a minimum birth weight of 2500 g were included in the analyses, sample size was reduced to $N = 397$. To allow estimation of morning and evening GI, GL, low-GI-CHO and higher-GI-CHO during adolescence (girls: 9–15 years, boys: 10–16 years), at least two 3-day weighed dietary records from three consecutive days were required ($N = 298$). Participants, who were identified to consistently underreport their energy intake were excluded from the study ($N = 12$, resulting in $N = 286$). In line with earlier publications [4,5] 'consistent underreporting' was defined to be present, when more than half of the available food records per participant were implausible. A 3-day weighed dietary record was considered implausible, when the total energy intake documented was inadequate in relation to the basal metabolic rate (estimated from Schofield equations [36]) using cut-offs from Goldberg et al. [37] modified for children and adolescents [38]. Finally, anthropometric measurements from adolescence and young adulthood as well as data on relevant covariates were required, resulting in analyses samples of $N = 253$ for liver steatosis outcomes, $N = 252$ for insulin sensitivity and $N = 249$ for inflammation-related outcomes. Sample sizes for insulin sensitivity and inflammation outcomes were lower because of fasting glucose concentrations below the threshold for calculation of HOMA2 sensitivity (reflecting hypoglycemia) or insufficient amounts of blood were available for determination of analytes.

2.8. Statistical Analysis

SAS procedures (SAS version 9.2, SAS Institute, Cary, NC, USA) were used for data analysis. p-values < 0.05 were considered significant. Tests for interaction indicated no sex differences for the primary outcomes, except for the relevance of evening GL for the pro-inflammatory score. Since stratified analyses for this association yielded similar non-significant results for males and females, all associations are from pooled analyses.

Characteristics of the study population are presented as medians (25th, 75th percentiles) for continuous variables and as absolute (relative) frequencies for categorical variables.

The prospective associations of morning and evening GI, GL, low-GI-CHO and higher-GI-CHO with the risk markers of type 2 diabetes were analyzed using multivariable linear regression models. To achieve normal distribution in the outcome variables, they were transformed prior to analysis using log, double-log, square root or reciprocal transformations, depending on the outcome. In addition, individual outliers which substantially interfered with normal distribution or regression modeling were winsorized, i.e., outliers were replaced by the sex-specifically closest value fitting a normal distribution. The procedure concerned IL-6 ($N = 4$), adiponectin ($N = 1$) and IL-1ra ($N = 2$). Exposures were energy-adjusted for morning and evening energy intake, respectively—except for dietary GI-using the residual method [39]. To account for sex- and age-dependent differences in nutritional intake, all variables were standardized (mean = 0, SD = 1) by sex and age (year) and averaged over the time period of adolescence. Crude models (model A) included the exposure variable as well as sex and age at blood withdrawal in adulthood. In a further step, adjusted models (model B) were constructed by individual examination of potentially influencing covariates and hierarchical inclusion [40] of those which substantially modified the exposure's regression coefficient by $\geq$10% [41] or independently predicted the outcome variable [42]. Potential confounding covariates considered for inclusion in the different hierarchical levels were (1) early life characteristics (gestational weight gain (kg), mother's age at birth (years), duration of pregnancy (weeks) and birth weight (g), first-born child (yes/no), full breastfeeding ($\geq$4 months yes/no)), (2) family and socio-economic characteristics (parental diabetes (yes/no), maternal overweight ($\geq$25 kg/m^2 yes/no), maternal educational status ($\geq$12 year of schooling yes/no), smoking in the household (yes/no)), (3) baseline characteristics (adolescent BMI-SDS, intake of saturated fatty acids (SFA, E%) and intake of animal protein (E%)). To ensure comparability, models were adjusted identically according to the strongest exposure-outcome associations for closely related outcomes (i.e., for (i) insulin sensitivity, (ii) hepatic steatosis markers (HSI, FLI, fetuin A, FGF-21) and (iii) inflammatory markers (pro-inflammatory score, IL-1ra, omentin)). For significant associations (model B), we additionally ran conditional models including waist circumferences to examine whether the observed associations are partly attributable to effects of carbohydrate nutrition on body composition. As HSI and FLI do by definition already include adult BMI and/or waist circumference, no conditional models were run for these outcomes.

3. Results

Characteristics of the study population at baseline and in young adulthood are shown in Tables 1 and 2, respectively (see Section 2.7. for selection of the sample). During adolescence, the GI and GL as well as the relative contribution of carbohydrates from low- or higher-GI sources were broadly comparable between morning and evening intake. Note that the carbohydrate content of morning intake was higher than the carbohydrate content of evening intake. In young adulthood, median age at blood withdrawal was 21 years (range 18–39 years).

Overall, **morning** GI and GL as well as morning carbohydrate intake from low- or higher-GI sources were not related to insulin sensitivity (Table S1), the primary hepatic steatosis outcomes HSI and FLI (Tables S2 and S3) or the pro-inflammatory score (Table 3, top) in young adulthood (all $p > 0.1$). Of note, low-GI-CHO intake during the morning was related to HSI in model A ($p = 0.041$), however, upon further adjustment this association was no longer statistically significant (Table S2, model B, $p = 0.24$). Morning exposures were neither related to the secondary outcomes fetuin A (Table S4), FGF-21 (Table S5), and IL-1ra (Table S6) (all $p > 0.08$). However, a higher morning GI during adolescence was associated with an increased level of the secondary outcome omentin in young adulthood ($p = 0.011$, Table S7); an association that persisted in the conditional model adjusting for adult waist circumference ($p = 0.003$).

In contrast, a higher **evening** carbohydrate intake from higher-GI sources during adolescence was associated with lower insulin sensitivity in young adulthood ($p = 0.046$, Figure 1). Additional adjustment for waist circumference rendered this association non-significant ($p = 0.11$). A higher evening GI ($p = 0.003$) and a higher evening higher-GI-CHO intake ($p = 0.006$) were related to an increased HSI, whereas higher evening low-GI-CHO intake ($p = 0.009$) was associated with a lower HSI (Figure 2). Similarly, a higher evening GL ($p = 0.005$) and higher evening higher-GI-CHO intake ($p = 0.029$) were associated with increased concentrations of the secondary outcome fetuin A (Table S4); neither of these relations was explained by adult waist circumference ($p = 0.006$ and $p = 0.040$ respectively). No prospective associations of evening intakes were observed with the primary outcomes FLI (Table S3) and the pro-inflammatory score (Table 3, bottom), or with the secondary outcomes FGF-21 (Table S5), IL-1ra (Table S6) and omentin (Table S7) (all $p > 0.01$).

Table 1. Baseline sample characteristics [1] ($N = 252$).

General Characteristics	
Sex ♀ (n (%))	130 (51.6)
Mean age (years)	12.4 (12.0; 13.0)
Early Life Factors	
Gestational weight gain (kg)	12 (10; 15)
Mothers age at gestation (years)	30.6 (28.2; 33.3)
Birth weight (g)	3450 (3130; 3810)
Duration of gestation (weeks)	40 (39; 41)
First born child (n (%))	152 (60.3)
Fully breastfed, ≥4 months (n (%))	124 (49.2)
Family Characteristics	
Parental diabetes (n (%))	9 (3.6)
Maternal overweight, ≥25 kg/m^2 (n (%))	101 (40.1)
Maternal educational status, ≥12 years of schooling (n (%))	136 (54.0)
Smoking in the household (n (%))	72 (28.6)
Body Composition during Adolescence [2]	
BMI (kg/m^2)	18.6 (16.8; 20.2)
BMI Standard Deviation Score	−0.13 (−0.87; 0.37)
FMI (kg/m^2)	3.2 (2.4; 4.5)
Overweight (n (%)) [3]	31 (12.3)
Nutrition Parameters during Adolescence [2]	
Number of 3-day dietary records per participant	7 (6; 7)
Daily energy intake (kcal)	1922 (1658; 2158)
Total carbohydrates (E% [4])	51.0 (48.4; 54.3)
Total protein (E% [4])	13.0 (12.0; 14.1)
Animal protein (E% [4])	8.1 (7.2; 9.1)
Total fat (E% [4])	35.9 (32.9; 38.1)
SFA (E% [4])	15.7 (14.1; 17.1)

Table 1. *Cont.*

Nutrition Parameters during Adolescence [2]	
Energy intake **before 11 a.m.** (kcal)	506 (418; 603)
Energy intake **before 11 a.m.** (E% [4])	26.7 (22.7; 30.7)
GI	56.2 (53.6; 58.8)
GL (g)	38.0 (32.5; 47.1)
Carbohydrates with low-GI [5] (E% [6])	21.2 (16.8; 26.6)
Carbohydrates with higher-GI [5] (E% [6])	32.6 (26.8; 37.3)
Total carbohydrates (E% [6])	54.5 (49.9; 59.6)
Total protein (E% [6])	12.0 (10.6; 13.6)
Animal protein (E% [6])	6.8 (5.3; 8.4)
Total fat (E% [6])	32.7 (28.3; 36.3)
SFA (E% [6])	15.0 (12.7; 17.6)
Energy intake **after 6 p.m.** (kcal)	580 (471; 691)
Energy intake **after 6 p.m.** (E% [4])	30.3 (26.7; 34.1)
GI	56.6 (54.3; 59.2)
GL (g)	40.2 (31.5; 49.1)
Carbohydrates with low-GI [5] (E% [6])	18.6 (14.7; 23.1)
Carbohydrates with higher-GI [5] (E% [6])	30.2 (24.8; 34.0)
Total carbohydrates (E% [6])	48.7 (44.8; 52.9)
Total protein (E% [6])	14.0 (12.3; 15.3)
Animal protein (E% [6])	9.0 (7.3; 10.5)
Total fat (E% [6])	37.1 (33.5; 40.5)
SFA (E% [6])	15.6 (14.3; 17.5)

Values are *n* (%) for categorical variables or medians (25th, 75th percentiles) for continuous variables. [1] General characteristics are shown for the sample used for diabetic risk markers only (N = 252), since samples used for risk marker of hepatic steatosis (N = 253) and inflammation (N = 249) are very similar; [2] mean over six years (♀: 9–15 years, ♂: 10–16 years); [3] includes overweight and obesity as defined by IOTF in Cole 2000 [28]; [4] % of daily energy intake; [5] distinction between carbohydrate intake from low- and higher-GI food sources with a GI of 55 as cut-off; [6] % of energy intake before 11 a.m./after 6 p.m. BMI—body mass index, FMI—fat mass index, GL—glycemic load, GI—glycemic index, SFA—saturated fatty acids.

Table 2. Sample characteristics for young adulthood [1].

	N	**Value**
General Characteristic		
Mean age at blood withdrawal (years)	252	21.0 (18.1; 24.0)
Lifestyle		
Alcohol consumption (g) [2]	197	0.3 (0.0; 6.0)
Smokers (*n* (%))	237	65 (27.4)
Body composition		
BMI (kg/m^2)	252	22.1 (20.6; 24.6)
FMI (kg/m^2)	252	5.7 (3.8; 7.2)
Overweight (*n* (%)) [3]	252	55 (21.8)
Waist circumference (cm)	252	75.9 (70.8; 80.9)
Risk markers of type 2 diabetes		
HOMA2 sensitivity (%)	252	77.1 (61.2; 99.0)
Hepatic steatosis index (HSI)	253	29.8 (27.8; 32.8)
Fatty liver index (FLI)	253	7.3 (4.6; 15.4)
Fetuin A (mg/L)	253	273 (241; 306)
FGF-21 (pg/mL)	253	83.4 (39.7; 156.6)
Pro-inflammatory score	249	−0.11 (−0.38; 0.32)
IL-1ra (pg/mL)	249	218 (169; 295)
Omentin (ng/mL)	249	379 (317; 458)

Values are *n* (%) for categorical variables and median (25th, 75th percentiles) for continuous variables. [1] General characteristics are shown for the sample used for diabetic risk markers only (N = 252), since samples used for risk marker of hepatic steatosis (N = 253) and inflammation (N = 249) are very similar; [2] estimation is based on N = 197 participants who had provided a 3-day weighed dietary record in young adulthood; [3] including all BMI $\geq$ 25.0; BMI—body mass index, FGF-21—*Fibroblast growth factor 21*, FMI—fat mass index, HOMA2—updated homeostasis model assessment for insulin sensitivity, IL-1ra—Interleukin 1 receptor antagonist.

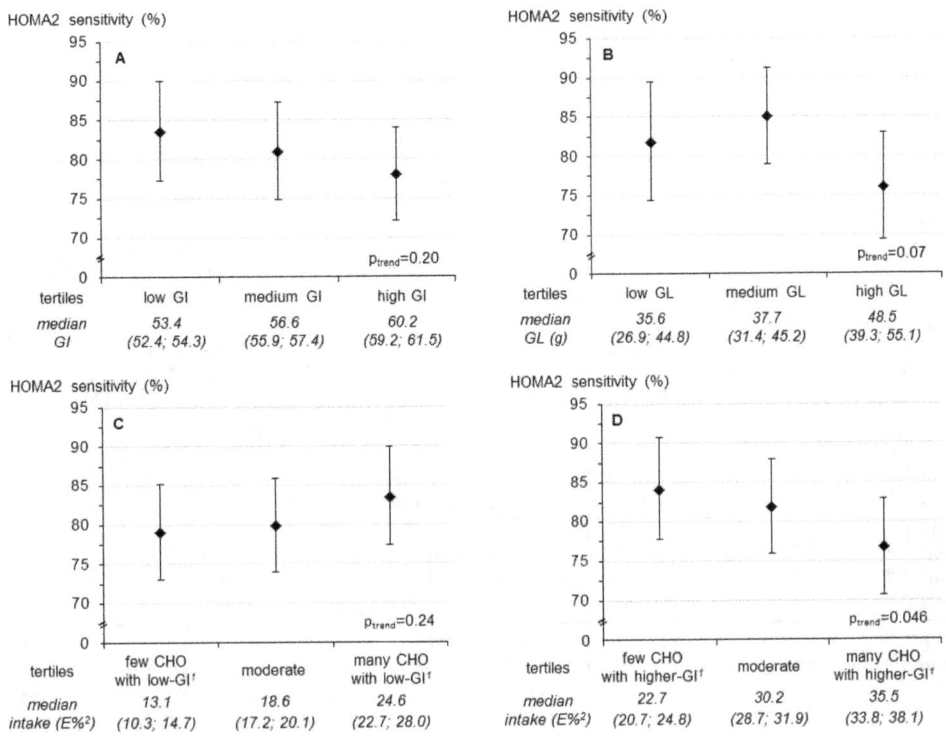

Figure 1. Predicted least square means (95% confidence interval) of **HOMA2 sensitivity** by tertiles of (**A**) glycemic index (GI) after 6 p.m., (**B**) glycemic load (GL) after 6 p.m., (**C**) intake of low-GI-CHO [1] after 6 p.m. and (**D**) intake of higher-GI-CHO [1] after 6 p.m. Values are least-square means for tertiles obtained from linear regression models. p-values are based on models using the continuous exposure variables. Models were adjusted for first born child (yes/no), baseline BMI-SDS, baseline evening intake of saturated fatty acids and animal protein ($N = 252$). Values below the figure refer to median intakes (25th; 75th percentiles) in each tertile of the respective exposure. [1] Distinction between carbohydrate intake from low- and higher-GI food sources with a GI of 55 as cut-off; [2] % of energy intake after 6 p.m.

Table 3. Prospective relation of GI and GL of morning (before 11 a.m.) and evening (after 6 p.m.) intake as well as morning and evening intake from low- and higher-GI food sources during adolescence to **pro-inflammatory score** in young adulthood ($N = 249$).

	Predicted Means [1] of Pro-Inflammatory Score by Exposure Tertiles (*Exposures: Morning and Evening GI, GL, Low-GI-CHO, Higher-GI-CHO*)			p for Trend [2]
	Low Exposure (*T1*)	Average Exposure (*T2*)	High Exposure (*T3*)	
		MORNING		
Glycemic Index (GI)				
Median GI	*52.2 (50.2; 53.8)*	*56.2 (55.2; 57.0)*	*59.5 (58.5; 60.6)*	
Model A [3]	−0.10 (−0.22; 0.03)	−0.03 (−0.15; 0.10)	−0.04 (−0.16; 0.08)	0.15
Model B [4]	−0.10 (−0.21; 0.02)	−0.04 (−0.16; 0.08)	−0.02 (−0.13; 0.10)	0.18
Glycemic Load (GL)				
Median GL	*35.7 (30.4; 41.6)*	*35.9 (30.4; 42.9)*	*45.4 (37.1; 53.9)*	
Model A [3]	−0.08 (−0.20; 0.04)	−0.02 (−0.14; 0.10)	−0.06 (−0.18; 0.06)	0.40
Model B [4]	−0.11 (−0.23; 0.02)	0.00 (−0.12; 0.12)	−0.05 (−0.17; 0.08)	0.27
CHO with low-GI [5]				
Median low-GI-CHO (E%)	*15.4 (12.4; 17.3)*	*21.4 (19.5; 23.3)*	*28.8 (26.5; 32.7)*	
Model A [3]	0.01 (−0.12; 0.14)	−0.05 (−0.17; 0.08)	−0.13 (−0.25; 0.00)	0.16
Model B [4]	−0.01 (−0.13; 0.11)	−0.03 (−0.14; 0.09)	−0.11 (−0.23; 0.00)	0.39
CHO with higher-GI [5]				
Median higher-GI-CHO (E%)	*25.0 (22.5; 27.2)*	*32.9 (31.0; 34.3)*	*38.6 (36.5; 42.8)*	
Model A [3]	−0.15 (−0.26; −0.03)	−0.06 (−0.18; 0.07)	0.04 (−0.08; 0.17)	0.06
Model B [4]	−0.14 (−0.25; −0.02)	−0.04 (−0.16; 0.08)	0.03 (−0.10; 0.15)	0.12

Table 3. *Cont.*

	Predicted Means [1] of Pro-Inflammatory Score by Exposure Tertiles *(Exposures: Morning and Evening GI, GL, Low-GI-CHO, Higher-GI-CHO)*			*p* for Trend [2]
	Low Exposure *(T1)*	Average Exposure *(T2)*	High Exposure *(T3)*	
		EVENING		
Glycemic Index (GI)				
Median GI	*53.3 (52.4; 54.3)*	*56.6 (55.9; 57.4)*	*60.2 (59.1; 61.5)*	
Model A [3]	0.04 (−0.09; 0.17)	−0.05 (−0.17; 0.08)	−0.15 (−0.27; −0.03)	0.30
Model B [4]	0.01 (−0.11; 0.13)	−0.04 (−0.16; 0.08)	−0.12 (−0.23; 0.00)	0.75
Glycemic Load (GL)				
Median GL	*34.4 (26.9; 44.8)*	*37.1 (31.3; 44.6)*	*48.5 (40.0; 55.1)*	
Model A [3]	−0.01 (−0.14; 0.12)	−0.17 (−0.29; −0.05)	0.02 (−0.10; 0.15)	0.66
Model B [4]	−0.05 (−0.18; 0.09)	−0.13 (−0.24; −0.01)	0.03 (−0.10; 0.16)	0.46
CHO with low-GI [5]				
Median low-GI-CHO (E%)	*13.1 (10.3; 14.7)*	*18.5 (17.2; 20.0)*	*24.6 (22.8; 28.2)*	
Model A [3]	−0.07 (−0.19; 0.06)	−0.06 (−0.18; 0.06)	−0.04 (−0.16; 0.09)	0.56
Model B [4]	−0.05 (−0.17; 0.08)	−0.06 (−0.18; 0.06)	−0.05 (−0.17; 0.07)	0.84
CHO with higher-GI [5]				
Median higher-GI-CHO (E%)	*22.5 (20.8; 24.9)*	*30.2 (28.8; 32.0)*	*35.4 (33.7; 38.1)*	
Model A [3]	−0.09 (−0.21; 0.03)	−0.07 (−0.19; 0.05)	0.00 (−0.12; 0.13)	0.69
Model B [4]	−0.11 (−0.23; 0.01)	−0.06 (−0.17; 0.06)	0.02 (−0.10; 0.14)	0.44

Values in italic refer to median intakes (25th, 75th percentiles) in each tertile of the respective exposure. [1] Model-values are least square means (95% confidence intervals) of pro-inflammatory score; [2] *p*-values for models are based on linear regression analyses using continuous exposure variables; [3] Model A (crude model) adjusted for sex and age at blood withdrawal; [4] Model B additionally adjusted for gestational weight gain, maternal educational status (≥12 years of schooling yes/no), baseline BMI-SDS, baseline morning or evening intake of animal protein; [5] Distinction between carbohydrate intake from low- and higher-GI food sources with a GI of 55 as cut-off.

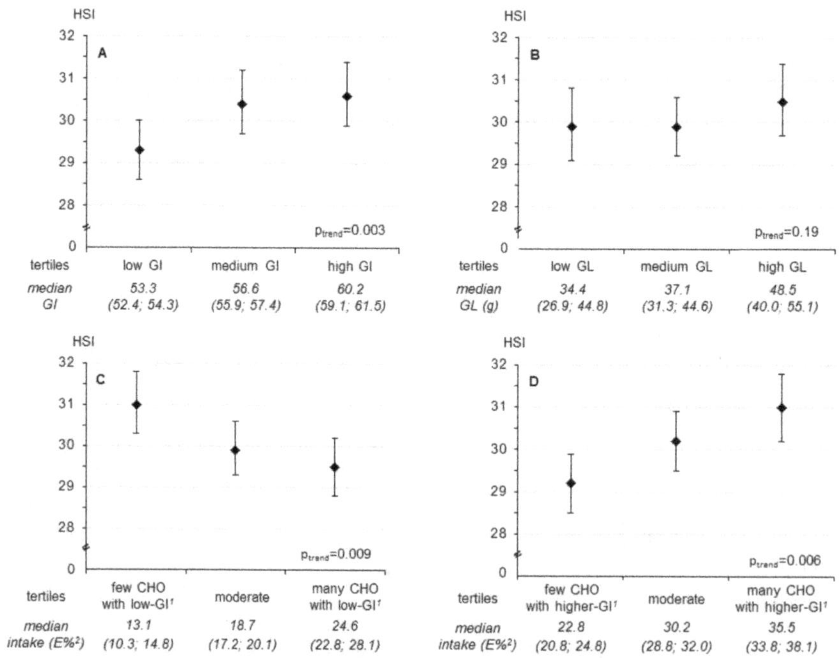

Figure 2. Predicted least square means (95% confidence interval) of **hepatic steatosis index (HSI)** by tertiles of **(A)** glycemic index (GI) after 6 p.m., **(B)** glycemic load (GL) after 6 p.m., **(C)** intake of low-GI-CHO [1] after 6 p.m. and **(D)** intake of higher-GI-CHO [1] after 6 p.m. Values are least-square means for tertiles obtained from linear regression models. *p*-values are based on models using the continuous exposure variables. Models were adjusted for sex, age at blood withdrawal, gestational weight gain, duration of pregnancy and birth weight, maternal educational status (≥12 years of schooling yes/no), maternal overweight (≥25 kg/m^2 yes/no), baseline BMI-SDS, and baseline evening intake of saturated fatty acids (*N* = 253). Values below the figure refer to median intakes (25th; 75th percentiles) in each tertile of the respective exposure. [1] Distinction between carbohydrate intake from low- and higher-GI food sources with a GI of 55 as cut-off; [2] % of energy intake after 6 p.m.

4. Discussion

The present study provides novel evidence that adverse longer-term metabolic effects of recurring postprandial glycemic excursions may be specific to evening carbohydrate consumption. Specifically, adolescents who habitually consumed more carbohydrates from higher-GI food sources in the evening had a lower insulin sensitivity and a higher HSI in young adulthood. By contrast, such adverse prospective associations were not observed for morning intakes. The absence of associations with the pro-inflammatory score suggests that day-time specific intake pattern in adolescence may not be of longer-term relevance for low-grade inflammation among young, healthy adults.

Our observation linking evening higher-GI-CHO to insulin sensitivity is in line with our hypothesis that evening rather than morning intake of higher-GI foods is potentially detrimental for risk factors of type 2 diabetes. A diurnal pattern of insulin sensitivity has been confirmed for both healthy persons [11] and participants with prediabetes [12]. The observed decrease in insulin sensitivity over the course of the day offers a plausible mechanism for our results. In line with our findings, a recent study measuring 20-h day-time profiles from 6 healthy volunteers (4 females, 2 males) reported that estimated postprandial insulin sensitivity was lowest when participants consumed 60% of their daily energy intake in the form of high-GI foods at supper [43]. In an earlier study from the same group, 8-h daytime profiles were collected from 17 middle-aged men with overweight or obesity and at least one cardiac risk factor [44]. Results revealed higher postprandial glucose and insulin responses following high-GI lunch and afternoon tea, but not high-GI breakfast compared to the corresponding low-GI meals. Upon adherence to the assigned diet over 24 days, postprandial insulin resistance had increased in the high-GI diet group compared to the low-GI diet group; thus, there was no metabolic adaptation to the high-GI diet. Our results expand on these findings in that they suggest that higher-GI-CHO habitually consumed in the evening by adolescents may have longer-term adverse consequences for adult insulin sensitivity. Our conditional model suggests that this association may be partly mediated by adult body composition. This is supported by the fact that lower glycogen synthesis over night was observed in subjects with diabetes mellitus type 2 compared to insulin-sensitive subjects [45], so that high evening higher-GI-CHO intake may shift glucose metabolites to de-novo lipogenesis and subsequent fat storage among adolescents experiencing physiological insulin resistance. Hence, future studies should also address the relevance of higher-GI-CHO consumed in the evening for body composition.

Glucose metabolism is closely linked to fatty acid metabolism; therefore insulin resistance and accumulation of fat in the liver are tightly interrelated [46]. Two studies, although heterogeneous in their methods (intervention vs observational study, extreme (dietary GI 32 vs. 84) vs. habitual low/high-GI diets and determination of liver steatosis severity by ^{1}H magnetic resonance spectroscopy and liver ultrasonography scanning, respectively), suggest that the dietary GI may be related to liver function [47,48]. However, it should be noted that imaging methods as used in these studies are time- and cost-intensive and therefore often infeasible in observational studies.

Our study used validated indices, which are preferable over the use of single liver enzyme activities in that they include more than one metabolic parameter predictive of hepatic steatosis. Our results extend existing evidence [47,48] suggesting that a higher-GI diet and an increased intake of higher-GI-CHO are both of longer-term relevance for hepatic steatosis and that these associations are specific to evening intakes.

It is important to note that HSI was shown to reflect the presence as well as the degree of hepatic steatosis [24]. The cut-off value to rule-out hepatic steatosis is 30, while the cut-off value to postulate the presence of hepatic steatosis is 36. In our healthy sample, only those in the lowest tertile of higher-GI-CHO intake had HSI levels clearly below 30, whereas those in the middle and highest tertiles had mean HSI values between 30 and 31 (Figure 2).

Similarly, albeit non-significant associations were observed with the FLI. Both HSI and FLI have similar efficacy to detect steatosis compared to an imaging method and were described as appropriate surrogate markers for epidemiological studies [49]. The two main differences between HSI and FLI are that the latter considers the activity of GGT instead of ALT and AST activities as well as TG and waist circumference in addition to BMI. In an earlier analysis of ours, dietary GI during adolescence had been related to both GGT and ALT in young adulthood [4], but a recent meta-analysis does not support an independent effect of the GI-level of diets on TG concentrations [50]. Therefore, the FLI could by definition be less responsive to the exposures under consideration in the present analysis. Yet, chance must be considered as a possible explanation as well. However, it was noted that results for fetuin A—one of our secondary outcomes, which is closely related to hepatic steatosis [16]—are in line with the findings for HSI and were independent of waist circumference.

We did not observe a relation of morning or evening GI, GL, or intake of low-GI-CHO or higher-GI-CHO to the pro-inflammatory score. In an earlier study of ours, a higher dietary GL as well as higher daily intakes of higher-GI-CHO during adolescence were associated with increased levels of IL-6, but not with hs-CRP, IL-18 or adiponectin in young adulthood [5]. Individual analyses of parameters which are included in the score confirmed these results for the current sample, albeit without an indication of a day-time specificity: Both a higher morning and a higher evening GL as well as higher intakes of morning and evening higher-GI-CHO were associated with increased adult levels of IL-6 (data not shown).

Conversely, a day-time specificity emerged for omentin. Here, higher morning GI during adolescence was associated with increased young adult omentin levels. The association was unaffected by additional adjustment for adult waist circumference. Consistent with our results, data from healthy normal weight children showed higher insulin levels and lower insulin sensitivity in children in the highest as compared to the lowest tertile of omentin [51]. As omentin is discussed to exert anti-inflammatory actions [17], we speculate that our findings may reflect an upregulation due to a habitual counter-regulatory omentin increase in response to regular pro-inflammatory signals. Indeed, a high-GI diet—regularly provoking postprandial glycemic spikes—induces increased oxidative stress [52]. In terms of the day-time specificity, it is worth noting that postprandial glycemic spikes following high GI meals are highest after breakfast compared to lunch and tea times [44].

If confirmed by other studies, our findings have several potential implications: First, the time of day when higher-GI foods are consumed is of relevance, so that a shift in focus is needed from 'what we eat' also to 'when do we eat what'. Second, our observations are based on habitual dietary intake data and reveal that the analyzed population consumed on average more than half of their morning and evening carbohydrates from higher-GI food sources, which translates into a third of their morning and evening energy intake from higher-GI food sources. Of note, those who consumed less than a quarter of their evening energy intake from higher-GI-CHO (i.e., those in the lowest tertile) had a mean HSI below 30. Hence, our data suggest that reducing higher-GI-CHO intake from a third to a quarter of energy intake in the evening offers preventive potential for adult type 2 diabetes risk. Third, the absence of a relation with morning GI, GL, low-GI-CHO or higher-GI-CHO does not justify a recommendation to shift high evening intake of high-GI foods to morning hours, as there is a possibility of adverse longer-term effects for chronic subclinical inflammation in response to habitual postprandial spikes induced in the morning. Moreover, due to the fact that the delay in chronotype (i.e., the preference for a delayed timing of sleep on free days) peaks approximately at the age of 20 years [13], encouraging morning food intake may augment circadian misalignment and would therefore be counterproductive for metabolic health in adolescents and young adults.

Our study is limited by the availability of one blood sample in young adulthood only; the use of surrogate markers of diabetes risk instead of hard end points can be considered as further limitation. However, our population was too young to have established type 2 diabetes. Moreover, it needs to be assumed that the analyzed outcomes themselves follow individual circadian rhythms [53,54] so that measurement of risk markers takes place in blood samples potentially withdrawn during the acrophase (i.e., the maximum value of one rhythm cycle) of one parameter and the bathyphase (i.e., the minimum value of one rhythm cycle) of another parameter. However, withdrawing all blood samples at the approximately same day-time, i.e., during morning hours in our study, results in a standardization of all outcome parameters to day-time. Consequently, differences in the circadian rhythm between the analytes do not affect the calculated indices (HOMA2 sensitivity, HSI, FLI, pro-inflammatory score). Concerning our dietary predictors, the GI concept is still contentious. Recent criticism relates to methodological aspects [55] and GI extrapolation to mixed meals [56]. However, the validity of dietary GI has been demonstrated repeatedly using different methodological approaches [15,57] and ISO-standardization will further reduce methodological errors in measuring the GI of foods [58]. It could be criticized that we excluded only participants who regularly under-reported their energy intake from our analyses. However, exclusion of under-reporters is controversial [59] and it should be noted that in our study only a further $N = 77$ participants had ever underreported their energy intake in any of their protocols (median: 7 protocols). Additional exclusion of these participants did not affect our results. Only the association of higher-GI-CHO with HOMA2 sensitivity was attenuated towards a trend ($p = 0.08$), which is likely attributable to the lower number of participants included in this sensitivity analysis (data not shown). Overall, our results could be subject to concerns about multiple testing. However, three separate sets of primary outcomes were considered (insulin sensitivity, hepatic steatosis, subclinical chronic inflammation) and different mechanisms are discussed for the relevance of GI, GL or CHO from low- or higher-GI sources for these outcomes. Moreover, we abstained from stressing and/or discussing findings that tended to be associated (p-values between 0.05 and <0.1). Generally, the DONALD population is characterized by a socio-economic status that is above average [18], so that extremes in nutritional behavior might not be represented. Consequently, a selection bias is likely introduced. However, the relatively homogeneous sample decreases the vulnerability of the results to residual confounding.

The overall strengths of the study are its prospective design and the detailed repeated dietary data including day-time specific nutritional information during adolescence. Due to the recruitment of study participants during infancy and the annually repeated data collection, 3-day weighed dietary records are documented by participants accustomed to the procedure. Moreover, availability of data on several important potential confounders, i.e., early-life characteristics, anthropometrics, familial and socio-economic factors strengthen our analyses.

5. Conclusions

In conclusion, our data suggest that young adult insulin sensitivity and hepatic steatosis markers are responsive to higher evening, but not morning intakes of higher-GI-CHO during adolescence, whereas there was no association with adult subclinical inflammation. Avoidance of large amounts of higher-GI-CHO in the evening and/or their replacement by low-GI-CHO during adolescence may present a promising preventive strategy to reduce risk of type 2 diabetes in adulthood.

Supplementary Materials:
Table S1: Prospective relation of GI and GL of morning (before 11 a.m.) intake as well as morning carbohydrate intake from low- and higher-GI food sources during adolescence to HOMA2 sensitivity in young adulthood ($N = 252$), Table S2: Prospective relation of GI and GL of morning (before 11 a.m.) intake as well as morning carbohydrate intake from low- and higher-GI food sources during adolescence to hepatic steatosis index (HSI) in young adulthood ($N = 253$), Table S3: Prospective relation of GI and GL of morning (before 11 a.m.) and evening (after 6 p.m.) intake as well as morning and evening intake from low- and higher-GI food sources during adolescence to fatty liver index (FLI) in young adulthood ($N = 253$), Table S4: Prospective relation of GI and GL of morning (before 11 a.m.) and evening (after 6 p.m.) intake as well as morning and evening intake from low- and higher-GI food sources during adolescence to fetuin A (mg/L) in young adulthood ($N = 253$), Table S5: Prospective relation of GI and GL of morning (before 11 a.m.) and evening (after 6 p.m.) intake as well as morning and evening intake from low- and higher-GI food sources during adolescence to fibroblast growth factor 21 (FGF-21, pg/mL) in young adulthood ($N = 253$), Table S6: Prospective relation of GI and GL of morning (before 11 a.m.) and evening (after 6 p.m.) intake as well as morning and evening intake from low- and higher-GI food sources during adolescence to interleukin 1 receptor antagonist (IL-1ra, pg/mL) in young adulthood ($N = 249$), Table S7: Prospective relation of GI and GL of morning (before 11 a.m.) and evening (after 6 p.m.) intake as well as morning and evening intake from low- and higher-GI food sources during adolescence to omentin (ng/mL) in young adulthood ($N = 249$).

Acknowledgments: This research project is funded by the German Research Foundation (Bu1807/3-1). The DONALD Study is supported by the Ministry of Science and Research of North Rhine Westphalia, Germany. With respect to the co-authorship of C.H. and M.R., the following applies: The German Diabetes Center is funded by the German Federal Ministry of Health and the Ministry of Innovation, Science, Research and Technology of the State North Rhine-Westphalia. Their participation in this project was supported in part by a grant from the German Federal Ministry of Education and Research to the German Center for Diabetes Research (DZD e.V.). We thank the staff of the DONALD study for carrying out the anthropometric measurements as well as for collecting and coding dietary records and all participants of the study for providing their data.

Author Contributions: A.E.B., U.A., C.H.: conceived the project; T.D.: conducted the statistical analysis and wrote the manuscript; A.E.B.: supervised the study, provided detailed assistance in the drafting process and had primary responsibility for the final content; C.H., M.R., S.A.W.: supervised laboratory measurements of blood analytes; all authors: made substantial contributions and read and approved the final manuscript.

References

1. Bhupathiraju, S.N.; Tobias, D.K.; Malik, V.S.; Pan, A.; Hruby, A.; Manson, J.E.; Willett, W.C.; Hu, F.B. Glycemic index, glycemic load, and risk of type 2 diabetes: Results from 3 large US cohorts and an updated meta-analysis. *Am. J. Clin. Nutr.* **2014**, *100*, 218–232. [CrossRef] [PubMed]
2. Augustin, L.S.A.; Kendall, C.W.C.; Jenkins, D.J.A.; Willett, W.C.; Astrup, A.; Barclay, A.W.; Bjorck, I.; Brand-Miller, J.C.; Brighenti, F.; Buyken, A.E.; et al. Glycemic index, glycemic load and glycemic response: An International Scientific Consensus Summit from the International Carbohydrate Quality Consortium (ICQC). *Nutr. Metab. Cardiovasc. Dis.* **2015**, *25*, 795–815. [CrossRef] [PubMed]
3. Buyken, A.E.; Mitchell, P.; Ceriello, A.; Brand-Miller, J. Optimal dietary approaches for prevention of type 2 diabetes: A life-course perspective. *Diabetologia* **2010**, *53*, 406–418. [CrossRef] [PubMed]
4. Goletzke, J.; Herder, C.; Joslowski, G.; Bolzenius, K.; Remer, T.; Wudy, S.A.; Roden, M.; Rathmann, W.; Buyken, A.E. Habitually higher dietary glycemic index during puberty is prospectively related to increased risk markers of type 2 diabetes in younger adulthood. *Diabetes Care* **2013**, *36*, 1870–1876. [CrossRef] [PubMed]
5. Goletzke, J.; Buyken, A.E.; Joslowski, G.; Bolzenius, K.; Remer, T.; Carstensen, M.; Egert, S.; Nothlings, U.; Rathmann, W.; Roden, M.; et al. Increased intake of carbohydrates from sources with a higher glycemic index and lower consumption of whole grains during puberty are prospectively associated with higher IL-6 concentrations in younger adulthood among healthy individuals. *J. Nutr.* **2014**, *144*, 1586–1593. [CrossRef] [PubMed]
6. Saponaro, C.; Gaggini, M.; Gastaldelli, A. Nonalcoholic fatty liver disease and type 2 diabetes: Common pathophysiologic mechanisms. *Curr. Diabetes Rep.* **2015**, *15*, 607. [CrossRef] [PubMed]
7. Bailey, S.M.; Udoh, U.S.; Young, M.E. Circadian regulation of metabolism. *J. Endocrinol.* **2014**, *222*, R75–R96. [CrossRef] [PubMed]
8. Scheer, F.A.J.L.; Hilton, M.F.; Mantzoros, C.S.; Shea, S.A. Adverse metabolic and cardiovascular consequences of circadian misalignment. *Proc. Natl. Acad. Sci. USA* **2009**, *106*, 4453–4458. [CrossRef] [PubMed]
9. Merikanto, I.; Lahti, T.; Puolijoki, H.; Vanhala, M.; Peltonen, M.; Laatikainen, T.; Vartiainen, E.; Salomaa, V.; Kronholm, E.; Partonen, T. Associations of chronotype and sleep with cardiovascular diseases and type 2 diabetes. *Chronobiol. Int.* **2013**, *30*, 470–477. [CrossRef] [PubMed]
10. Roenneberg, T.; Allebrandt, K.V.; Merrow, M.; Vetter, C. Social jetlag and obesity. *Curr. Boil.* **2012**, *22*, 939–943. [CrossRef] [PubMed]
11. Saad, A.; Dalla Man, C.; Nandy, D.K.; Levine, J.A.; Bharucha, A.E.; Rizza, R.A.; Basu, R.; Carter, R.E.; Cobelli, C.; Kudva, Y.C.; et al. Diurnal pattern to insulin secretion and insulin action in healthy individuals. *Diabetes* **2012**, *61*, 2691–2700. [CrossRef] [PubMed]
12. Sonnier, T.; Rood, J.; Gimble, J.M.; Peterson, C.M. Glycemic control is impaired in the evening in prediabetes through multiple diurnal rhythms. *J. Diabetes Complicat.* **2014**, *28*, 836–843. [CrossRef] [PubMed]
13. Roenneberg, T.; Kuehnle, T.; Pramstaller, P.P.; Ricken, J.; Havel, M.; Guth, A.; Merrow, M. A marker for the end of adolescence. *Curr. Boil.* **2004**, *14*, R1038–R1039. [CrossRef] [PubMed]
14. Goran, M.I.; Gower, B.A. Longitudinal study on pubertal insulin resistance. *Diabetes* **2001**, *50*, 2444–2450. [CrossRef] [PubMed]
15. Kochan, A.M.; Wolever, T.M.S.; Chetty, V.T.; Anand, S.S.; Gerstein, H.C.; Sharma, A.M. Glycemic index predicts individual glucose responses after self-selected breakfasts in free-living, abdominally obese adults. *J. Nutr.* **2012**, *142*, 27–32. [CrossRef] [PubMed]

16. Iroz, A.; Couty, J.-P.; Postic, C. Hepatokines: Unlocking the multi-organ network in metabolic diseases. *Diabetologia* **2015**, *58*, 1699–1703. [CrossRef] [PubMed]
17. Herder, C.; Carstensen, M.; Ouwens, D.M. Anti-inflammatory cytokines and risk of type 2 diabetes. *Diabetes Obes. Metab.* **2013**, *15*, 39–50. [CrossRef] [PubMed]
18. Kroke, A.; Manz, F.; Kersting, M.; Remer, T.; Sichert-Hellert, W.; Alexy, U.; Lentze, M.J. The DONALD Study. History, current status and future perspectives. *Eur. J. Nutr.* **2004**, *43*, 45–54. [CrossRef] [PubMed]
19. Sichert-Hellert, W.; Kersting, M.; Chahda, C.; Schäfer, R.; Kroke, A. German food composition database for dietary evaluations in children and adolescents. *J. Food Compos. Anal.* **2007**, *20*, 63–70. [CrossRef]
20. Herder, C.; Bongaerts, B.W.C.; Rathmann, W.; Heier, M.; Kowall, B.; Koenig, W.; Thorand, B.; Roden, M.; Meisinger, C.; Ziegler, D. Association of subclinical inflammation with polyneuropathy in the older population: KORA F4 study. *Diabetes Care* **2013**, *36*, 3663–3670. [CrossRef] [PubMed]
21. Herder, C.; Ouwens, D.M.; Carstensen, M.; Kowall, B.; Huth, C.; Meisinger, C.; Rathmann, W.; Roden, M.; Thorand, B. Adiponectin may mediate the association between omentin, circulating lipids and insulin sensitivity: Results from the KORA F4 study. *Eur. J. Endocrinol.* **2015**, *172*, 423–432. [CrossRef] [PubMed]
22. Hatziagelaki, E.; Herder, C.; Tsiavou, A.; Teichert, T.; Chounta, A.; Nowotny, P.; Pacini, G.; Dimitriadis, G.; Roden, M. Serum Chemerin Concentrations Associate with Beta-Cell Function, but Not with Insulin Resistance in Individuals with Non-Alcoholic Fatty Liver Disease (NAFLD). *PLoS ONE* **2015**, *10*, e0124935. [CrossRef] [PubMed]
23. Wallace, T.M.; Levy, J.C.; Matthews, D.R. Use and abuse of HOMA modeling. *Diabetes Care* **2004**, *27*, 1487–1495. [CrossRef] [PubMed]
24. Lee, J.-H.; Kim, D.; Kim, H.J.; Lee, C.-H.; Yang, J.I.; Kim, W.; Kim, Y.J.; Yoon, J.-H.; Cho, S.-H.; Sung, M.-W.; et al. Hepatic steatosis index: A simple screening tool reflecting nonalcoholic fatty liver disease. *Dig. Liver Dis.* **2010**, *42*, 503–508. [CrossRef] [PubMed]
25. Bedogni, G.; Bellentani, S.; Miglioli, L.; Masutti, F.; Passalacqua, M.; Castiglione, A.; Tiribelli, C. The Fatty Liver Index: A simple and accurate predictor of hepatic steatosis in the general population. *BMC Gastroenterol.* **2006**, *6*, 33. [CrossRef] [PubMed]
26. Calder, P.C. Feeding the immune system. *Proc. Nutr. Soc.* **2013**, *72*, 299–309. [CrossRef] [PubMed]
27. Robert-Koch-Institut. *Beiträge zur Gesundheitsberichterstattung des Bundes: Referenzperzentile für anthropometrische* Maßzahlen und Blutdruck aus der Studie zur Gesundheit von Kindern und Jugendlichen in Deutschland (KiGGS) 2003 bis 2006, 1st ed.; Robert-Koch-Institut: Berlin, Germany, 2011.
28. Cole, T.J.; Bellizzi, M.C.; Flegal, K.M.; Dietz, W.H. Establishing a standard definition for child overweight and obesity worldwide: International survey. *BMJ* **2000**, *320*, 1240–1243. [CrossRef] [PubMed]
29. Slaughter, M.H.; Lohman, T.G.; Boileau, R.A.; Horswill, C.A.; Stillman, R.J.; van Loan, M.D.; Bemben, D.A. Skinfold equations for estimation of body fatness in children and youth. *Hum. Boil.* **1988**, *60*, 709–723.
30. Durnin, J.V.; Womersley, J. Body fat assessed from total body density and its estimation from skinfold thickness: Measurements on 481 men and women aged from 16 to 72 years. *Br. J. Nutr.* **1974**, *32*, 77–97. [CrossRef] [PubMed]
31. Rossbach, S.; Diederichs, T.; Bolzenius, K.; Herder, C.; Buyken, A.E.; Alexy, U. Age and time trends in eating frequency and duration of nightly fasting of German children and adolescents. *Eur. J. Nutr.* **2016**. [CrossRef]
32. Diederichs, T.; Rossbach, S.; Herder, C.; Alexy, U.; Buyken, A.E. Relevance of Morning and Evening Energy and Macronutrient Intake during Childhood for Body Composition in Early Adolescence. *Nutrients* **2016**, *8*, 716. [CrossRef] [PubMed]
33. University of Sydney (Sydney, Australia). The Official Website of the Glycemic Index and GI Database. Available online: http://www.glycemicindex.com.
34. Atkinson, F.S.; Foster-Powell, K.; Brand-Miller, J.C. International tables of glycemic index and glycemic load values: 2008. *Diabetes Care* **2008**, *31*, 2281–2283. [CrossRef] [PubMed]
35. Buyken, A.E.; Dettmann, W.; Kersting, M.; Kroke, A. Glycaemic index and glycaemic load in the diet of healthy schoolchildren: Trends from 1990 to 2002, contribution of different carbohydrate sources and relationships to dietary quality. *BJN* **2005**, *94*, 796–803. [CrossRef]

36. Schofield, W.N. Predicting basal metabolic rate, new standards and review of previous work. *Hum. Nutr. Clin. Nutr.* **1985**, *39*, 5–41. [PubMed]
37. Goldberg, G.R.; Black, A.E.; Jebb, S.A.; Cole, T.J.; Murgatroyd, P.R.; Coward, W.A.; Prentice, A.M. Critical evaluation of energy intake data using fundamental principles of energy physiology: 1. Derivation of cut-off limits to identify under-recording. *Eur. J. Clin. Nutr.* **1991**, *45*, 569–581. [PubMed]
38. Sichert-Hellert, W.; Kersting, M.; Schoch, G. Underreporting of energy intake in 1 to 18 year old German children and adolescents. *Z. Ernahrungswiss.* **1998**, *37*, 242–251. [CrossRef] [PubMed]
39. Willett, W.C.; Howe, G.R.; Kushi, L.H. Adjustment for total energy intake in epidemiologic studies. *Am. J. Clin. Nutr.* **1997**, *65*, 1220S–1228S; discussion 1229S–1231S. [PubMed]
40. Victora, C.G.; Huttly, S.R.; Fuchs, S.C.; Olinto, M.T. The role of conceptual frameworks in epidemiological analysis: A hierarchical approach. *Int. J. Epidemiol.* **1997**, *26*, 224–227. [CrossRef] [PubMed]
41. Maldonado, G.; Greenland, S. Simulation study of confounder-selection strategies. *Am. J. Epidemiol.* **1993**, *138*, 923–936. [CrossRef] [PubMed]
42. Kirkwood, B.R.; Sterne, J.A.C. *Essential Medical Statistics*, 2nd ed.; Blackwell Science: Malden, MA, USA, 2003; pp. 315–342.
43. Morgan, L.M.; Shi, J.-W.; Hampton, S.M.; Frost, G. Effect of meal timing and glycaemic index on glucose control and insulin secretion in healthy volunteers. *Br. J. Nutr.* **2012**, *108*, 1286–1291. [CrossRef] [PubMed]
44. Brynes, A.E.; Mark Edwards, C.; Ghatei, M.A.; Dornhorst, A.; Morgan, L.M.; Bloom, S.R.; Frost, G.S. A randomised four-intervention crossover study investigating the effect of carbohydrates on daytime profiles of insulin, glucose, non-esterified fatty acids and triacylglycerols in middle-aged men. *Br. J. Nutr.* **2003**, *89*, 207–218. [CrossRef] [PubMed]
45. Krssak, M.; Brehm, A.; Bernroider, E.; Anderwald, C.; Nowotny, P.; Dalla Man, C.; Cobelli, C.; Cline, G.W.; Shulman, G.I.; Waldhausl, W.; et al. Alterations in postprandial hepatic glycogen metabolism in type 2 diabetes. *Diabetes* **2004**, *53*, 3048–3056. [CrossRef] [PubMed]
46. Sanders, F.W.B.; Griffin, J.L. De novo lipogenesis in the liver in health and disease: More than just a shunting yard for glucose. *Biol. Rev. Camb. Philos. Soc.* **2016**, *91*, 452–468. [CrossRef] [PubMed]
47. Valtuena, S.; Pellegrini, N.; Ardigo, D.; Del Rio, D.; Numeroso, F.; Scazzina, F.; Monti, L.; Zavaroni, I.; Brighenti, F. Dietary glycemic index and liver steatosis. *Am. J. Clin. Nutr.* **2006**, *84*, 136–142. [PubMed]
48. Bawden, S.; Stephenson, M.; Falcone, Y.; Lingaya, M.; Ciampi, E.; Hunter, K.; Bligh, F.; Schirra, J.; Taylor, M.; Morris, P.; et al. Increased liver fat and glycogen stores after consumption of high versus low glycaemic index food: A randomized crossover study. *Diabetes Obes. Metab.* **2017**, *19*, 70–77. [CrossRef] [PubMed]
49. Kahl, S.; Strassburger, K.; Nowotny, B.; Livingstone, R.; Kluppelholz, B.; Kessel, K.; Hwang, J.-H.; Giani, G.; Hoffmann, B.; Pacini, G.; et al. Comparison of liver fat indices for the diagnosis of hepatic steatosis and insulin resistance. *PLoS ONE* **2014**, *9*, e94059. [CrossRef] [PubMed]
50. Goff, L.M.; Cowland, D.E.; Hooper, L.; Frost, G.S. Low glycaemic index diets and blood lipids: A systematic review and meta-analysis of randomised controlled trials. *Nutr. Metab. Cardiovasc. Dis.* **2013**, *23*, 1–10. [CrossRef] [PubMed]
51. Prats-Puig, A.; Bassols, J.; Bargallo, E.; Mas-Parareda, M.; Ribot, R.; Soriano-Rodriguez, P.; Berengui, A.; Diaz, M.; de Zegher, F.; Ibanez, L.; et al. Toward an early marker of metabolic dysfunction: Omentin-1 in prepubertal children. *Obesity* **2011**, *19*, 1905–1907. [CrossRef] [PubMed]
52. Hu, Y.; Block, G.; Norkus, E.P.; Morrow, J.D.; Dietrich, M.; Hudes, M. Relations of glycemic index and glycemic load with plasma oxidative stress markers. *Am. J. Clin. Nutr.* **2006**, *84*, 70–76. [PubMed]
53. Rivera-Coll, A.; Fuentes-Arderiu, X.; Díez-Noguera, A. Circadian Rhythms of Serum Concentrations of 12 Enzymes of Clinical Interest. *Chronobiol. Int.* **2009**, *10*, 190–200. [CrossRef]
54. Rahman, S.A.; Castanon-Cervantes, O.; Scheer, F.A.J.L.; Shea, S.A.; Czeisler, C.A.; Davidson, A.J.; Lockley, S.W. Endogenous circadian regulation of pro-inflammatory cytokines and chemokines in the presence of bacterial lipopolysaccharide in humans. *Brain Behav. Immun.* **2015**, *47*, 4–13. [CrossRef] [PubMed]
55. Matthan, N.R.; Ausman, L.M.; Meng, H.; Tighiouart, H.; Lichtenstein, A.H. Estimating the reliability of glycemic index values and potential sources of methodological and biological variability. *Am. J. Clin. Nutr.* **2016**, *104*, 1004–1013. [CrossRef] [PubMed]
56. Meng, H.; Matthan, N.R.; Ausman, L.M.; Lichtenstein, A.H. Effect of macronutrients and fiber on postprandial glycemic responses and meal glycemic index and glycemic load value determinations. *Am. J. Clin. Nutr.* **2017**, *105*, 842–853. [CrossRef] [PubMed]

57. Fabricatore, A.N.; Ebbeling, C.B.; Wadden, T.A.; Ludwig, D.S. Continuous glucose monitoring to assess the ecologic validity of dietary glycemic index and glycemic load. *Am. J. Clin. Nutr.* **2011**, *94*, 1519–1524. [CrossRef] [PubMed]
58. International Organization for Standardization. *Food Products—Determination of the Glycaemic Index (GI) and Recommendation for Food Classification (ISO 26642:2010)*; ISO: Geneva, Switzerland, 2010.
59. Castro-Quezada, I.; Ruano-Rodriguez, C.; Ribas-Barba, L.; Serra-Majem, L. Misreporting in nutritional surveys: Methodological implications. *Nutr. Hospitalaria* **2015**, *31*, 119–127.

Effect of *n*-3 Polyunsaturated Fatty Acid Supplementation on Metabolic and Inflammatory Biomarkers in Type 2 Diabetes Mellitus Patients

M. Gorety Jacobo-Cejudo [1], Roxana Valdés-Ramos [1,*], Ana L. Guadarrama-López [1], Rosa-Virgen Pardo-Morales [2], Beatriz E. Martínez-Carrillo [1] and Laurence S. Harbige [3]

[1] Faculty of Medicine, Universidad Autónoma del Estado de México, Paseo Tollocan esq. Jesús Carranza, Col. Moderna de la Cruz, Toluca 50180, Mexico; ln_gorejace@yahoo.com.mx (M.G.J.-C.); anag3075@hotmail.com (A.L.G.-L.); martinez_elina9@hotmail.com (B.E.M.-C.)

[2] Instlituto Materno-Infantil del Estado de México, Paseo Colón s/n, Col. Villa Hogar, Toluca 50170, Mexico; rvpardo@gmail.com

[3] Faculty of Life Sciences and Computing, London Metropolitan University, 166-220 Holloway Road, London N7 8DB, UK; L.Harbige@londonmet.ac.uk

* Correspondence: rvaldesr@uaemex.mx

Abstract: Background: Type 2 diabetes mellitus (T2DM) is accompanied by chronic low-grade inflammation, with an imbalance in the secretion of adipokines and, worsening insulin resistance. Supplementation with *n*-3 PUFA in T2DM decreases inflammatory markers, the purpose of the study was to investigate the effect of *n*-3 PUFA supplementation on adipokines, metabolic control, and lipid profile in T2DM Mexican adults. Methods: In a randomized, single-blind, placebo-controlled pilot study, 54 patients with T2DM received 520 mg of DHA + EPA-enriched fish-oil (FOG) or a placebo (PG) daily. Baseline and 24-week anthropometric and biochemical measurements included glucose, insulin, glycosylated hemoglobin (Hb1Ac), leptin, adiponectin, resistin, and lipid profile; *n*-3 PUFA intake was calculated in g/day. Results: Waist circumference and blood glucose showed significant reductions in the FOG group ($p = 0.001$ and $p = 0.011$, respectively). Hb1Ac ($p = 0.009$ and $p = 0.004$), leptin ($p < 0.000$ and $p < 0.000$), and leptin/adiponectin ratio ($p < 0.000$ and $p < 0.000$) decreased significantly in both groups after 24 weeks (FOG and PG respectively). Serum resistin (FOG $p < 0.000$ and PG $p = 0.001$), insulin (FOG $p < 0.000$ and PG $p < 0.000$), and HOMA-IR (FOG $p = 0.000$ and PG $p < 0.000$) increased significantly in both groups. FOG had an overall improvement in the lipid profile with a significant decrease in triacylgycerols ($p = 0.002$) and atherogenic index ($p = 0.031$); in contrast, the PG group had increased total cholesterol ($p < 0.000$), non-HDL cholesterol ($p < 0.000$), and atherogenic index ($p = 0.017$). Conclusions: We found a beneficial effect of *n*-3 PUFA supplementation on waist circumference, glucose, Hb1Ac, leptin, leptin/adiponectin ratio, and lipid profile, without significant changes in adiponectin, and increases in resistin, insulin, and HOMA-IR in both groups.

Keywords: type 2 diabetes mellitus; adipokines; lipid profile; *n*-3 PUFAs

---

1. Introduction

Type 2 diabetes mellitus (T2DM) is one of the most prevalent chronic diseases around the world, with an increase in its prevalence due to the increase in its risk factors such as obesity and physical inactivity [1]. According to the National Health and Nutrition Survey, in 2012, in Mexico there were 6.4 million people with T2DM, which means an increase in prevalence from 7% in 2006 to 9.2% in 2012 [2]. T2DM is characterized by impaired pancreatic β-cell function that causes impaired insulin secretion and insulin resistance (IR) mainly in liver, muscle, and adipose tissue [3].

It is well recognized that the actively secreted products of adipose tissue known as adipokines can modulate different functions [4]; adipokines play a pivotal role in the regulation of whole-body metabolism, as well as in inflammatory and immune responses, and are considered a link between obesity and the development of T2DM [5].

Adiponectin is a collagen-like protein exclusively expressed in adipose tissue [6], which possesses potent antidiabetic and anti-inflammatory properties [7]. In humans, plasma adiponectin levels are closely related to whole-body insulin sensitivity [8] and are correlated negatively with IR and T2DM. Prospective and longitudinal studies have indicated that lower adiponectin levels are associated with a higher incidence of T2DM [4]. Adiponectin regulates glucose and lipid metabolism through the reduction of fat storage (lipogenesis) and the promotion of fat utilization (fatty acid oxidation) [9].

Leptin is a cytokine-like molecule secreted by adipose tissue which regulates adipose tissue mass and body weight by inhibiting food intake and stimulating energy expenditure [6], thus maintaining energy homeostasis. Leptin correlates directly with adipose tissue mass. Obesity and T2DM are associated with increased plasma leptin levels, which fail to correct hyperglycemia in these patients because of the presence of leptin resistance [5], and these elevated plasma leptin levels are associated with IR, independent of obesity and insulin sensitivity [10].

In humans, resistin is mainly secreted by macrophages and monocytes and by organs such as spleen and bone marrow [11]. Since its discovery, resistin has been related to obesity and IR in many animal experiments, but the application of these findings to human studies has been difficult to determine. However, studies in humans have shown that serum resistin levels are higher in obese patients with T2DM compared with non-diabetic obese and that mRNA levels of resistin are higher in female patients with T2DM compared to healthy women [12].

Dyslipidemias are very common in type 2 diabetes mellitus and are the cause of cardiovascular disease in uncontrolled patients. Hypertriacylglyceridemia as well as low HDL-cholesterol concentrations, together with high LDL- and non-HDL-cholesterol is a common lipid profile pattern observed in subjects with diabetes [13–16].

Eicosapentaenoic acid (EPA) and docosahexaenoic acid (DHA) are polyunsaturated fatty acids found at high levels in fish oils [17]. Accumulating evidence suggests that n-3 PUFAs from fish oil may counteract the adipokine dysregulation that occurs in obesity and its related diseases like T2DM [9], but it is not well established if the consumption of n-3 PUFAs affects circulating adiponectin, resistin, and leptin in humans; the results are inconclusive [18]. Furthermore, research in humans and animal models show a lipid normalizing effect of PUFA supplementation [19,20].

For these reasons, we undertook a pilot study with the aim of investigating the effect of a six-month supplementation trial with n-3 PUFAs on adiponectin, resistin, leptin, and the lipid profile in adults with T2DM from Toluca, Mexico.

2. Materials and Methods

2.1. Study Design

This study was a randomized, single-blind and placebo-controlled pilot study conducted in eight Urban Public Health Centers (UPHC) in Toluca, Mexico, from February to September 2015. The inclusion criteria were the following: men and women with T2DM, between 25 and 60 years, without other chronic diseases such as hypertension, arthritis, kidney disease, cancer, and HIV, with a BMI $\leq$ 29.9, without fish allergies or insulin treatment, and not lactating or pregnant.

2.2. Methods

Sixty-five Mexican subjects with T2DM were enrolled from the eight UPHC in Toluca as follows: Capultitlán (n = 1), Emiliano Zapata (n = 6), Nueva Oxtototitlán (n = 2), Reforma (21), Seminario (3), Tlacotepec (1), San Diego de los Padres (n = 16), and Ejido de la Y (n = 15). The 65 subjects were randomly and blindly separated into an experimental group (fish oil group: FOG) of 34 patients

(10 males, 24 females) and a control group (placebo group: PG) of 31 patients (5 males, 26 females). The majority of patients were medicated with Glibenclamide plus Metformin or Metformin alone and were controlled by their family practitioner, we did not give them additional dietary or lifestyle advice; we only asked them to continue with their regular medication and diet.

Written informed consent was given to all participants. The study was approved by the Research and Ethics Committee of the Universidad Autónoma del Estado de Mexico and the Institute for Health of the State of Mexico's Research and Education Coordination. The protocol was conducted following the regulations of the Helsinki Declaration of 1975 and its amendment of 2013, as well as the principles for experiments with human beings from the Nüremberg Code for medical ethics. Individual data is being maintained confidential.

Once obtained the sample, the baseline evaluation was performed as follows:

Anthropometric evaluation:

All measurements were recorded with light clothes and height without shoes by a trained nutritionist who was previously standardized. Weight was measured in a TANITA® scale (Mod. 1631) and was registered in kg; height was measured in cm using a portable SECA 206 stadiometer; the percentage of body fat was obtained by electrical bioimpedance with the same TANITA scale; body mass index (BMI) was calculated as body weight in kilograms divided by the square of height in meters. Waist and hip circumferences were measured with a Gülick™ fiberglass tape and the waist/hip ratio was calculated.

Biochemical evaluation:

After an overnight fast ($\geq$12 h), collection of a venous blood sample into an 8.5 mL tiger-top tube containing gel and clotting activator for the subsequent biochemical analysis of glucose, insulin, adipokines, and lipid profile was undertaken. Another venous blood sample in a 3 mL tube with EDTA for the analysis of glycosylated hemoglobin was also obtained.

Serum was obtained after centrifugation at 900 *g* or 3400 rpm for 10 min at 4 °C, within 30 min after blood sample collection; serum samples for glucose and lipid profile were processed within one hour, and the rest of the samples were aliquoted and stored at −80 °C until assayed.

Serum glucose, triacylglycerols, total cholesterol, HDL-cholesterol, LDL-cholesterol, and glycosylated hemoglobin levels (in total blood) were measured by enzymatic colorimetric assays in the auto-analyzer Selectra II (ROCHE™), using reagents from RANDOX™ (Cat. GL1611, Cat. Tr213, Cat. CHO215, Cat. CH3811A, Cat. CH3811B and Cat. HA3830A). Non-HDL-cholesterol was calculated by difference (total cholesterol − HDL-cholesterol).

Serum levels of insulin were measured with a Human Insulin ELISA kit from EMD Millipore Corporation® (Cat. # EZHI-14K) according to the manufacturer´s instructions. We evaluated IR with glucose and insulin concentrations using the Homeostatic model assessment as follows:

$$\text{HOMA-IR} = (\text{fasting insulin } (\mu\text{U/mL})) \times (\text{fasting glucose } (\text{mg/dL}))/405\ [21].$$

Commercially available kits from Merck Millipore® (Cat. # HADK1MAG-61K and HADK2MAG-61K) were used to measure the serum levels of adiponectin, resistin, and leptin in the Luminex® 100™ analyzer by luminometry according to the manufacturer's recommended protocols.

2.3. Supplementation

The supplementation period started after basal evaluation. Patients took two softgels per day of the assigned supplement for 24 weeks. Each 1.4 g *n*-3 PUFAs softgel contained a combination of 160 mg of eicosapentaenoic acid (EPA) with 100 mg of docosahexaenoic acid (DHA) from fish oil, so the total daily oral dose was 520 mg of *n*-3 PUFAs (320 mg of EPA and 200 mg of DHA, 2 g of total fat, 1.2 mg of vitamin E, gelatin and glycerine) during the six months of intervention. PUFA supplements were purchased from General Nutrition Centers™. The placebo softgels were identical to the *n*-3 PUFAs softgels in appearance and contained cornstarch (1 g carbohydrates and 1.7 mg of sodium per softgel).

2.4. Follow-up

After basal evaluation, patients were monitored by 6 monthly visits, in which they received their corresponding supplement and were followed-up every two weeks by telephone to make sure that they were taking their capsules, as well as to remind them not to change their habitual diet, medication, or physical activity regimes.

2.5. Diet Analysis

A trained nutritionist performed 24-h recalls, one at the beginning and one at the end of the study to analyze the diet. The dietary nutrient intake and the consumption of polyunsaturated fatty acids were calculated in grams and percentages using DIAL® (ver 3.3.2., Universidad Complutense, Madrid, Spain) software. In the final 24 h recalls of the FOG, we added the nutritional composition of *n*-3 PUFA softgels.

2.6. Statistical Analysis

Data were expressed as mean ± SD. To compare differences in the same group after intervention, paired *t*-test was used for parametric variables and Wilcoxon signed rank test for non-parametric variables. In the diet analysis, unpaired two-sample *t*-test was used to compare differences between groups in a parametric way and a Mann–Whitney U-test for non-parametric data. Normality of data was assessed by the Kolmogorov–Smirnoff test. All analyses were performed using the statistical software SPSS (version 19.0; SPSS Inc., Chicago, IL, USA). A p-value < 0.05 was considered statistically significant.

3. Results

During the study, 10 subjects, 4 in the omega-3 group and 6 in the placebo group, were eliminated for not completing the six-month supplementation for personal reasons, and the drop-out rate in both groups was less than 20%. When analyzing the causes for drop-out, it is important to note that all patients had low-education and socioeconomic levels, and even though we tried to reach them by phone or house-visits, they were not located either to follow-up or to obtain data at the end of the trial. We analyzed basal data for differences between those who dropped out and those who stayed, and there were no significant differences between groups that indicated that they stopped attending due to the variables we were evaluating.

Age, gender distribution, and diabetes duration were similar between groups without significant differences; in the FOG, 7 subjects were males, and 22 were females; in the PG, 5 subjects were males and 20 were females. The mean age of the FOG was of 50.4 ± 6.3 years, while in the PG it was 48.1 ± 6.8 years (p = 0.208), and the average time of diabetes duration was of 6.6 ± 5.0 years in the FOG and of 6.5 ± 5.8 years in the PG (p = 0.954).

In anthropometric measurements, only the FOG showed a significant decrease in waist circumference after supplementation (p = 0.001) (Table 1). No significant changes in body weight (p = 0.250 and 0.578), BMI (p = 0.278 and 0.485), body fat (p = 0.889 and 0.614), and waist/hip ratio (p = 0.288 and 0.076) were observed in FOG and PG, respectively, after intervention.

At baseline, there was only a significant difference between groups in serum resistin levels (p = 0.006). The results of biochemical analysis are summarized in Table 2. Glucose serum levels only showed a significant decrease in FOG (p = 0.001), and there were significant reductions in glycosylated hemoglobin (p = 0.009 and p = 0.004), leptin (p = 0.000 and p = 0.000), and leptin/adiponectin ratio in both groups (FOG and PG, respectively). Adiponectin did not show significant changes (p = 0.177 for FOG and p = 0.563 for PG). Contrary to expected, resistin showed a significant increase in both groups (p = 0.000 for FOG and p = 0.001 for PG). With respect to IR, there were significant increases in insulin serum levels ($p = 0.000$ for FOG and $p = 0.000$ for PG) and in HOMA-IR ($p = 0.000$ for FOG and $p = 0.000$ for PG).

Table 1. Anthropometric measurements.

	Fish Oil Group (n = 29)			Placebo Group (n = 25)		
Variables	**Basal**	**Final**	p	**Basal**	**Final**	p
Body weight (kg)	63.0 ± 9.3	62.7 ± 9.4	0.250	60.2 ± 6.4	60.0 ± 7.3	0.578
BMI (kg/m^2)	25.6 ± 2.4	25.4 ± 2.7	0.278	26.0 ± 1.6	25.9 ± 2.0	0.485
Body fat (%)	30.9 ± 9.1	31.1 ± 7.2	0.889	29.9 + 5.3	30.4 ± 6.1	0.614
Waist circumference (cm)	86.4 ± 7.6	83.1 ± 6.2	0.001	83.2 ± 5.3	83.1 ± 6.1	0.893
Waist/hip ratio	0.89 ± 0.05	0.90 ± 0.05	0.288	0.90 ± 0.05	0.92 ± 0.04	0.076

BMI: body mass index. Paired t-test was performed to compare differences in time (before and after supplementation). A p-value < 0.05 was considered statistically significant, marked in bold numbers.

Table 2. Biochemical measurements.

	Omega-3 (n = 29)			Placebo (n = 25)		
Variables	**Basal**	**Final**	p	**Basal**	**Final**	p
Glucose (mg/dL) ‡	177.2 ± 68.4	156.1 ± 69.4	0.011	184.6 ± 71.1	183.3 ± 53.3	0.326
Glycosylated hemoglobin (%) †	9.6 ± 3.1	8.2 ± 1.9	0.009	10.0 ± 2.1	9.0 ± 1.8	0.004
Adiponectin (µg) ‡	23.6 ± 20.3	24.5 ± 13.0	0.177	22.8 ± 10.5	24.3 ± 13.3	0.563
Leptin (ng) †	21.7 ± 15.5	3.9 ± 2.5	0.000	18.4 ± 13.2	3.5 ± 2.3	0.000
Resistin (ng) ‡	30.2 ± 14.0	65.9 ± 23.4	0.000	39.2 ± 12.5	61.3 ± 20.6	0.000
Leptin/adiponectin ratio †	1.3 ± 1.2	0.24 ± 0.26	0.000	0.88 ± 0.68	0.17 ± 0.12	0.000
Insulin µU/mL ‡	7.6 ± 3.0	14.2 ± 8.2	0.000	6.5 ± 1.6	10.2 ± 3.3	0.000
HOMA-IR ‡	3.1 ± 1.3	5.3 ± 3.8	0.000	2.9 ± 1.2	4.4 ± 1.6	0.000
Total Cholesterol (mg/dL) †	203.38 ± 33.72	199.10 ± 47.63	0.542	180.32 ± 30.56	209.75 ± 36.80	0.000
Triacylglycerides (mg/dL) †	186.24 ± 85.58	137.28 ± 65.39	0.002	269.40 ± 169.30	251.20 ± 149.76	0.503
HDL-Cholesterol (mg/dL) †	43.52 ± 7.95	48.13 ± 14.59	0.076	38.35 ± 9.51	40.01 ± 9.28	0.384
LDL-Cholesterol (mg/dL) †	131.00 ± 34.66	129.82 ± 44.74	0.869	109.40 ± 34.22	127.26 ± 38.80	0.076
Non-HDL-Cholesterol (mg/dL) †	159.52 ± 31.28	150.97 ± 44.26	0.152	141.97 ± 24.98	169.74 ± 38.15	0.000
Atherogenic Index †	5.04 ± 1.77	4.37 ± 1.04	0.031	4.86 ± 1.06	5.52 ± 1.63	0.017

† Paired t-test was used for parametric variables and ‡ Wilcoxon signed rank test for non-parametric variables. A p-value ≤ 0.05 was considered statistically significant, marked in bold numbers.

Table 2 shows changes in lipid profile indicators, FOG significantly decreased triacylglycerides ($p < 0.01$) and the atherogenic index ($p < 0.05$), whereas the placebo group showed a statistically significant increase in total cholesterol ($p < 0.000$), non-HDL-cholesterol ($p < 0.000$), and the atherogenic index ($p < 0.05$).

The results of diet analysis are shown in Table 3. The FOG showed a significant increase in total omega-3 fatty acids ($p < 0.001$), particularly in EPA and DHA ($p < 0.000$); n-6 to n-3 ratio decreased from 16:1 to 10:1 ($p < 0.05$). The placebo group showed a statistically significant increase in protein and monounsaturated fatty acid intake ($p < 0.05$). No differences were found in any other nutrient analyzed.

Table 3. Diet analysis.

Variable	Omega-3 (n = 29)			Placebo (n = 25)		
	Basal	**Final**	p	**Basal**	**Final**	p
Energy (kcal/day)	1562.2 ± 387.4	1672.8 ± 665.2	0.476	1751.4 ± 479.9	1875.9 ± 698.5	0.276
Protein (g/day)	57.3 ± 17.2	59.4 ± 24.3	0.737	50.8 ± 19.4	60.5 ± 27.8	* 0.030
Carbohydrates (g/day)	192.1 ± 60.4	187.8 ± 68.8	0.729	258.2 ± 73.1	255.0 ± 104.7	0.905
Lipids (g/day)	59.5 ± 21.2	72.2 ± 38.4	0.097	54.2 ± 27.7	65.2 ± 31.1	0.092
Saturated fatty acids (g/day)	16.4 ± 7.2	19.3 ± 11.9	0.271	11.4 ± 9.0	14.7 ± 9.7	0.065
Monounsaturated fatty acids (g/day)	20.2 ± 8.2	24.6 ± 15.5	0.160	15.4 ± 10.6	22.6 ± 14.3	* 0.013
Polyunsaturated fatty acids (g/day)	13.2 ± 8.1	16.5 ± 12.7	0.197	13.2 ± 11.9	13.0 ± 6.4	0.367
Omega-3 fatty acids (g/day)	0.89 ± 0.76	1.32 ± 0.34	* 0.001	0.79 ± 1.12	0.75 ± 0.53	0.178
Omega-6 fatty acids (g/day)	10.5 ± 7.7	13.6 ± 12.0	0.221	9.4 ± 11.0	8.8 ± 5.2	0.382
$n6$:$n3$ Ratio	14:1	10:1	* 0.025	16:1	14:1	0.882
EPA (g/day)	0.077 ± 0.317	0.330 ± 0.018	* 0.000	0.016 ± 0.037	0.047 ± 0.177	0.837
DHA (g/day)	0.103 ± 0.236	0.287 ± 0.089	* 0.000	0.086 ± 0.109	0.155 ± 0.187	0.074

Mann–Whitney U test for differences between groups. * A p-value < 0.05 was considered significant, marked with bold numbers.

4. Discussion

In this study, we investigated the effect of supplementation with *n*-3 PUFAs on serum levels of adiponectin, resistin, and leptin in an adult Mexican population with T2DM.

The results of the anthropometric analysis (Table 1) are similar to the results observed in previous similar studies such as a study of supplementation with *n*-3 PUFAs in diabetic patients [22]; patients with impaired fasting glucose (IFG) or impaired glucose tolerance (IGT) [23]; and two more in women with polycystic ovarian syndrome [24,25], which regularly present insulin resistance. All of these studies showed no significant change in body weight, BMI, body fat, waist circumference, or waist/hip ratio after the supplementation period, even at higher doses of *n*-3 PUFAs and longer periods of supplementation. However, in a crossover model in which 16 T2DM patients were assigned to one of two consecutive 3.5-week periods of diabetic diets (foods rich in *n*-6 or *n*-3 PUFAs), the authors found a slight but significant reduction in body weight and BMI in both dietary periods [26]. This suggests that *n*-3 PUFAs from food are more effective in controlling body weight than *n*-3 PUFAs from supplements. In our study, supplementation with *n*-3 PUFAs for 24 weeks only helped to significantly reduce waist circumference and did not help control body weight or reduce BMI, body fat percentage, or waist/hip ratio. Furthermore, one of the studies in women with polycystic ovarian syndrome reported that effects of *n*-3 PUFAs on anthropometric measurements might be dependent on gender, age, and BMI of subjects at baseline [25].

The effect of *n*-3 PUFAs on glucose and glycosylated hemoglobin is not clear. A study of supplementation with DHA-rich fish oil in an Iranian diabetic population [27] and reviews of clinical trials of supplementation with *n*-3 PUFAs in different diabetic populations, have not found significant positive effects on glycemic control [17,28]. However, a recent study [23] showed that *n*-3 PUFA supplementation with high doses for 18 months was effective in reducing glycemia and IR in patients affected by IFG or IGT and that the regression of the condition of impaired glycemia to normoglycemia seems to be helpful in delaying the development of T2DM. Flanchs et al. showed in a review that the beneficial effects of *n*-3 PUFAs on insulin sensitivity and glucose metabolism in people with IR are dependent on factors such as disease progression and age [29]. In this study, we found a significant positive effect of *n*-3 PUFA supplementation on glycemic control (glucose and glycosylated hemoglobin), but more studies are needed to test this hypothesis because most of the beneficial effects have been shown in epidemiologic studies based on a habitual fish diet consumed for years [28].

As expected, there were significant reductions in leptin serum levels and hence in leptin/adiponectin ratio, which has been demonstrated to be related to obesity and T2DM [29]. Contrary to expectation, adiponectin did not increase significantly, while resistin increased significantly. Our results are not in line with the results observed in similar studies of supplementation with *n*-3 PUFAs in diabetes [8] and in healthy subjects with a high consumption of fish, which has shown significant increases in adiponectin serum levels after various supplementation periods [30]. As the changes in adipokine profile were similar in both groups, we cannot affirm that higher doses of *n*-3 PUFAs would have led to a decrease in leptin and leptin/adiponectin ratio because there was no lead tendency toward lower leptin concentrations in subjects with the *n*-3 PUFA supplement than in subjects with the placebo.

Our study population showed higher basal adiponectin and leptin serum levels than have been reported in other similar studies, for example, in German [31], Finnish [32], Japanese [8], Asian Indian [33], and Arabic diabetic populations [34], which is likely to be due to ethnicity. Resistin showed similar results compared with serum resistin levels of Egyptians and Japanese although slightly lower [35,36].

It has been demonstrated that weight reduction increases plasma adiponectin concentrations and improves IR [10], but in this study, possibly because there were no significant changes in body weight, there were no significant increases in serum adiponectin levels. In a study with *ob/ob* mice, the administration of recombinant adiponectin, even after the development of diabetes, significantly ameliorated hyperglycemia [37], and it has been reported that serum adiponectin levels correlate inversely with IR [5]. Plasma adiponectin levels have also been demonstrated to be negatively correlated to IR [4], but in this study, we did not find a negative correlation because adiponectin (non-significant) and HOMA-IR increased.

Leptin correlates directly with adipose tissue mass; [5] however, we did not observe a significant reduction in body weight, BMI, and body fat, despite the reduction in serum leptin levels. When we used a bivariate correlation analysis, we found that serum leptin levels showed a positive correlation with BMI ($R = 0.353$ and $p = 0.009$) and body fat percentage ($R = 0.518$ and $p = 0.000$), which is in line with the results of a similar study [5].

Leptin/adiponectin ratio showed a significant reduction in both groups related to the significant decrease in leptin levels. Leptin/adiponectin ratio was a useful measure of IR in non-diabetic white adults [38], but we did not observe a positive correlation between HOMA-IR and leptin serum levels; despite the reduction in this ratio, there was no reduction in HOMA-IR. However, these findings suggest the use of the leptin/adiponectin ratio as a useful tool to detect IR. On the other hand, resistin has been linked to obesity and IR since its discovery [12], but our results are not consistent with these findings because we found a weak negative correlation between resistin levels and HOMA-IR ($R = -0.274$ and $p = 0.045$).

Obesity is the most significant factor contributing to IR and T2DM [39], and although our patients were not obese, we found a weak but significant positive correlation between body fat percentage and HOMA-IR ($R = 0.275$ and $p = 0.046$). This factor might explain the significant increase in HOMA-IR in both groups because there was a non-significant increase in body fat percentage.

Our results are not in accordance with those of Yamamoto et al., who showed in a supplementation study with EPA in hyperlipidemic patients that IR determined by the HOMA-IR was significantly improved in the supplemented group, compared with the placebo [21]. In our study, both groups showed an increase in HOMA-IR, more studies are therefore necessary to evaluate only the EPA effect in the IR of individuals with T2DM.

Our data show an overall improvement in the lipid profile through the atherogenic index in the *n*-3 PUFA supplemented group, with an overall deterioration in the placebo group. Derosa et al. found an increase in HDL-cholesterol and a decrease in triacylglycerides after 18 months of supplementation with *n*-3 PUFA, in patients with impaired glucose metabolism [23]. While in subjects with type 2 diabetes supplemented with DHA-rich fish oil, Mansoori et al. found a decrease in triacylglycerides independently of their initial values [27]. However, several trials of supplementation with *n*-3 PUFA have not found an effect on lipid profile in adults with T2DM [40,41].

Non-HDL-cholesterol has been recommended as a sensitive proxy of the atherogenic metabolic lipid status; importantly, its values in our study population showed a non-significant decrease in the supplemented group but a highly significant increase in the placebo group. This may be considered a protective effect of *n*-3 PUFA supplementation on the lipid metabolic deterioration caused by T2DM [15,16].

With respect to diet analysis, our results are in line with those of a previous study of this group that showed that a Mexican population with T2DM had a very low intake of *n*-3 PUFAs and a high consumption of lipids, particularly saturated fatty acids [42]. According to the recommendations of the Mexican Official Standard NOM-015-SSA2-2010, for prevention, treatment, and control of diabetes mellitus [43], the mean daily energy intake of all groups was adequate, though protein and *n*-3 PUFA intake in both groups and carbohydrate intake in FOG were lower than recommendations, while the total lipid intake and saturated fatty acid intake were higher than recommendations in FOG.

It is well known that the quality of dietary fat is a key determinant of IR and that saturated and trans fatty acids decrease insulin secretion and worsen insulin sensitivity [10]; a factor which could explain the higher increase in HOMA-IR in FOG because of their higher intake of saturated fatty acids.

The quality of fat may have a significant influence on adiponectin concentrations. The data from 13 studies in a systematic review showed a modest and significant effect of *n*-3 PUFA supplementation on adiponectin concentrations [44]. Because of the very low intake of *n*-3 PUFAs in both our groups, we may not have been able to observe significant changes in adiponectin levels. *In vitro* human adipocyte studies found that EPA and DHA (100 μM) treatment for 48 h, increases adiponectin secretion, and that only EPA led to higher cellular adiponectin being introduced into the adipocytes, suggesting that the regulation of adiponectin by *n*-3 PUFAs is dose- and time-dependent and that it can be affected by the maturation stage of adipocytes [9]. However, another study of supplementation with *n*-3 PUFAs in Mexican children and adolescents with obesity and insulin resistance, showed that for *n*-3 PUFAs, the duration of treatment is not associated with the effects observed and that the dosage could be more important, which in this case would suggest that in our study the *n*-3 PUFA dose we used can be considered low [45].

It has been demonstrated that diets high in fish and flaxseed oil lower the serum phospholipid ratio of omega-6/omega-3 fatty acids and that *n*-3 PUFAs are beneficial in patients affected by inflammatory diseases. The omega 6/omega 3 ratio is of importance in health and disease; during the Paleolithic period of human evolution, there was a different balance between *n*-6 and *n*-3, but the last 150 years have seen a significant increase, as in Western diets this ratio is now in the range of 15–20:1 [46]. Because of the low intake of *n*-3 PUFAs and the increased amounts of the *n*-6 PUFA linoleic acid (and high levels found in plasma phospholipids to be published elsewhere) in our study population, the omega 6/omega 3 ratios were of 11:1 and of 13:1 in FOG and PG, respectively, very similar to Western diets [47].

Although we found a beneficial effect of EPA + DHA supplementation on waist circumference, glucose, glycosylated hemoglobin, leptin, and leptin/adiponectin ratio in this population, these beneficial effects may not have been due to the supplement alone because we observed similar results in some of these parameters between patients who took the *n*-3 PUFA supplement and those that took the placebo. Similarly, there were significant increases in resistin, serum insulin, and HOMA-IR in both groups. It is possible that some of the beneficial effects observed in both groups were due to metformin and that the combined use of *n*-3 PUFA and metformin gave rise to better outcome measures. However, the significant increase in monounsaturated fatty acids and protein in the placebo group may also have contributed to the decrease in glycosylated hemoglobin, leptin, and leptin/adiponectin ratio and the increase in resistin, insulin, and HOMA-IR in this group. Interestingly, Schwingshack et al., 2001, and McAllan et al., 2014, have reported that macronutrient quality and composition, i.e. monounsaturated fat and protein can affect some of the parameters we have measured (leptin and glycosylated hemoglobin) and in the same direction we observed for the placebo group [48,49].

5. Conclusions

Additional research is required to fully understand the associated mechanisms between *n*-3 PUFA-rich fish oil consumption and adipokine secretion/expression. The small sample size and use of metformin may have limited our findings as well as the use of a relatively low dose of *n*-3 PUFAs, so larger studies with higher doses of *n*-3 PUFAs are required to confirm and extend our findings. It would be important to measure serum levels of other adipokines related to IR and T2DM, such as visfatin and apelin, to determine if the beneficial effects of PUFA *n*-3 are sustained after the cessation of therapy and to determine if negative effects on insulin sensitivity are actually caused by the supplement. The different effects of EPA and DHA observed in some studies highlight the need to study their actions separately.

In summary and despite the limitations, our study is the first to report serum concentrations of adiponectin, resistin, and leptin and show a beneficial effect of *n*-3 PUFA supplementation on waist circumference, glucose, glycosylated hemoglobin, leptin, and leptin/adiponectin ratio and lipid profile in a group of Mexican individuals with T2DM. Supplementation with *n*-3 PUFA and *n*-3 PUFA combined with metformin both warrant further investigation in Mexican T2DM.

Acknowledgments: The project from which this article derives was funded by the Consejo Nacional de Ciencia y Tecnología (CONACyT), Scientific Development Proposals for the Attention of National Problems No. 212946. México.

Author Contributions: R.V.-R., A.L.G.-L., B.E.M.-C., and L.S.H. participated in the design and implementation of the study protocol. M.G.J.-C., R.V.-R., A.L.G.-L., and B.E.M.-C. underwent all the fieldwork, biochemical and anthropometric measurements. All authors participated in data analysis, contributed in writing the manuscript, and read and approved the final version. The present manuscript is part of the Master in Health Sciences research thesis of M.G.J.-C.

References

1. Whiting, D.R.; Guariguata, L.; Weil, C.; Shaw, J. IDF Diabetes Atlas: Global estimates of the prevalence of diabetes for 2011 and 2030. *Diabetes Res. Clin. Pract.* **2011**, *94*, 311–321. [CrossRef] [PubMed]
2. Gutiérrez, J.P.; Rivera-Dommarco, J.; Shamah-Levy, T.; Villalpando-Hernández, S.; Franco, A.C.-N.L.; Romero-Martínez, M.H.-Á.M. Encuesta Nacional de Salud y Nutrición 2012. Resultados Nacionales (Internet). Cuernavaca Morelos, México. 2012. Available online: http://ensanut.insp.mx/informes/ENSANUT2012ResultadosNacionales.pdf (accessed on 5 June 2014).
3. Kwon, H.; Pessin, J.E. Adipokines mediate inflammation and insulin resistance. *Front. Endocrinol.* **2013**, *4*, 71. [CrossRef] [PubMed]
4. Rabe, K.; Lehrke, M.; Parhofer, K.G.; Broedl, U.C. Adipokines and insulin resistance. *Mol. Med.* **2008**, *14*, 741–751. [CrossRef] [PubMed]
5. Catalán, V.; Gómez-Ambrosi, J.; Rodríguez, A.; Salvador, J.; Frühbeck, G. Adipokines in the treatment of diabetes mellitus and obesity. *Expert Opin. Pharmacother.* **2009**, *10*, 239–254. [CrossRef] [PubMed]
6. Zhang, M.; Zhao, X.; Li, M.; Cheng, H.; Hou, D.; Wen, Y.; Katherine, C.; Mi, J. Abnormal adipokines associated with various types of obesity in Chinese children and adolescents. *Biomed. Environ. Sci.* **2011**, *24*, 12–21. [PubMed]
7. Hampe, L.; Radjainia, M.; Xu, C.; Harris, P.W.; Bashiri, G.; Goldstone, D.C.; Brimble, M.A.; Wang, Y.; Mitra, A.K. Regulation and quality control of adiponectin assembly by endoplasmic reticulum chaperone ERp44. *J. Biol. Chem.* **2015**, *290*, 18111–18123. [CrossRef] [PubMed]
8. Nomura, S.; Shouzu, A.; Omoto, S.; Inami, N.; Ueba, T.; Urase, F.; Maeda, Y. Effects of eicosapentaenoic acid on endothelial cell-derived microparticles, angiopoietins and adiponectin in patients with type 2 diabetes. *J. Atheroscler. Thromb.* **2009**, *2*, 83–90. [CrossRef]
9. Martínez-Fernández, M.L.; Laiglesia, L.M.; Huerta, A.E.; Martínez, J.A.; Moreno-Aliaga, M.J. Omega-3 fatty acids and adipose tissue function in obesity and metabolic syndrome. *Prostaglandins Other Lipid Mediat.* **2015**, *121*, 24–41. [CrossRef] [PubMed]
10. Bhaswant, M.; Poudyal, H.; Brown, L. Mechanisms of enhanced insulin secretion and sensitivity with *n*-3 unsaturated fatty acids. *J. Nutr. Biochem.* **2015**, *26*, 571–584. [CrossRef] [PubMed]
11. Son, Y.M.; Ahn, S.M.; Kim, G.R.; Moon, Y.S.; Kim, S.H.; Park, Y.M.; Lee, W.K.; Min, T.S.; Han, S.H.; Yun, C.H. Resistin enhances the expansion of regulatory T cells through modulation of dendritic cells. *BMC Immunol.* **2010**, *11*, 33. [CrossRef] [PubMed]
12. Jamaluddin, M.S.; Weakley, S.M.; Yao, Q.; Chen, C. Resistin: Functional roles and therapeutic considerations for cardiovascular disease. *Br. J. Pharmacol.* **2012**, *165*, 622–632. [CrossRef] [PubMed]
13. Subramanian, S.; Chait, A. Hypertriglyceridemia secondary to obesity and diabetes. *Biochim. Biophys. Acta* **2012**, *1821*, 819–825. [CrossRef] [PubMed]
14. Wu, L.; Parhofer, K.G. Diabetic dyslipidemia. *Metabolism* **2014**, *63*, 1469–1479. [CrossRef] [PubMed]
15. Kuryan, R.E.; Jacobson, M.S.; Frank, G.R. Non-HDL-cholesterol in an adolescent diabetes population. *J. Clin. Lipidol.* **2014**, *8*, 194–198. [CrossRef] [PubMed]
16. Ram, N.; Ahmed, B.; Hashmi, F.; Jabbar, A. Importance of measuring non-HDL cholesterol in type 2 diabetes patients. *J. Pak. Med. Assoc.* **2014**, *64*, 124–128. [PubMed]
17. Nettleton, J.A.; Katz, R. *n*-3 long-chain polyunsaturated fatty acids in type 2 diabetes: A Review. *J. Am. Diet. Assoc.* **2005**, *105*, 428–440. [CrossRef] [PubMed]
18. Wu, J.H.-Y.; Cahill, L.E.; Mozaffarian, D. Effect of fish oil on circulating adiponectin: A systematic review and meta-analysis of randomized controlled trials. *J. Clin. Endocrinol. Metab.* **2013**, *98*, 2451–2459. [CrossRef] [PubMed]

19. Kamat, S.G.; Roy, R. Evaluation of the effect of *n*-3 PUFA-rich dietary fish oils on lipid profile and membrane fluidity in alloxan-induced diabetic mice (*Mus musculus*). *Mol. Cell. Biochem.* **2016**, *416*, 117–129. [CrossRef] [PubMed]
20. Christou, G.A.; Rizos, E.C.; Mpechlioulis, A.; Penzo, C.; Pacchioni, A.; Nikas, D.N. Confronting the residual cardiovascular risk beyond statins: The role of fibrates, omega-3 fatty acids, or niacin, in diabetic patients. *Curr. Pharm. Des.* **2014**, *20*, 3675–3688. [CrossRef] [PubMed]
21. Yamamoto, T.; Kajikawa, Y.; Otani, S.; Yamada, Y.; Takemoto, S.; Hirota, M.; Ikeda, M.; Iwagaki, H.; Saito, S.; Fujiwara, T. Protective effect of eicosapentaenoic acid on insulin resistance in hyperlipidemic patients and on the postoperative course of cardiac surgery patients: The possible involvement of adiponectin. *Acta Med. Okayama* **2014**, *68*, 349–361. [PubMed]
22. Malekshahi, M.A.; Saedisomeolia, A.; Djalali, M.; Djazayery, A.; Pooya, S.; Sojoudi, F. Efficacy of omega-3 fatty acid supplementation on serum levels of tumour necrosis factor alpha, C-reactive protein and interleukin-2 in type 2 diabetes mellitus patients. *Singap. Med. J.* **2012**, *53*, 615–619.
23. Derosa, G.; Cicero, A.F.; D'Angelo, A.; Borghi, C.; Maffioli, P. Effects of *n*-3 PUFAs on fasting plasma glucose and insulin resistance in patients with impaired fasting glucose or impaired glucose tolerance. *Biofactors* **2016**, *42*, 316–322. [PubMed]
24. Vargas, M.L.; Almario, R.U.; Buchan, W.; Kim, K.; Karakas, S.E. Metabolic and endocrine effects of long chain vs. essential omega-3 polyunsaturated fatty acids in polycystic ovary syndrome. *Metabolism* **2011**, *60*, 1711–1718. [CrossRef] [PubMed]
25. Mohammadi, E.; Rafraf, M.; Farzadi, L.; Asghari-Jafarabadi, M.; Sabour, S. Effects of omega-3 fatty acids supplementation on serum adiponectin levels and some metabolic risk factors in women with polycystic ovary syndrome. *Asia Pac. J. Clin. Nutr.* **2012**, *21*, 511–518. [PubMed]
26. Karlström, B.E.; Järvi, A.E.; Byberg, L.; Berglund, L.G.; Vessby, B.O. Fatty fish in the diet of patients with type 2 diabetes: Comparison of the metabolic effects of foods rich in *n*-3 and *n*-6 fatty acids. *Am. J. Clin. Nutr.* **2011**, *94*, 26–33. [CrossRef] [PubMed]
27. Mansoori, A.; Sotoudeh, G.; Djalali, M.; Eshraghian, M.R.; Keramatipour, M.; Nasli-Esfahani, E.; Shidfar, F.; Alvandi, E.; Toupchian, O.; Koohdani, F. Effect of DHA-rich fish oil on PPARγ target genes related to lipid metabolism in type 2 diabetes: A randomized, double-blind, placebo-controlled clinical trial. *J. Clin. Lipidol.* **2015**, *9*, 770–777. [CrossRef] [PubMed]
28. Hendrich, S. (*n*-3) Fatty acids: clinical trials in people with type 2 diabetes. *Adv. Nutr.* **2010**, *1*, 3–7. [CrossRef] [PubMed]
29. Flachs, P.; Rossmeisl, M.; Kopecky, J. The effect of *n*-3 fatty acids on glucose homeostasis and insulin sensitivity. *Physiol. Res.* **2014**, *63*, S93–S118. [PubMed]
30. Al-Hamodi, Z.; AL-Habori, M.; Al-Meeri, A.; Saif-Ali, R. Association of adipokines, leptin/adiponectin ratio and C-reactive protein with obesity and type 2 diabetes mellitus. *Diabetol. Metab. Syndr.* **2014**, *6*, 99. [CrossRef] [PubMed]
31. Lara, J.J.; Economou, M.; Wallace, A.M.; Rumley, A.; Lowe, G.; Slater, C.; Caslake, M.; Sattar, N.; Lean, M.E. Benefits of salmon eating on traditional and novel vascular risk factors in young, non-obese healthy subjects. *Atherosclerosis* **2007**, *193*, 213–221. [CrossRef] [PubMed]
32. Stirban, A.; Nandrean, S.; Götting, C.; Stratmann, B.; Tschoepe, D. Effects of *n*-3 polyunsaturated fatty acids (PUFAs) on circulating adiponectin and leptin in subjects with type 2 diabetes mellitus. *Horm. Metab. Res.* **2014**, *46*, 490–492. [CrossRef] [PubMed]
33. Saltevo, J.; Kautiainen, H.; Vanhala, M. Gender differences in adiponectin and low-grade inflammation among individuals with normal glucose tolerance, prediabetes, and type 2 diabetes. *Gend. Med.* **2009**, *6*, 463–470. [CrossRef] [PubMed]
34. Snehalatha, C.; Mukesh, B.; Simon, M.; Viswanathan, V.; Haffner, S.M.; Ramachandran, A. Plasma adiponectin is an independent predictor of type 2 diabetes in Asian Indians. *Diabetes Care* **2003**, *26*, 3226–3229. [CrossRef] [PubMed]
35. Alfadda, A.A. Circulating adipokines in healthy versus unhealthy overweight and obese subjects. *Int. J. Endocrinol.* **2014**, *2014*, 170434. [CrossRef] [PubMed]
36. Azab, N.; Abdel-Aziz, T.; Ahmed, A.; El-deen, I.M. Correlation of serum resistin level with insulin resistance and severity of retinopathy in type 2 diabetes mellitus. *J. Saudi Chem. Soc.* **2016**, *20*, 272–277. [CrossRef]

37. Tokuyama, Y.; Osawa, H.; Ishizuka, T.; Onuma, H.; Matsui, K.; Egashira, T.; Makino, H.; Kanatsuka, A. Serum resistin level is associated with insulin sensitivity in Japanese patients with type 2 diabetes mellitus. *Metabolism* **2007**, *56*, 693–698. [CrossRef] [PubMed]
38. Deng, Y.; Scherer, P.E. Adipokines as novel biomarkers and regulators of the metabolic syndrome. *Ann. N. Y. Acad. Sci.* **2010**, *1212*, E1–E19. [CrossRef] [PubMed]
39. Finucane, F.M.; Luan, J.; Wareham, N.J.; Sharp, S.J.; O'Rahilly, S.; Balkau, B.; Flyvbjerg, A.; Walker, M.; Hojlund, K.; Nolan, J.J.; et al. Correlation of the leptin: Adiponectin ratio with measures of insulin resistance in non-diabetic individuals. *Diabetologia* **2009**, *52*, 2345–2349. [CrossRef] [PubMed]
40. Müllner, E.; Plasser, E.; Brath, H.; Waldschütz, W.; Forster, E.; Kundi, M.; Wagner, K.H. Impact of polyunsaturated vegetable oils on adiponectin levels, glycaemia and blood lipids in individuals with type 2 diabetes: a randomised, double-blind intervention study. *J. Hum. Nutr. Diet.* **2014**, *27*, 468–478. [CrossRef] [PubMed]
41. Wong, C.Y.; Yiu, K.H.; Li, S.W.; Lee, S.; Tam, S.; Lau, C.P.; Tse, H.F. Fish-oil supplement has neutral effects on vascular and metabolic function but improves renal function in patients with Type 2 diabetes mellitus. *Diabet. Med.* **2010**, *27*, 54–60. [CrossRef] [PubMed]
42. Via, M.A.; Mechanick, J.I. Nutrition in Type 2 Diabetes and the Metabolic Syndrome. *Med. Clin. N. Am.* **2016**, *100*, 1285–1302. [CrossRef] [PubMed]
43. Guadarrama-López, A.L.; Valdés-Ramos, R.; Kaufer-Horwitz, M.; Harbige, L.S.; Contreras, I.; Martínez-Carrillo, B.E. Relationship between fatty acid habitual intake and early inflammation biomarkers in individuals with and without type 2 diabetes in Mexico. *Endocr. Metab. Immune Disord. Drug Targets* **2015**, *15*, 234–241. [CrossRef] [PubMed]
44. NORMA Oficial Mexicana NOM-015-SSA2-2010, Para la Prevención, Tratamiento y Control de la Diabetes Mellitus. Available online: http://www.salud.gob.mx/unidades/cdi/nom/m015ssa24.html (accessed on 5 June 2014).
45. Von Frankenberg, A.D.; Silva, F.M.; de Almeida, J.C.; Piccoli, V.; do Nascimento, F.V.; Sost, M.M.; Leitao, C.B.; Remonti, L.L.; Umpierre, D.; Reis, A.F.; et al. Effect of dietary lipids on circulating adiponectin: A systematic review with meta-analysis of randomised controlled trials. *Br. J. Nutr.* **2014**, *112*, 1235–1250. [CrossRef] [PubMed]
46. Juárez-López, C.; Klünder-Klünder, M.; Madrigal-Azcárate, A.; Flores-Huerta, S. Omega-3 polyunsaturated fatty acids reduce insulin resistance and triglycerides in obese children and adolescents. *Pediatr. Diabetes* **2013**, *14*, 377–383. [CrossRef] [PubMed]
47. Simopoulos, A.P. The importance of the Omega-6/Omega-3 fatty acid ratio in cardiovascular disease and other chronic diseases. *Exp. Biol. Med.* **2008**, *233*, 674–688. [CrossRef] [PubMed]
48. Schwingshackl, L.; Strasser, B.; Hoffmann, G. Effects of Monounsaturated Fatty Acids on Glycaemic Control in Patients with Abnormal Glucose Metabolism: A Systematic Review and Meta-Analysis. *Ann. Nutr. Metab.* **2011**, *58*, 290–296. [CrossRef] [PubMed]
49. McAllan, L.; Skuse, P.; Cotter, P.D.; O' Connor, P.; Cryan, J.F.; Ross, R.P.; Fitzgerald, G.; Roche, H.M.; Nilaweera, K.N. Protein Quality and the Protein to Carbohydrate Ratio within a High Fat Diet Influences Energy Balance and the Gut Microbiota in C57BL/6J Mice. *PLoS ONE* **2014**, *9*, e88904. [CrossRef] [PubMed]

13

PREVIEW: Prevention of Diabetes through Lifestyle Intervention and Population Studies in Europe and around the World: Design, Methods and Baseline Participant Description of an Adult Cohort Enrolled into a Three-Year Randomised Clinical Trial

Mikael Fogelholm [1,*], Thomas Meinert Larsen [2], Margriet Westerterp-Plantenga [3], Ian Macdonald [4], J. Alfredo Martinez [5,6], Nadka Boyadjieva [7], Sally Poppitt [8], Wolfgang Schlicht [9], Gareth Stratton [10], Jouko Sundvall [11], Tony Lam [12], Elli Jalo [1], Pia Christensen [2], Mathijs Drummen [3], Elizabeth Simpson [4], Santiago Navas-Carretero [5,6], Teodora Handjieva-Darlenska [7], Roslyn Muirhead [13], Marta P. Silvestre [8], Daniela Kahlert [14], Laura Pastor-Sanz [2], Jennie Brand-Miller [13] and Anne Raben [2]

1 Department of Food and Environmental Sciences, University of Helsinki, 00014 Helsinki, Finland; elli.jalo@helsinki.fi
2 Department of Nutrition, Exercise and Sports, Faculty of Science, University of Copenhagen, Rolighedsvej 30, Frederiksberg C, DK-1958 Copenhagen, Denmark; tml@nexs.ku.dk (T.M.L.); piach@nexs.ku.dk (P.C.); laura.pastor@adm.ku.dk (L.P.-S.); ara@nexs.ku.dk (A.R.)
3 Department of Human Biology, Maastricht University, P.O. Box 616, 6200 MD Maastricht, The Netherlands; m.westerterp@maastrichtuniversity.nl (M.W.-P.); m.drummen@maastrichtuniversity.nl (M.D.)
4 School of Life Sciences, Faculty of Medicine and Health Sciences, University of Nottingham, Nottingham NG7 2UH, UK; Ian.Macdonald@nottingham.ac.uk (I.M.); liz.simpson@nottingham.ac.uk (E.S.)
5 Center for Nutrition Research, University of Navarra, 31008 Pamplona, Spain; jalfmtz@unav.es (J.A.M.); snavas@unav.es (S.N.-C.)
6 CIBERobn, Instituto de Salud Carlos III, 28029 Madrid, Spain
7 Department of pharmacology and toxicology, Medical University of Sofia, 1431 Sofia, Bulgaria; nadkaboyadjieva@gmail.com (N.B.); teodorah@abv.bg (T.H.-D.)
8 Human Nutrition Unit, School of Biological Sciences, University of Auckland, Auckland 1024, New Zealand; s.poppitt@auckland.ac.nz (S.P.); m.silvestre@auckland.ac.nz (M.P.S.)
9 Department of Exercise and Health Sciences, University of Stuttgart, 70569 Stuttgart, Germany; wolfgang.schlicht@inspo.uni-stuttgart.de
10 School of Sport and Exercise Sciences, A.STEM Research Centre, Swansea University, Swansea SA1 8EN, UK; g.stratton@swansea.ac.uk
11 National Institute for Health and Welfare THL, 00300 Helsinki, Finland; jouko.sundvall@thl.fi
12 NetUnion sarl, Ave des Figuires 20, 1007 Lausanne, Switzerland; lam@netunion.com
13 Charles Perkins Centre, University of Sydney, Sydney 2006, Australia; roslyn.muirhead@sydney.edu.au (R.M.); jennie.brandmiller@sydney.edu.au (J.B.-M.)
14 Department of Health Science, University of Education Schwäbisch Gmünd, 73525 Gmünd, Germany; daniela.kahlert@ph-gmuend.de
* Correspondence: mikael.fogelholm@helsinki.fi

Abstract: Type-2 diabetes (T2D) is one of the fastest growing chronic diseases worldwide. The PREVIEW project has been initiated to find the most effective lifestyle (diet and physical activity) for the prevention of T2D, in overweight and obese participants with increased risk for T2D. The study is a three-year multi-centre, 2 × 2 factorial, randomised controlled trial. The impact of a high-protein, low-glycaemic index (GI) vs. moderate protein, moderate-GI diet in combination with moderate or high-intensity physical activity on the incidence of T2D and the related clinical end-points are investigated. The intervention started with a two-month weight reduction using a low-calorie diet, followed by a randomised 34-month weight maintenance phase comprising four treatment arms. Eight intervention centres are participating (Denmark, Finland, United Kingdom, The Netherlands, Spain, Bulgaria, Australia, and New Zealand). Data from blood specimens, urine, faeces, questionnaires, diaries, body composition assessments, and accelerometers are collected at months 0, 2, 6, 12, 18, 24, and 36. In total, 2326 adults were recruited. The mean age was 51.6 (SD 11.6) years, 67% were women. PREVIEW is, to date, the largest multinational trial to address the prevention of T2D in pre-diabetic adults through diet and exercise intervention. Participants will complete the final intervention in March, 2018.

Keywords: diet; protein; carbohydrate; glycaemic index; physical activity; obesity

1. Introduction

Type-2 diabetes (T2D) is a disease associated with serious comorbidities, including microvascular (retinopathy, nephropathy, neuropathy) and macrovascular (cardiovascular) events [1]. The estimated global prevalence is approximately 8% and a prediction suggests that this will increase by 55% up to the year 2035 [2,3]. An important risk factor for T2D is obesity (BMI > 30 kg/m^2) predicting a more than 10-fold increase in incidence compared to normal weight [4]. Weight gain during adulthood is also an independent risk factor for T2D [5], as are genetic inheritance, unhealthy dietary habits, and insufficient physical activity [6–8].

Long-term studies have shown benefits of a lifestyle intervention (diet and exercise), on T2D incidence in China [9], USA [10], and Finland [11]. Lifestyle change (diet, physical activity, weight loss) may reduce the incidence of T2D by 28–59% [12]. The American Diabetes Prevention Program (DPP) [13], the Finnish Diabetes Prevention Study (DPS) [14], and the Chinese Da Qing Diabetes Prevention Study [15] were all designed to produce weight loss by prescribing a higher carbohydrate (CHO) (>50 percent of energy (E%) from CHO), low-fat (<30 E%) diet approach, which reflected the understanding of a prudent diet 20 years ago. No attention was paid to glycaemic index (GI), per se, and, to date, no studies have investigated the role of GI for prevention of type-2 diabetes.

Other dietary prescriptions that produce significant and sustainable weight loss may also be effective in T2D prevention. Current international recommendations include lower ranges for CHO intake [16] and a recommendation to choose lower GI foods [17]. A combination of lower CHO (45 E%), higher protein, together with lower GI, might be the optimal diet for prevention of T2D [18], perhaps related to sustained weight loss as shown in medium term trials [19]. To date these hypotheses have not been tested in large trials of long duration [20].

The program for physical activity in the trials described above followed the international public health recommendations, that is, a total of approximately 150 min per week of moderate-intensity aerobic activities or 75 min of vigorous intensity activity [10,14]. A question, not examined in earlier studies, is whether the metabolic responses are different between higher- and lower-intensity exercise programs. Moderate-intensity exercise relies relatively more on fat oxidation, whereas vigorous-intensity exercise relies more on CHO oxidation and use of intramuscular substrates [21]. Houmard et al. found that total exercise time, not intensity or exercise energy expenditure, was associated with the greatest improvement of insulin sensitivity in obese participants [22]. However, the hypothesis that physical activity with different intensity levels may differentially affect T2D prevention has yet to be tested in any large-scale intervention.

Since obesity is a strong risk factor for T2D, any successful prevention program should be able to prevent weight regain in individuals after a significant weight loss. The high heterogeneity of dietary intervention design prevents firm conclusions being drawn regarding preferred macronutrient composition [23]. Notably a recent multi-centre trial 'DiOGenes' (Diet, Obesity, and Genes) identified a higher-protein, moderate-CHO, and low-GI diet as superior to other diets of varying macronutrient composition in preventing weight regain over six months [19] and in a smaller subset over 12 months [24], after two months of rapid weight loss.

Despite the evidence that a lifestyle program combining prudent diet, increased physical activity and weight loss reduces the risk for T2D in susceptible individuals [12], important details remain unanswered. These include the long-term effects and sustainability of diets higher in protein with a lower glycaemic load, combined with the effects of higher intensity exercise. The present paper describes PREVention of diabetes through lifestyle Intervention and population studies in Europe and around the World (PREVIEW), a large multi-centre international randomised controlled trial in adults designed to answer these questions.

2. Methods

2.1. *Aims of the Study*

The aim is to determine the effects and interactions of two diets and two physical activity programmes on the prevention of T2D in overweight, pre-diabetic adults, who have undergone a short period of significant weight loss. Our primary hypothesis is that a higher protein, lower CHO/low GI diet (based on the DiOGenes study [19]) will be superior in preventing T2D when compared with a moderate protein, higher CHO/moderate GI diet (based on the DPS and DPP studies [10,14]). We also hypothesise that high-intensity physical activity will be superior compared to moderate-intensity physical activity [25].

Each participant receives one of the two dietary programs, and one of the two physical activity programs, thus, we have four groups (high protein diet and high-intensity physical activity; moderate protein diet and high-intensity physical activity; high protein diet and moderate-intensity physical activity; moderate-protein diet and moderate-intensity physical activity). The majority of outcomes will be analysed by using these four arms. The primary endpoint and statistical power calculations are based on a two-arm design (diets compared against each other).

2.2. *Primary and Secondary Endpoints*

The primary endpoint is incidence of T2D in high vs. moderate protein diet measured over a 36-month intervention period, based on the WHO criteria [26] of either (i) oral glucose tolerance test (OGTT) with fasting plasma glucose (FPG) > 7.0 mmol/L and/or 2-h post prandial (75 g glucose load) plasma glucose $\geq$11.1 mmol/L; or (ii) T2D diagnosed by a medical doctor between the clinical investigation days (CID) of PREVIEW, by using random plasma glucose $\geq$11.1 mmol/L in the presence of symptoms of diabetes, OGTT, or glycated haemoglobin (HbA1c). Asymptomatic individuals with a single abnormal value will have to repeat the test within 2–4 weeks to confirm the T2D diagnosis. The secondary endpoints include changes in HbA1c, body weight, body mass index (BMI), waist, and thigh circumference, body composition, insulin sensitivity, including Matsuda Index [27], glucose tolerance assessed by the area under the curve during OGTT, blood pressure, serum lipids, C-reactive protein, liver enzymes, perceived quality of life and work ability, habitual well-being, sleep, chronic stress, and subjective appetite sensations.

Other endpoints assessed by sub-group studies include liver fat content using magnetic resonance imaging (MRI) and proton magnetic resonance spectroscopy (H-MRS); colorectal cancer risk assessed from faecal markers; gut microbiome community assessment from faecal collections; maximal oxygen uptake capacity (VO_2 max); urine metabolite profiles using metabolomic techniques and food reward outcomes.

2.3. *Study Setting and Design*

The PREVIEW intervention study for adult participants has eight study sites: University of Copenhagen (Denmark), University of Helsinki (Finland), University of Maastricht (The Netherlands), University of Nottingham (UK), University of Navarra (Spain), Medical University of Sofia (Bulgaria), University of Sydney (Australia), and University of Auckland (New Zealand).

The 36-month intervention consists of two phases (Figure 1): a two-month period of rapid weight reduction achieved using a commercial low-calorie diet (about 800 kcal/day), followed by a 34-month randomised lifestyle (diet and physical activity) intervention phase for weight loss maintenance.

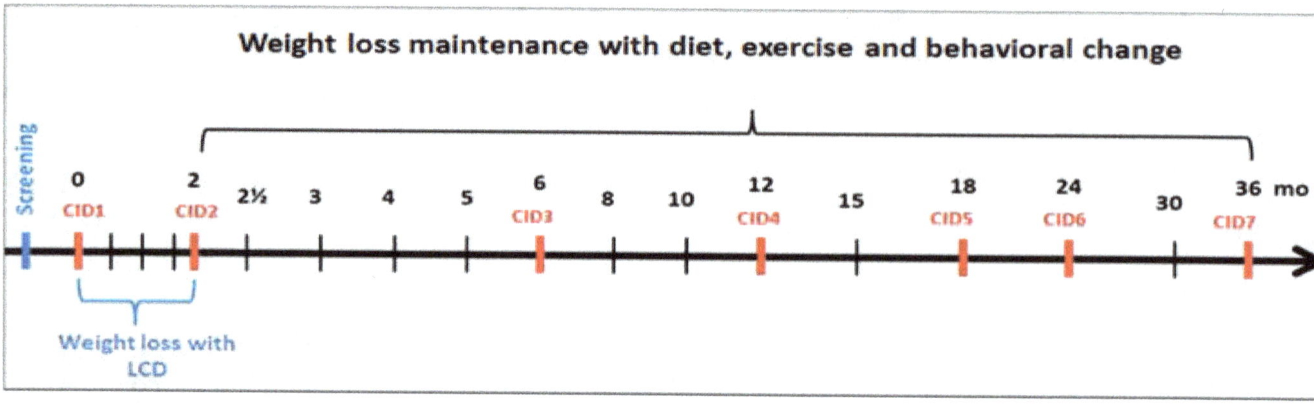

Figure 1. PREVIEW intervention: the general study design.

Clinical investigation days (CID) are conducted throughout the intervention, from CID1 (baseline) to CID7 (end of trial). At CID visits, anthropometry, blood tests, and questionnaires are performed and collection of completed diet records, accelerometers, and 24-h urine samples is done. Adverse (AE) and serious adverse events (SAE) and concomitant medications are recorded. In addition, a total of 17 group visits, leaded by instructors, are held throughout the trial to support lifestyle modification.

The CID assessments and group visits are conducted within University settings or associated Clinics. Participants follow the diet and physical activity counselling advice in a "real-life" setting without daily supervision from researchers.

2.4. Participants, Recruitment, and Randomisation

The inclusion criteria were: age 25–70 years (from mid-2013 to mid-2014 individuals aged 25–45 and 55–70 years were enrolled, and from mid-2014 onwards additionally age-group 45–54 years); BMI > 25 kg/m^2; pre-diabetes confirmed by an OGTT using the American Diabetes Association (ADA) criteria (13): (i) increased fasting glucose (IFG), with venous plasma glucose concentration of 5.6–6.9 mmol/L when fasted; and/or (ii) impaired glucose tolerance (IGT), with venous plasma glucose concentration of 7.8–11.0 mmol/L at 2 h after oral administration of standard 75 g glucose dose, and fasting plasma glucose <7.0 mmol/L. The main exclusion criteria were T2D, and any illness and/or medication with known or potential effect on compliance (e.g., unable to follow the physical activity program) or the main outcomes. A complete list of inclusion and exclusion criteria is presented as Supplementary Table S1.

Participants were recruited using multiple methods across the eight study sites, e.g., newspaper advertisements, newsletters, radio and television advertisements/interviews, and direct contact with primary and occupational health care providers. Interested individuals were contacted for the pre-screening. In the interview, inclusion and exclusion criteria were queried, including the Finnish Diabetes Risk Score [28] assessment. Potential participants were given written and oral information. Signed informed consent was required prior to commencement of laboratory screening.

The laboratory screening comprised measurements of weight, height, resting blood pressure, electrocardiography (in those aged 55 years or more), and an OGTT. A fasting blood sample was collected from the ante-cubital vein for later assessment of full inclusion and exclusion criteria, whilst glucose concentration was immediately analysed at each study site (HemoCue™, Angelholm, Sweden; Reflotron™, Roche diagnostics, Switzerland; or EML105 Radiometer, Copenhagen). Participants were then given a standard glucose drink (75 g glucose, dissolved in 300 mL water), which they had to take within 3–5 min, and a second venous blood sample was collected after 2 h. No other food or drinks or smoking were allowed and participants were required to remain sedentary during the test. The 0 and 2 h glucose concentration were used to identify those with pre-diabetes. Potentially eligible participants had fasting blood samples analysed to assess safety with haemoglobin, creatinine and alanine (ALT)/aspartate transaminase (AST).

Upon confirmation of eligibility, participants were enrolled into the trial and randomised to one of the four treatment groups. Randomisation was stratified by gender and age group (25–45, 46–54, and 55–70 years of age), and sequentially assigned from each stratum to different interventions, hence, securing an even distribution of gender and age group over the four intervention arms in each centre.

2.5. Description of Interventions

2.5.1. Low-Calorie Diet (LCD)

The trial started with a two-month (eight-week) weight reduction program using a commercial LCD, with a requirement to lose $\geq$ 8% initial body weight in order to continue to the weight maintenance phase. The LCD consisted of 3.4 MJ (800 kcal), 15–20 E% fat, 35–40 E% protein (84 g protein), and 45–50 E% CHO. The daily diet comprised of 4 $\times$ 40 g Cambridge Weight Plan® meal replacement sachets (Cambridge Weight Plan Ltd., Corby, UK), three of which were dissolved in 250 mL low fat milk ,or similar lactose-free alternatives, and one in 250 mL water. Energy-free drinks were permitted. Moreover, a maximum of 400 g of non-starchy, low-CHO vegetables, such as lettuce, asparagus, broccoli, celery, cucumber, mushrooms, radish, tomato, and watercress could be consumed.

During the LCD, participants attended group visits at weeks 2, 4, 6, and 8. Body weight, AE, SAE, and concomitant medications were recorded, LCD sachets dispensed, and dietary and behavioural instructions given. No specific instructions on physical activity were given during the LCD weight-reduction phase. Upon completion of the two months (CID2), participants who failed to reach the target weight reduction (i.e., $\geq$ 8% of initial body weight) were excluded from the intervention.

2.5.2. Weight Maintenance Phase: Intervention Diets

The two intervention diets are described in Table 1. The moderate protein (MP) diet is based on the DPS-dietary advice [14] aiming to reach a moderate protein (15 E%) and higher CHO (55 E%) macronutrient distribution with at least moderate dietary GI (>56), following current recommendations for prevention of T2D [17]. The (HP) diet has a higher protein (25 E%) and moderate CHO (45 E%) distribution with lower dietary GI (<50), based on the most successful weight-loss maintenance diet in the DiOGenes study [19]. Protein intake is higher and CHO intake is lower than the recommended range for prevention of T2D [16,17].

Both intervention diets are moderate in fat (30 E%) and the target macronutrient profile and food choices are supported by evidence for prevention of weight gain and/or T2D [8,23]. Notably, increased intake of sugar-rich foods or refined grains is not encouraged as a means to reach the higher CHO level, nor is increased consumption of red meat encouraged within the higher protein diet.

The diets are consumed ad libitum with respect to energy, with no provision of an individual target for daily energy intake. Self-monitoring of total energy consumption is not required. However, participants are instructed about controlling portion sizes of specific food types in order to achieve the macronutrient and GI prescriptions, and in self-monitoring and adjustment of portion sizes in general, in order to maintain their body weight loss. They are also encouraged to follow a regular meal pattern. Additional weight reduction is allowed, but without anything other than adherence to the maintenance diet and physical activity regimens.

The participants are given examples of daily eating plans with foods in appropriate proportions to reflect the macronutrient and GI requirements of the two interventions. A food-exchange list assists in self-selected variety, whilst preserving the required macronutrient and GI levels. Cooking books (one for each diet) with recipes suitable for all countries were specifically prepared for PREVIEW.

Table 1. Description of the PREVIEW dietary interventions.

	Higher Protein (25 E% [a]) Moderate Carbohydrate (45 E%) Low GI [b] (≤50) Diet	Moderate Protein (15 E%) Higher Carbohydrate (55 E%) Medium GI (≥56) Diet
Comparison between the groups	• Protein intake higher • Carbohydrate intake lower • GI lower	• Protein intake lower • Carbohydrate intake higher • GI medium
Food items with increased use (relative to the other group)	• Whole-grain cereals with low GI • Pasta • Low-fat dairy products • Poultry • Fish • Legumes	• Whole-grain cereals with moderate/high GI, e.g., bread • Potatoes, sweet potatoes, couscous, rice • Bananas
Similar use	• Most fruits and vegetables • Vegetable oils, margarine • Red meat (decreased in both) • Sugar-sweetened beverages (decreased in both)	

[a] E%, percentage of energy; [b] GI, glycaemic index.

2.5.3. Weight Maintenance Phase: Physical Activity Programmes

The trial has two physical activity interventions with a similar target for energy expenditure (>4.2 MJ/week, >1000 kcal/week), comprising high-intensity (HI) exercise or moderate-intensity (MI) exercise, as shown in Table 2. Measured heart rate using a heart rate monitor or wrist palpation, and/or perceived exertion using the Borg scale [29], are the principal methods of controlling the intensity. The participants may choose from several exercise options with similar level of metabolic turnover (energy expenditure divided by resting metabolic rate, i.e., MET values). The specific advice is based on the U.S. Centres for Disease Control and Prevention (CDC) recommendations of 75 min high-intensity (HI) or 150 min moderate-intensity (MI) physical activity weekly [30]. We developed a leaflet and other written instruction materials for the two PA groups. Physical activity is generally not supervised by the PREVIEW team, but participants are allowed to join supervised exercise groups of their own choice.

Table 2. Description of the physical activity interventions.

	High-Intensity Physical Activity (HI)	Moderate-Intensity Physical Activity (MI)
Heart rate	• 76–90% HRmax [a] or 61–80% HRR [b]	• 60–75% HRmax or 45–60% HRR
Examples of activities (these may vary depending on the fitness level of the participant)	• Bicycling, vigorous effort • Strenuous ball games • Aerobics with very vigorous effort, e.g., with extra weights • Jogging > 8 km/h • Swimming, vigorous effort • Cross-country skiing	• Bicycling, moderate effort • Leisurely ball games • Most conditioning exercises (aerobic, power yoga, etc.) • Brisk walking (4–6 km/h) • Swimming, recreational • Downhill skiing
Weekly duration (in total)	• at least 75 min	• at least 150 min
Recommended weekly frequency	• 2–3 times	• 3–5 times
Daily duration (guideline)	• 25–40 min	• 30–50 min (may be broken down into shorter sessions)
Additional exercises	• Muscle conditioning exercises, by using own weight: twice weekly at home, 15–20 min per session. • Stretching: twice weekly, 15–20 min per session	

[a] HRmax = max heart rate, defined as 220—age (220 in children under 16 years of age); [b] HRR = heart rate reserve, defined as the difference between measured resting HR and estimated HRmax.

A critical issue in PREVIEW is that many participants may be morbidly obese (BMI > 40) and, therefore, their ability to cope with a high-intensity exercise program is likely to be limited, and even risky. We addressed this point during the recruitments by specifically asking about perceived competence in coping with our program, and by ECG in all volunteers aged >55 years. Moreover, significant weight reduction ($\geq$ 8% of baseline body weight) during the first two months' LCD period will also simultaneously decrease the cardiovascular risks. The flexibility of our exercise program (only target energy expenditure is specified, the modes of exercise are due to the participant) is also likely to improve safety and adherence.

2.5.4. Group Visits and the Behavioural Modification Program

Group visits (8–12 individuals), are conducted throughout the three year intervention to deliver the behaviour modification information in relation to diet and physical activity [31]. There are 17 group visits, each 1–2 h, with decreasing frequency as the trial progresses. The behaviour modification programme is developed based on theories and evidence from health psychology and behaviour change [32–34]. For example, participants' beliefs about the consequences of behaviour (i.e., outcome expectancies), their intention to change their behaviour in the long run, and their belief in their ability to achieve the behaviour change goals (self-efficacy) are relevant predictors of successful behaviour change. Counsellors may apply respective behaviour change techniques [35] that are scheduled to common stages of behaviour change [36].

At the beginning of the weight-maintenance phase (i.e., month 2), the participants are instructed on how to plan, to start, and to follow the physical activity programme. In the group sessions, the participants are also instructed on basic principles of increasing physical activity and in motivational and self-regulative behaviour techniques to overcome barriers to exercise and behaviour modification. Stretching and home-based muscle-conditioning exercises are also supervised in a group-based session accompanied with written educational material [31].

2.6. Collection of Data and Description of Analyses

Data are collected from biological specimens (blood, urine, faecal), self-administered records and questionnaires, and an activity-monitoring device (ActiGraph GT3X accelerometer; ActiGraph, Pensacola, FL, USA) (see Table 3 with a description of timing). The CIDs are scheduled for a specific week and the aim is to make the measurements as precisely as scheduled. To accommodate as complete a data collection as possible we allow the following visit windows: month 2: -3 to +5 days; month 6: ± 1 weeks; month 12: ± 2 weeks; the remaining measurement points: ± 4 weeks.

Blood samples are initially stored locally at $-80\,^{\circ}$C, then transported and analysed centrally at the National Institution for Health and Welfare (THL) in Helsinki, Finland. Diet records are analysed at each site using local food composition data and software. If available, local GI data for individual food items are used, and when not available, generic global GI data are used. Accelerometer data are downloaded at local sites, and collated and analysed centrally at the Swansea University, Wales, UK.

All questionnaires used in PREVIEW were prepared in English, then translated into the local language in Finland, Denmark, The Netherlands, Spain, and Bulgaria using authorized translators. A second authorized translator then back-translated the local versions to English, with this iterative process repeated until a final version of sufficient quality was obtained.

Table 3. Overview of main data collection methods at different clinical investigation days (CID) in PREVIEW.

Outcome	Data Collection Method	Assessment Time-Points (Month)						
		0	2	6	12	18	24	36
		CID1	CID2	CID3	CID4	CID5	CID6	CID7
Glucose tolerance/diagnosis of T2D	75 g oral glucose tolerance test	×		×	×		×	×
Blood chemistry (lipid metabolism, glucose metabolism, inflammation markers, etc.)	Fasting venous blood specimen	×	×	×	×	×	×	×
Urinary nitrogen	24-h urine collection	×		×	×		×	×
Risk markers for colon cancer (e.g., Short Chain Fatty Acids)	3-day faecal collection [a]	×			×			
Gut microbiota	Faecal spot sample [a]	×			×			
Weight, height, BMI and anthropometrics	Weight; height (week 0 and 156); waist and hip circumference	×	×	×	×	×	×	×
Body composition	Body composition by DXA, BodPod or Bioelectrical impedance (BIA)	×	×	×	×		×	×
Blood pressure and resting heart rate	Resting blood pressure and heart rate	×	×	×	×	×	×	×
Nutrient intakes, dietary GI and food consumption	4-day food record	×		×	×		×	×
Physical activity	7-day accelerometer, 7-day physical activity log, Baecke questionnaire	×		×	×		×	×
Maximal oxygen uptake	VO_2 max test by ergometer or treadmill [b]	×		×			×	
Psycho-social mediators and moderators health behaviour	Several questionnaires (listed with references in Supplementary Table S2)	×	×	×	×		×	×
Eating behaviour	Three Factor Eating Questionnaire (TFEQ)	×	×	×	×		×	×
Sleeping	Epworth Sleepiness Scale (ESS), Pittsburgh Sleep Quality Index (PSQI)	×	×	×	×		×	×
Stress and mood	Perceived Stress Scale (PSS), Profile of Mood Scale (POMS)	×	×	×	×		×	×
Quality of life	WHO Quality of Life questionnaire	x			x		x	x
Work ability	Work Ability Index questionnaire	x			x		x	x
Cost-effectiveness	Questionnaire designed by the PREVIEW research group	x			x		x	x

[a] In a subgroup (n = 250) in Helsinki and Auckland; [b] In a subgroup (n = 120) in Copenhagen, Maastricht, Navarra and Nottingham.

2.7. Data Management

All data are stored in a central project database at the University of Copenhagen. The central database ensures standardized handling and storing of data and the possibility for easy extraction and delivery of data both within and after the official project period (2013–2018).

Currently, the database receives input from four data sources on a regular basis: (1) All immediate data measured (e.g., anthropometrics, blood glucose) and interviewed (e.g., use of medication) during the CIDs and entered into OpenClinica server (electronic case report form); (2) data on social-cognitive determinants of behaviour, on cultural and socio-demographics, as well as socio-economic components, are collected by the questionnaire delivery platform (QDP), designed for PREVIEW by NetUnion. The participants enter their own data into the QDP. A paper version of the questionnaires is also available; (3) physical activity is reported using the Baecke inventory, and an electronic physical activity log (PAL), designed by Swansea University, University of Stuttgart, and implemented by NetUnion; (4) the Central Lab at the National Institute for Health and Welfare (THL) enters all laboratory analyses into the data hub. Data from analyses of the ActiGraph data accelerometers, from food diaries, and from the maximal oxygen uptake (VO_2 max) analyses are imported from all sites.

2.8. Governance and Quality Management

The intervention trial is led by Prof. Fogelholm at the University of Helsinki, in collaboration with the project coordinator, Prof. Raben at the University of Copenhagen. In this large, international multi-centre trial, we are collaborating intensively to ensure data collection of high-quality and consistency of the intervention across all sites.

Specific working groups were formed with relevant site representatives. The purpose of these working groups is to discuss and agree on questions related to dietary topics, physical activity, data management, and other methodological and medical issues.

During the recruitment phase, principal investigators from each centre participated in a monthly teleconference, which continues at regular intervals throughout the intervention.

The core personnel for each site meet annually at a three-day general assembly for the full PREVIEW consortium. PREVIEW has a website [37] with both public access and a restricted area for the PREVIEW researchers.

An electronic trial master file with relevant documents has been designed and is maintained by the University of Copenhagen within the private part of the PREVIEW website. All written study material is uploaded and made available at the PREVIEW website private area, including the protocol and amendments, standard operating procedures (SOPs), and instruction materials for the intervention subjects, in order ensure that comparable methods are followed across individual sites. The SOPs are reviewed and revised as needed and also new SOPs are prepared, if necessary.

Representatives from each intervention site participated in two training sessions, each of 2–3 days duration, in 2013. One session focussed on the main study protocol, the CID protocols, and all outcome measurements (University of Copenhagen). The other session focused on instructor training in group counselling (behaviour change) methods (University of Stuttgart). Attendees then trained their local staff.

2.9. Statistical Power and Basic Analyses

The anticipated three-year incidence of T2D in the PREVIEW trial is 21%, based on data from the Finnish DPS and US DPP [10,11]. The power calculation was derived for comparison of the two dietary interventions (HP vs. MP).

It was hypothesized that a risk reduction of one quarter (1/4) in the MP group would reduce the incidence of T2D incidence from 21% to 16%, and that a risk reduction of one half (1/2) in the HP group would reduce the incidence of T2D from 21% to 10.5%. Consequently, the sample size required to detect this difference in T2D incidence (16% vs. 10.5%) was at least 649 per diet group or 1298 participants in total (for a two-sided comparison with a power (1-ß) of 80% and $p < 0.05$), with a 10% drop-out during the first 10 months from month 2 (CID2) onwards, and another 20% drop-out between months 12 (CID4) and 36 (CID7). Thus, the number of participants needed for the intervention was 1802. To allow an estimated drop-out of 25% as a result of failure to lose >8% of initial body weight during the two-month LCD period, the number of participants required to be enrolled into PREVIEW was initially estimated to be 2403.

The primary data are analysed statistically using the principle of 'intention-to-treat' (ITT cohort) and also as a completers' cohort. A 'completer' is defined as a participant who has remained in the trial for the full three year intervention period, or who has been diagnosed with T2D before the end of the intervention.

The primary outcome in the adults' trial is incidence of T2D. For statistical analysis assessing the effect of the two diets on the T2D is a 'semi-parametric Cox proportional hazards regression model'. Missing data are addressed using hot-deck imputation. Missing covariate information is addressed using multiple imputation. Sensitivity analyses (e.g., complete-case analyses without drop-outs) will be carried out to assess if censoring was informative or non-informative.

For statistical analysis of the continuous secondary outcomes (e.g., blood chemistry, anthropometrics, etc.) a 'linear mixed model' is used. For the categorical outcomes (e.g., sex, educational attainment, proportion of subjects maintaining a defined weight loss, etc.), the type of statistical analysis is 'logistic' or 'ordinal mixed-effects model'. The parameter of interest is the difference in odds ratio between the intervention groups. Although the main statistical analyses will be done by using the entire cohort, one of the most important stratified analyses will use an age-group (e.g., above and below 65 years) stratification. By comparing older against younger participants we might obtain new insight on whether dietary protein content in this respect has different effects on, e.g., body composition, weight, and clinical variables.

2.10. Ethical Issues

The study protocol and amendments were reviewed and approved by local Human Ethics Committees at all study sites. The work of PREVIEW is carried out in full compliance with the relevant requirements of the latest version of the Declaration of Helsinki (59th WMA General Assembly, Seoul, Korea, October 2008), and the ICH-GCP, The International Conference on Harmonisation (ICH) for Good Clinical Practice to the extent that this is possible and relevant. All participants provided written informed consent prior to commencing screening procedures in clinic. All information obtained during the trial is handled according to local regulations and the European Directive 95/46/CE (directive on protection of individuals with regard to the processing of personal data and on the free movement of such data). The trial is registered with ClinicalTrials.gov, NCT01777893.

3. Results

As PREVIEW is an on-going trial, only results obtained from participant screening and baseline phases are presented here. Screening was conducted from June 2013 to February 2015. On average, 35% of the pre-screened individuals were eligible for the laboratory screening. Further, 43% of the screened participants were found to be eligible for the trial. In total, 2326 overweight, pre-diabetic adults were enrolled and randomised into the trial. This was 97% of the original pre-specified target (Figure 2). Approximately half of the participants were 55–70 years at baseline (Table 4).

Baseline characteristics from blood biochemistry and anthropometric assessments are shown assigned to each intervention group in Table 5. The basic characteristics of the groups are similar. A notable feature of the participants is that the mean baseline fasting glucose concentration was approximately at the mid of the eligibility range, whereas the mean 2-h glucose concentration was at the lower cut-off point. According to the OGTT laboratory data, 1389 (62%) of all participants had increased fasting glucose at baseline, 506 (23%) had impaired glucose tolerance and 286 (13%) had both of these pre-diabetic indicators. At baseline (CID1), 25 participants (1%)—who all had been diagnosed with pre-diabetes at screening—were not diagnosed with pre-diabetes anymore. The prevalence of pre-diabetes described above were not significantly different between the four study groups.

Table 4. Number and age distribution of participants recruited for the PREVIEW intervention trial.

Site	Pre-Screened	Screened	Randomised (*n*)	Men (*n*)	Women (*n*)	Age 25–45 Years (*n*)	Age 46–54 Years (*n*)	Age 55–70 Years (*n*)	Mean Age Years (SD)
UCPH	2061	908	379	159	220	86	62	233	54.2 (10.9)
HEL	1269	633	289	88	201	39	33	221	58.2 (8.9)
UM	675	553	203	94	109	42	17	145	56.6 (10.0)
UNOTT	3914	979	264	102	162	95	42	133	51.6 (12.0)
UNAV	1740	732	307	93	214	145	82	93	47.5 (10.6)
MU	1190	488	368	87	281	190	7	158	47.8 (12.0)
UNSYD	3108	595	195	56	139	59	36	102	53.0 (10.8)
UOA	1654	584	321	77	244	156	47	103	47.0 (11.4)
Total	15,611	5472	2326	756	1570	812	326	1188	51.6 (11.6)

Abbreviations for study sites: UCPH = University of Copenhagen (Denmark); HEL = University of Helsinki (Finland); UM = Maastricht University (The Netherlands); UNOTT = University of Nottingham (UK); UNAV = University of Navarra (Spain); MU = Medical University of Sofia (Bulgaria); UNSYD = University of Sydney (Australia); UOA = University of Auckland (New Zealand).

Table 5. Number of participants, age, anthropometric results, blood chemistry, and blood pressure for all intervention groups, assessed at baseline (CID1) before weight reduction. The results are shown as the mean (±SD).

	HP: Higher Protein (25 E%) Moderate Carbohydrate (45 E%) Low GI (≤50) Diet		MP: Moderate Protein (15 E%) Higher Carbohydrate (55 E%) Medium GI (≥56) Diet	
	Moderate-Intensity Physical Activity	High-Intensity Physical Activity	Moderate-Intensity Physical Activity	High-Intensity Physical Activity
No. (men/women)	556 (184/372)	556 (177/379)	559 (180/379)	553 (179/374)
Age, years	51.6 ± 11.5	51.8 ± 11.7	51.4 ± 11.2	51.4 ± 11.8
Anthropometrics				
Height, cm	168 ± 9	168 ± 9	168 ± 9	168 ± 10
Weight, kg	99.3 ± 20.8	100.6 ± 21.0	101.6 ± 22.6	98.7 ± 20.9
Body Mass Index, kg/m^2	35.1 ± 6.5	35.6 ± 6.7	35.7 ± 6.6	35.0 ± 6.4
Waist circumference, cm	109.6 ± 15.2	111.0 ± 15.3	111.1 ± 15.4	109.6 ± 14.5
Hip circumference, cm	117.6 ± 14.5	118.8 ± 14.8	119.2 ± 13.9	117.8 ± 13.8
Body fat (% of weight)	43.0 ± 7.5	43.5 ± 7.5	43.5 ± 7.9	43.1 ± 7.8
Blood chemistry and blood pressure				
f P-glucose, mmol/L	6.2 ± 0.8	6.2 ± 0.6	6.2 ± 0.7	6.2 ± 0.8
2hP-glucose, mmol/L	7.8 ± 2.3	7.7 ± 2.25	7.5 ± 2.2	7.7 ± 2.1
fP-insulin, mU/L	13.6 ± 7.9	14.0 ± 8.7	13.2 ± 7.7	13.1 ± 7.2
HbA1c, mmol/mol	36.6 ± 3.9	36.8 ± 3.9	36.7 ± 4.2	36.7 ± 4.0
Cholesterol, mmol/L	5.2 ± 1.0	5.1 ± 1.0	5.3 ± 1.0	5.1 ± 1.0
LDL cholesterol, mmol/L	3.3 ± 0.9	3.2 ± 0.8	3.3 ± 0.9	3.2 ± 0.8
HDL cholesterol, mmol/L	1.3 ± 0.3	1.3 ± 0.3	1.3 ± 0.3	1.3 ± 0.3
Triglycerides, mmol/L	1.5 ± 0.8	1.5 ± 0.7	1.5 ± 0.9	1.5 ± 0.8
CRP, mg/L	5.3 ± 6.3	6.0 ± 8.7	5.2 ± 5.1	5.1 ± 7.5
Systolic BP, mmHg	128.5 ± 15.6	129.7 ± 16.2	128.7 ± 16.3	129.3 ± 15.5
Diastolic BP, mmHg	78.2 ± 10.9	77.6 ± 11.2	78.4 ± 11.5	78.3 ± 10.7

GI = glycaemic index; BP = blood pressure.

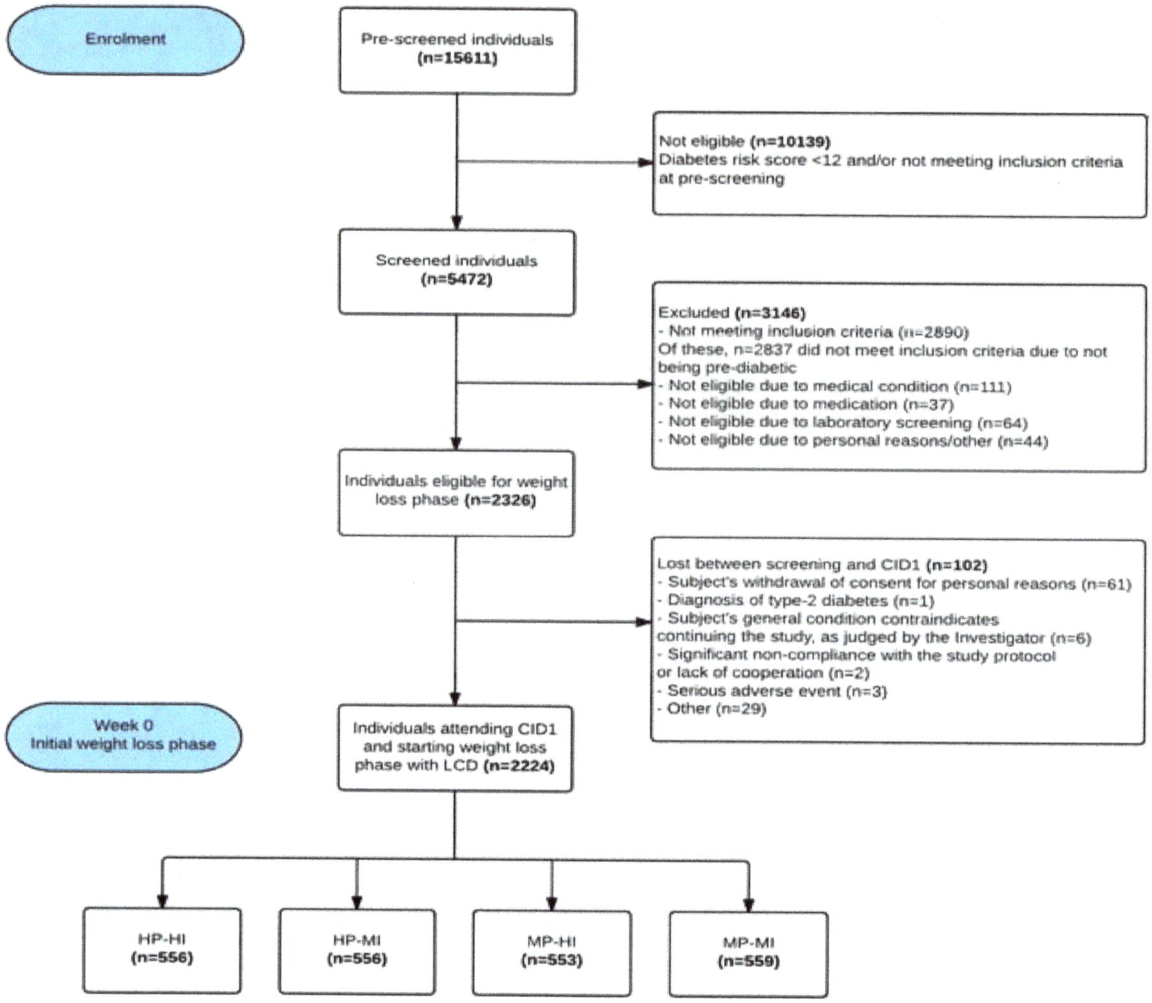

Figure 2. PREVIEW intervention: the subjects' flowchart.

4. Discussion

To our knowledge, PREVIEW is the first trial of its kind comparing two potentially effective interventions, a novel higher protein/low GI diet vs. current best practice moderate protein, higher CHO/moderate GI diet, in order to determine whether there is a more efficient lifestyle strategy to prevent T2D. Moreover, previous studies have neither used an effective weight-loss phase by LCD as a start of the intervention, nor a multi-country design.

Our inclusion criteria for "pre-diabetes" differed from the Finnish DPS. Here, IGT was an unconditional requirement without limits for IFG [14]. In the US DPP, both IGT and IFG were required [38] and the lower limit for IFG was 5.3 mmol/L (vs. 5.6 mmol/L in PREVIEW). It is unclear if the differences in diagnostic criteria between these studies have any major effects on the outcome. In addition to the diagnostic cut-offs, per se, and the distribution of results within the diagnostic criteria (i.e., above the lower and below the upper cut-off points) may have an effect on the outcome [39]. In PREVIEW, a majority of the subjects were eligible due to higher fasting blood glucose, rather than impaired glucose tolerance (higher 2-h value). A small proportion (1%) were no longer diagnosed with pre-diabetes at baseline. This may be explained by change of method (HemoCue™ or Reflotron™ at screening, or the laboratory assessment at baseline), to normal day-to-day variance in the assessed variables, or to a change in lifestyle after being accepted as a participant to PREVIEW. For future studies of T2D prevention, a single measurement of HbA1c, which is becoming the standard clinical practice in many countries may save both time and costs [40]. Still, there remains some controversy as to the utility of HbA1c when compared with standard OGTT as a diagnostic tool [41].

PREVIEW is a much larger trial than both the Finnish DPS (n = 522) [11] and Chinese Da Qing study (n = 577) [9], although smaller than the DPP (n = 3234) [10]. However, in the DPP a third of the participants received 'Metformin' in addition to dietary advice; hence, the number of participants without medical treatment, but adhering to lifestyle intervention (diet and physical activity) was 2161, which is similar to PREVIEW. Of the above interventions, the geographical and ethnic variation is greatest in PREVIEW. The age-range of participants in DPP and DPS was 33–67 years, slightly narrower than in PREVIEW, but the mean age of participants is similar across the studies (50–55 years). The large proportion of older participants in PREVIEW, (>55 years), was expected since the risk for T2D increases with age [2], and due to the growing health consciousness of this age group, many of whom are retired and have the time to participate in a demanding intervention. The smaller proportion of middle age-adults is also explained by later initiation of recruitment in this age group, compared with younger and older participants. In general, finding an adequate number of pre-diabetic subjects was a real challenge in most countries, given the "hidden" status of this condition. Thus, recruitment took about three times as long as planned from the beginning of the project.

One major challenge in PREVIEW is related to adherence to the diet and physical activity programs. The HP-diet is novel and, with the higher protein content, also somewhat outside the current boundaries of nutritional guidelines [42,43]. Whether the HP diet results in better adherence than the MP diet with high CHO and whole-grain cereal intakes is one of the key interests in PREVIEW. Nutrient intakes and food consumption patterns will be assessed in PREVIEW by repeated 4-d diet-records. The poor accuracy of dietary assessment is well known [44], but it is expected that the difference in dietary protein and CHO intakes should be sufficiently large to be detected using this method. Moreover, protein intake is verified using 24 h urinary nitrogen excretion [45].

It may be more difficult to create a verifiable difference for GI than for protein-to-CHO ratio. Whilst GI values of foods have been shown to provide a good summary of postprandial glycaemia [46], difficulties in attributing GI values to foods for which there are no validated data available may add to the variability [47], particularly in a multi-centre intervention such as PREVIEW. In DiOGenes, the reported observed difference in mean dietary GI was small (56 vs. 60 units) [19] which increases the requirements of precision.

The physical activity intervention in PREVIEW is not a supervised training programme. Participants are expected to integrate activity into their daily lives and use local opportunities to achieve their goals. To improve adherence, there is flexibility with the type of activities chosen. A combination of measures of physical activity is used to analyse the compliance to the type of intervention and our methods allow a description of activities that were used to achieve this.

It is probable that the HI-program will be more challenging in the long-term. Warming-up, cooling-down, muscular conditioning exercises, and stretching are carefully explained to the participants in order to decrease the risk for injuries. It should be noted that the HI-program in PREVIEW is not high-intensity interval-training (HIIT). While there are some data on potential benefits from HIIT on cardiovascular function and glucose metabolism [48], we considered the data on feasibility and long-term maintenance of this kind of training still too limited.

In addition to good compliance of the programmes, keeping the drop-out rate as low as possible will be challenging. Frequent contact with the research staff is one way to reduce the drop-out rate. However, PREVIEW has been planned to study how behavioural change is realized under 'real-life' conditions and, hence, the fading visit design where group visits are infrequent during years two and three of the intervention. Adherence is encouraged through a number of practices, including use of specific behavioural change techniques [31], such as implementation intentions, or Facebook groups, one for each randomised group, to promote attendance at group visits and CIDs. In addition, the sites can also conduct general information lectures, physical activity sessions, and/or send a newsletter to the participants, once or twice a year.

Compared to DPS and DPP studies, a particular feature of PREVIEW is related to the different settings in which the intervention is conducted, including not only genetic background, but also attitudes, norms, and socio-economic features. Although the participating countries are well-developed, considerable variations exist, e.g., regarding food attitudes and habits, as well as traditions of practicing physical activity.

The unique feature in the PREVIEW intervention is the direct comparison of two potentially efficacious diet and physical activity intervention programs. Hence, PREVIEW has a clear potential to identify a recommended optimal diet and physical activity programme to prevent T2D, a programme which is also suitable across different countries. It is also possible, however, that PREVIEW data will demonstrate that there are several, equally efficacious alternatives. Clearly, both answers are important from a public health viewpoint.

Acknowledgments: This study has received grants from the EU 7th Framework Programme (FP7-KBBE-2012), grant agreement No. 312057; the New Zealand Health Research Council, grant No. 14/191; and the NHMRC-EU Collaborative Grant, Australia. All LCD products were provided by Cambridge Weight Plan®, UK. This sponsorship is highly appreciated. We want to acknowledge, particularly, the following medical and scientific experts, who have helped us in building up the study: Arne Astrup (Copenhagen, Denmark), Stephen Collagiuri (Sydney, Australia), Peter Mansell (Nottingham, UK), and the PREVIEW Scientific Advisory Board, Louise Dye (Leeds, UK), Richard L. Atkinson (Richmond, VA, USA), Boyd Swinburn (Auckland, New Zealand), Lauren Lissner, (Gothenburg, Sweden), and Grethe Andersen (Copenhagen, Denmark). Moreover, we want to acknowledge the great staff who have worked and are currently working for PREVIEW, e.g., study nurses, lab technicians, nutritionists, physical activity experts, trainees, and post- and under-graduate students, involved in the recruitment of all participants and in planning and initiating the weight-reduction phase and intervention.

Author Contributions: A.R., J.B.-M. and M.F.M. were responsible for the initial study conception. T.M.L., M.W.-P., I.M., J.A.M.H., S.P., W.S., G.S., J.S., T.L., T.H.-D., D.K., J.B.-M. and A.R. were involved in development of the study design. All authors, but particularly E.J., P.C., M.D., E.S., S.N.-C., N.B., R.M., M.P.S. and L.P.-S. were involved in the development of the practical implementation of the study. M.F.M. wrote the draft version of the manuscript and all authors were involved in critically revising the paper. All authors have also seen and accepted the submitted version.

References

1. American Diabetes Association. Standards of medical care in diabetes—2011. *Diabetes Care* **2011**, *34* (Suppl. 1), S11–S61.
2. Guariguata, L.; Whiting, D.R.; Hambleton, I.; Beagley, J.; Linnenkamp, U.; Shaw, J.E. Global estimates of diabetes prevalence for 2013 and projections for 2035. *Diabetes Res. Clin. Pract.* **2014**, *103*, 137–149. [CrossRef] [PubMed]
3. Tamayo, T.; Rosenbauer, J.; Wild, S.H.; Spijkerman, A.M.W.; Baan, C.; Forouhi, N.G.; Herder, C.; Rathmann, W. Diabetes in Europe: An update. *Diabetes Res. Clin. Pract.* **2014**, *103*, 206–217. [CrossRef] [PubMed]
4. Guh, D.P.; Zhang, W.; Bansback, N.; Amarsi, Z.; Birmingham, C.L.; Anis, A.H. The incidence of co-morbidities related to obesity and overweight: A systematic review and meta-analysis. *BMC Public Health* **2009**, *9*, 88. [CrossRef] [PubMed]
5. Morimoto, Y.; Schembre, S.M.; Steinbrecher, A.; Erber, E.; Pagano, I.; Grandinetti, A.; Kolonel, L.N.; Maskarinec, G. Ethnic differences in weight gain and diabetes risk: The Multiethnic Cohort Study. *Diabetes Metab.* **2011**, *37*, 230–236. [CrossRef] [PubMed]
6. Aune, D.; Norat, T.; Leitzmann, M.; Tonstad, S.; Vatten, L.J. Physical activity and the risk of type 2 diabetes: A systematic review and dose-response meta-analysis. *Eur. J. Epidemiol.* **2015**, *30*, 529–542. [CrossRef] [PubMed]
7. Bhupathiraju, S.N.; Tobias, D.K.; Malik, V.S.; Pan, A.; Hruby, A.; Manson, J.E.; Willett, W.C.; Hu, F.B. Glycemic index, glycemic load, and risk of type 2 diabetes: Results from 3 large US cohorts and an updated meta-analysis. *Am. J. Clin. Nutr.* **2014**, *100*, 218–232. [CrossRef] [PubMed]
8. Ley, S.H.; Hamdy, O.; Mohan, V.; Hu, F.B. Prevention and management of type 2 diabetes: Dietary components and nutritional strategies. *Lancet* **2014**, *383*, 1999–2007. [CrossRef]
9. Li, G.; Zhang, P.; Wang, J.; An, Y.; Gong, Q.; Gregg, E.W.; Yang, W.; Zhang, B.; Shuai, Y.; Hong, J.; et al. Cardiovascular mortality, all-cause mortality, and diabetes incidence after lifestyle intervention for people with impaired glucose tolerance in the Da Qing Diabetes Prevention Study: A 23-year follow-up study. *Lancet Diabetes Endocrinol.* **2014**, *2*, 474–480. [CrossRef]

10. Knowler, W.C.; Barrett-Connor, E.; Fowler, S.E.; Hamman, R.F.; Lachin, J.M.; Walker, E.A.; et al. Reduction in the incidence of type 2 diabetes with lifestyle intervention or metformin. *N. Engl. J. Med.* **2002**, *346*, 393–403. [PubMed]
11. Tuomilehto, J.; Lindström, J.; Eriksson, J.G.; Valle, T.T.; Hämäläinen, H.; Ilanne-Parikka, P.; Keinänen-Kiukaanniemi, S.; Laakso, M.; Louheranta, A.; Rastas, M.; et al. Prevention of type 2 diabetes mellitus by changes in lifestyle among subjects with impaired glucose tolerance. *N. Engl. J. Med.* **2001**, *344*, 1343–1350. [CrossRef] [PubMed]
12. Walker, K.Z.; O'Dea, K.; Gomez, M.; Girgis, S.; Colagiuri, R. Diet and exercise in the prevention of diabetes. *J. Hum. Nutr. Diet.* **2010**, *23*, 344–352. [CrossRef] [PubMed]
13. Mayer-Davis, E.J.; Sparks, K.C.; Hirst, K.; Costacou, T.; Lovejoy, J.C.; Regensteiner, J.G.; Hoskin, M.A.; Kriska, A.M.; Bray, G.A.; Diabetes Prevention Program Research Group. Dietary intake in the diabetes prevention program cohort: Baseline and 1-year post randomization. *Ann. Epidemiol.* **2004**, *14*, 763–772. [CrossRef] [PubMed]
14. Eriksson, J.; Lindström, J.; Valle, T.; Aunola, S.; Hämäläinen, H.; Ilanne-Parikka, P.; Keinänen-Kiukaanniemi, S.; Laakso, M.; Lauhkonen, M.; Lehto, P.; et al. Prevention of Type II diabetes in subjects with impaired glucose tolerance: The Diabetes Prevention Study (DPS) in Finland. Study design and 1-year interim report on the feasibility of the lifestyle intervention programme. *Diabetologia* **1999**, *42*, 793–801. [CrossRef] [PubMed]
15. Pan, X.R.; Li, G.W.; Hu, Y.H.; Wang, J.X.; Yang, W.Y.; An, Z.X.; Hu, Z.X.; Lin, J.; Xiao, J.Z.; Cao, H.B.; et al. Effects of diet and exercise in preventing NIDDM in people with impaired glucose tolerance. The Da Qing IGT and Diabetes Study. *Diabetes Care* **1997**, *20*, 537–544. [CrossRef] [PubMed]
16. Mann, J.I.; De Leeuw, I.; Hermansen, K.; Karamanos, B.; Karlström, B.; Katsilambros, N.; Riccardi, G.; Rivellese, A.A.; Rizkalla, S.; Slama, G.; et al. Evidence-based nutritional approaches to the treatment and prevention of diabetes mellitus. *Nutr. Metab. Cardiovasc. Dis.* **2004**, *14*, 373–394. [CrossRef]
17. Ajala, O.; English, P.; Pinkney, J. Systematic review and meta-analysis of different dietary approaches to the management of type 2 diabetes. *Am. J. Clin. Nutr.* **2013**, *97*, 505–516. [CrossRef] [PubMed]
18. Buyken, A.E.; Mitchell, P.; Ceriello, A.; Brand-Miller, J. Optimal dietary approaches for prevention of type 2 diabetes: A life-course perspective. *Diabetologia* **2010**, *53*, 406–418. [CrossRef] [PubMed]
19. Larsen, T.M.; Dalskov, S.-M.; van Baak, M.; Jebb, S.A.; Papadaki, A.; Pfeiffer, A.F.H.; Martinez, J.A.; Handjieva-Darlenska, T.; Kunešová, M.; Pihlsgård, M.; et al. Diets with high or low protein content and glycemic index for weight-loss maintenance. *N. Engl. J. Med.* **2010**, *363*, 2102–2113. [CrossRef] [PubMed]
20. Astrup, A.; Raben, A.; Geiker, N. The role of higher protein diets in weight control and obesity-related comorbidities. *Int. J. Obes.* **2015**, *39*, 721–726. [CrossRef] [PubMed]
21. Romijn, J.A.; Coyle, E.F.; Sidossis, L.S.; Gastaldelli, A.; Horowitz, J.F.; Endert, E.; Wolfe, R.R. Regulation of endogenous fat and carbohydrate metabolism in relation to exercise intensity and duration. *Am. J. Physiol.* **1993**, *265 Pt 1*, E380–E391. [PubMed]
22. Houmard, J.A.; Tanner, C.J.; Slentz, C.A.; Duscha, B.D.; McCartney, J.S.; Kraus, W.E. Effect of the volume and intensity of exercise training on insulin sensitivity. *J. Appl. Physiol.* **2004**, *96*, 101–106. [CrossRef] [PubMed]
23. Fogelholm, M.; Anderssen, S.; Gunnarsdottir, I.; Lahti-Koski, M. Dietary macronutrients and food consumption as determinants of long-term weight change in adult populations: A systematic literature review. *Food Nutr. Res.* **2012**, *56*. [CrossRef] [PubMed]
24. Aller, E.E.J.G.; Larsen, T.M.; Claus, H.; Lindroos, A.K.; Kafatos, A.; Pfeiffer, A.; Martinez, J.A.; Handjieva-Darlenska, T.; Kunesova, M.; Stender, S.; et al. Weight loss maintenance in overweight subjects on ad libitum diets with high or low protein content and glycemic index: The DIOGENES trial 12-month results. *Int. J. Obes.* **2014**, *38*, 1511–1517. [CrossRef] [PubMed]
25. Watt, M.J.; Heigenhauser, G.J.; Spriet, L.L. Effects of dynamic exercise intensity on the activation of hormone-sensitive lipase in human skeletal muscle. *J. Physiol.* **2003**, *547 Pt 1*, 301–308. [CrossRef] [PubMed]
26. WHO. Definition and Diagnosis of Diabetes Mellitus and Intermediate Hyperglycaemia. Available online: http://www.who.int/diabetes/publications/diagnosis_diabetes2006/en/ (accessed on 19 July 2017).
27. Matsuda, M.; DeFronzo, R.A. Insulin sensitivity indices obtained from oral glucose tolerance testing: Comparison with the euglycemic insulin clamp. *Diabetes Care* **1999**, *22*, 1462–1470. [CrossRef] [PubMed]
28. Silventoinen, K.; Pankow, J.; Lindström, J.; Jousilahti, P.; Hu, G.; Tuomilehto, J. The validity of the Finnish Diabetes Risk Score for the prediction of the incidence of coronary heart disease and stroke, and total mortality. *Eur. J. Cardiovasc. Prev. Rehabil.* **2005**, *12*, 451–458. [CrossRef] [PubMed]

29. Borg, G.A. Psychophysical bases of perceived exertion. *Med. Sci. Sports Exerc.* **1982**, *14*, 377–381. [CrossRef] [PubMed]
30. 2008 Physical Activity Guidelines for Americans. Available online: http://www.health.gov/paguidelines/guidelines/ (accessed on 19 July 2017).
31. Kahlert, D.; Unyi-Reicherz, A.; Stratton, G.; Meinert Larsen, T.; Fogelholm, M.; Raben, A.; Schlicht, W. PREVIEW Behavior Modification Intervention Toolbox (PREMIT): A Study Protocol for a Psychological Element of a Multicenter Project. *Front. Psychol.* **2016**, *7*, 1136. [CrossRef] [PubMed]
32. Michie, S.; Abraham, C.; Whittington, C.; McAteer, J.; Gupta, S. Effective techniques in healthy eating and physical activity interventions: A meta-regression. *Health Psychol.* **2009**, *28*, 690–701. [CrossRef] [PubMed]
33. Greaves, .C.J.; Sheppard, K.E.; Abraham, C.; Hardeman, W.; Roden, M.; Evans, P.H.; Schwarz, P.; IMAGE Study Group. Systematic review of reviews of intervention components associated with increased effectiveness in dietary and physical activity interventions. *BMC Public Health* **2011**, *11*, 119. [CrossRef] [PubMed]
34. Olander, E.K.; Fletcher, H.; Williams, S.; Atkinson, L.; Turner, A.; French, D.P. What are the most effective techniques in changing obese individuals' physical activity self-efficacy and behaviour: A systematic review and meta-analysis. *Int. J. Behav. Nutr. Phys. Act.* **2013**, *10*, 29. [CrossRef] [PubMed]
35. Michie, S.; Richardson, M.; Johnston, M.; Abraham, C.; Francis, J.; Hardeman, W.; Eccles, M.P.; Cane, J.; Wood, C.E. The behavior change technique taxonomy (v1) of 93 hierarchically clustered techniques: Building an international consensus for the reporting of behavior change interventions. *Ann. Behav. Med.* **2013**, *46*, 81–95. [CrossRef] [PubMed]
36. Prochaska, J.O.; DiClemente, C.C. Stages of change in the modification of problem behaviors. *Prog. Behav. Modif.* **1992**, *28*, 183–218. [PubMed]
37. PREVIEW. Available online: http://previewstudy.com (accessed on 19 July 2017).
38. The Diabetes Prevention Program: Baseline characteristics of the randomized cohort. The Diabetes Prevention Program Research Group. *Diabetes Care* **2000**, *23*, 1619–1629.
39. Edelstein, S.L.; Knowler, W.C.; Bain, R.P.; Andres, R.; Barrett-Connor, E.L.; Dowse, G.K.; Haffner, S.M.; Pettitt, D.J.; Sorkin, J.D.; Muller, D.C.; et al. Predictors of progression from impaired glucose tolerance to NIDDM: An analysis of six prospective studies. *Diabetes* **1997**, *46*, 701–710. [CrossRef] [PubMed]
40. Saudek, C.D.; Herman, W.H.; Sacks, D.B.; Bergenstal, R.M.; Edelman, D.; Davidson, M.B. A new look at screening and diagnosing diabetes mellitus. *J. Clin. Endocrinol. Metab.* **2008**, *93*, 2447–2453. [CrossRef] [PubMed]
41. Malkani, S.; Mordes, J.P. Implications of using hemoglobin A1C for diagnosing diabetes mellitus. *Am. J. Med.* **2011**, *124*, 395–401. [CrossRef] [PubMed]
42. Nordic Nutrition Recommendations Project Group. *Nordic Nutrition Recommendations 2012. Integrating Nutrition and Physical Activity*, 5th ed.; Nordic Council of Ministers: Copenhagen, Denmark, 2014.
43. Dietary Guidelines for Americans. Available online: http://www.cnpp.usda.gov/DietaryGuidelines (accessed on 19 July 2017).
44. Dhurandhar, N.V.; Schoeller, D.; Brown, A.W.; Heymsfield, S.B.; Thomas, D.; Sørensen, T.I.A.; Speakman, J.R.; Jeansonne, M.; Allison, D.B.; Energy Balance Measurement Working Group. Energy balance measurement: When something is not better than nothing. *Int. J. Obes.* **2015**, *39*, 1109–1113. [CrossRef] [PubMed]
45. Corella, D.; Ordovás, J.M. Biomarkers: Background, classification and guidelines for applications in nutritional epidemiology. *Nutr. Hosp.* **2015**, *31* (Suppl. 3), 177–188. [PubMed]
46. Brand-Miller, J.C.; Stockmann, K.; Atkinson, F.; Petocz, P.; Denyer, G. Glycemic index, postprandial glycemia, and the shape of the curve in healthy subjects: Analysis of a database of more than 1000 foods. *Am. J. Clin. Nutr.* **2009**, *89*, 97–105. [CrossRef] [PubMed]
47. Whelan, W.J.; Hollar, D.; Agatston, A.; Dodson, H.J.; Tahal, D.S. The glycemic response is a personal attribute. *IUBMB Life* **2010**, *62*, 637–641. [CrossRef] [PubMed]
48. Ramos, J.S.; Dalleck, L.C.; Tjonna, A.E.; Beetham, K.S.; Coombes, J.S. The impact of high-intensity interval training versus moderate-intensity continuous training on vascular function: A systematic review and meta-analysis. *Sports Med.* **2015**, *45*, 679–692. [CrossRef] [PubMed]

14

Nuts and Dried Fruits: An Update of Their Beneficial Effects on Type 2 Diabetes

Pablo Hernández-Alonso [1,2], Lucía Camacho-Barcia [1,2], Mònica Bulló [1,2,*] and Jordi Salas-Salvadó [1,2,*]

1 Human Nutrition Unit, Biochemistry and Biotechnology Department, Faculty of Medicine and Health Sciences, University Hospital of Sant Joan de Reus, IISPV, Universitat Rovira i Virgili, St/Sant Llorenç 21, 43201 Reus, Spain; pablo1280@gmail.com (P.H.-A.); marialucia.camacho@urv.cat (L.C.-B.)

2 CIBERobn Physiopathology of Obesity and Nutrition, Instituto de Salud Carlos III, 28029 Madrid, Spain

* Correspondence: monica.bullo@urv.cat (M.B.); jordi.salas@urv.cat (J.S.-S.);

Abstract: Nuts and dried fruit are essential foods in the Mediterranean diet. Their frequent consumption has been associated with the prevention and/or the management of such metabolic conditions as type 2 diabetes (T2D), metabolic syndrome and cardiovascular diseases. Several previous reviews of epidemiological studies and clinical trials have evaluated the associations of nuts and/or dried fruit with various metabolic disorders. However, no reviews have focused on the mechanisms underlying the role of nuts and/or dried fruit in insulin resistance and T2D. This review aims to report nut and dried-fruit nutritional interventions in animals and humans, and to focus on mechanisms that could play a significant role in the prevention and treatment of insulin resistance and T2D.

Keywords: diabetes; nuts; dried fruits; insulin resistance; mechanisms; clinical trials

1. Introduction

Nuts and traditional dried fruit (i.e., with no added sugar) are key food categories in the Mediterranean diet and other regional diets [1]. Several prospective studies, clinical trials and research in animals have reported beneficial effects after nut consumption [2]. However, the benefits of dried fruits (DF), mainly raisins, have been less explored [3].

Over time, food consumption has varied. More than 30 years ago, the consumption of nuts and DF was discouraged because of their high fat and sugar content, respectively. However, at the beginning of the 1990s, several randomized clinical trials (RCT) and animal experiments demonstrated their potential beneficial effect on cardiovascular diseases (CVD). Nuts and DF contain various macro and micronutrients together with other important bioactive compounds that may synergically contribute to modulate specific metabolic diseases such as hypercholesterolemia, hypertension and type 2 diabetes (T2D) (reviewed in [3,4]). Even so, the specific role of nuts and DF in the development and progression of insulin resistance (IR) and T2D are still controversial.

In this review, we focus on the role of nuts and DF in the prevention and treatment of T2D. We summarize published in vivo, in vitro, epidemiological and clinical studies, and we review the potential mechanisms that could explain the beneficial role of nut consumption on glucose and insulin metabolism, both of which are altered in T2D and in other glucose-impaired states. Given that the present article is not a systematic review, we may not have identified some studies and publication bias should be acknowledged. However, all authors independently conducted the literature search.

1.1. Nuts and Dried Fruits: The Concept

1.1.1. Nuts

Nuts have been part of the human diet since prehistoric times [5,6]. They are an independent food group and are one of the cornerstones of the Mediterranean diet (MedDiet) [7]. According to the botanical definition, a nut is simply a dried fruit with one seed (rarely two) in which the ovary walls are very hard (stony or woody) at maturity, and the seed is unattached or free within the ovary wall. However, the word "nut" is commonly used to refer to any large, oily kernel in a shell that can be eaten as food. In this review, we use the term "nuts" to refer to almonds, Brazil nuts, cashews, hazelnuts, macadamias, peanuts, pecans, pine nuts, pistachios and walnuts. Although peanuts are actually classified as legumes because of their similar nutrient composition and their proven cardiovascular health benefits, they are commonly regarded as being a nut.

1.1.2. Dried Fruits

To extend their shelf life, fresh fruits are processed by various techniques to become DFs [3]. Dried fruits are a concentrated form of fresh fruits with a lower moisture content. Fruits can be dried whole (e.g., apricots, berries and grapes), in halves, or in slices (e.g., kiwis, mangoes and papayas). In this form, they are easy to store and distribute, they can be available throughout the year, and they are a healthier alternative to salty or sugary snacks. Apples, apricots, currants, dates, figs, peaches, pears, prunes, and raisins are referred to as "conventional" or "traditional" DFs. Meanwhile, such fruits as blueberries, cranberries, cherries, strawberries and mangoes are commonly infused with different types of sugar solution (or fruit juice) concentrate before drying [8] so are not included in the aforementioned category. Moreover, we have also excluded dried tomato because although it is botanically a berry-type fruit, it is culinary considered a vegetable and it shares nutrient composition with this food category.

1.2. Nutritional Composition of Nuts and Dried Fruits

Nuts and DFs are a matrix of important bioactive compounds such as Vitamins (Vitamin E, niacin, choline and/or folic acid), minerals (magnesium, potassium, calcium and/or phosphorus), phenolic compounds, carotenoids and/or phytosterols [9]. Importantly, some nuts and DFs are among the 50 foods with the highest antioxidant capacity [10] and are also a known source of bioactive compounds, including plant sterols [11]. Pistachios are particularly rich in β-carotenes which have been widely associated with a protective T2D role [12,13]. In addition, pistachios are the only nuts that contain significant amounts of lutein and zeaxanthin [9]. Sun-dried raisins retain the minerals and most of the phytochemicals and antioxidants of the grape, including its resveratrol [14,15]. In fact, sun-drying enhances the antioxidant content of raisins. Because of the dehydration process, phytonutrients are more concentrated in raisins than in grapes. However, the concentration of some compounds is decreased by the sun-drying process in DFs and by dry roasting techniques in nuts [9]. Polyphenols and tocopherols from nuts and DF have proved to be rapidly accessible in the stomach, thus maximizing the possibility of absorption in the upper small intestine, and contributing to the beneficial relation between nut and DF consumption and health-related outcomes [8,16].

However, their macronutrient compositions are quite different, which means that their energy contents are also quite different. Nuts contain a high amount of total fat (Range (Re): 43.9–78.8%) with a high amount of unsaturated fat (monounsaturated fatty acids (MUFA) + polyunsaturated fatty acids (PUFA), Re: 31.6–62.4%), a relatively low amount of carbohydrates (CHOs) (Re: 11.7–30.2%) and vegetable protein (Re: 7.9–25.8%) (Table 1).

Conversely, DFs are mainly composed of CHOs (Re: 61.3–72.8%). They have a low content of protein (Re: 0.17–4.08%) and a fat content of less than 1% (Table 2). Importantly, both foods also contain a considerable amount of dietary fiber. Overall, their unique and varied nutrient composition makes them key foods to counteract various metabolic diseases.

Table 1. Nutrient composition of nuts (per 100 g of raw nut).

Nutrient	Almonds	Brazil Nuts [b]	Cashews	Hazelnuts	Macadamias	Peanuts	Pecans	Pine Nuts [b]	Pistachios	Walnuts [c]
Energy, Kcal	579	659	553	628	718	567	691	673	560	654
Water, g	4.4	3.4	5.2	5.3	1.4	6.5	3.5	2.3	4.4	4.1
Fat, g	49.9	67.1	43.9	60.8	75.8	49.2	72.0	68.4	45.3	65.2
SFA, g	3.8	16.1	7.8	4.5	12.1	6.3	6.2	4.9	5.9	6.1
MUFA, g	31.6	23.9	23.8	45.7	58.9	24.4	40.8	18.8	23.3	9.0
PUFA, g	12.3	24.4	7.8	7.9	1.5	15.6	21.6	34.1	14.4	47.2
Protein, g	21.2	14.3	18.2	15.0	7.9	25.8	9.2	13.7	20.2	15.2
CHO, g	21.6	11.7	30.2	16.7	13.8	16.1	13.9	13.1	27.2	13.7
Fiber, g	12.5	7.5	3.3	9.7	8.6	8.5	9.6	3.7	10.6	6.7
Ca, mg	269	160	37	114	85	92	70	16	105	98
Mg, mg	270	376	292	163	130	168	121	251	121	158
Na, mg	1	3	12	0	5	18	0	2	1	2
K, mg	733	659	660	680	368	705	410	597	1025	441
P, mg	481	725	593	290	188	376	277	575	490	346
Lutein-Zeaxanthin, μg	1	0	22	92	NA	0	17	9	2903	9
β-Carotene, μg	1	0	0	11	NA	0	29	17	305	12
α-Carotene, μg	0	0	0	3	NA	0	0	0	10	0
Phytosterols [a], mg	197	123.5	151	122	116	NA	158.8	236.1	214	110.2
Total phenols, mg	287	244	137	687	126	406	1284	32	867	1576
Vitamin E (α-tocopherol), mg	25.6	5.7	0.9	15.0	0.5	8.3	1.4	9.3	2.9	0.7

Nutrient information is taken from the United States Department of Agriculture (USDA) Nutrient Database Standard Reference, Release 28 [9]. CHO, carbohydrates; MUFA, monounsaturated fatty acids; NA: not available; PUFA, polyunsaturated fatty acids; SFA, saturated fatty acids. [a] Phytosterols, are the sum of stigmasterol, campesterol, β-sitosterol and other phytosterols; [b] dry roasted; [c] English variety.

Table 2. Nutrient composition of dried fruits (per 100 g).

Nutrient	Apples [a]	Apricots [a]	Currants (Zante)	Cranberries [b]	Dates [c]	Figs	Peaches [a]	Pears [a]	Plums/Prunes	Raisins [d]
Energy, Kcal	243	241	283	308	282	249	239	262	240	299
Water, g	31.76	30.89	19.21	15.79	20.53	30.05	31.80	26.69	30.92	15.43
Fat, g	0.32	0.51	0.27	1.09	0.39	0.93	0.76	0.63	0.38	0.46
CHO, g	65.89	62.64	74.08	82.80	75.03	63.87	61.33	69.70	63.88	79.18
Sugars, g	57.19	53.44	67.28	72.56	63.35	47.92	41.74	62.20	38.13	59.19
Fructose, g	NA	12.47	NA	26.96	19.56	22.93	13.49	NA	12.45	29.68
Protein, g	0.93	3.39	4.08	0.17	2.45	3.30	3.61	1.87	2.18	3.07
Fiber, g	8.7	7.3	6.8	5.3	8.0	9.8	8.2	7.5	7.1	3.7
Ca, mg	14	55	86	9	39	162	28	34	43	50
Fe, mg	1.40	2.66	3.26	0.39	1.02	2.03	4.06	2.10	0.93	1.88
Mg, mg	16	32	41	4	43	68	42	33	41	32
Na, mg	87	10	8	5	2	10	7	6	2	11
K, mg	450	1162	892	49	656	680	996	533	732	749
Cu, mg	0.19	0.34	0.47	0.06	0.21	0.29	0.36	0.37	0.28	0.32
β-carotene, μg	0	2163	43	27	6	6	1074	2	394	0
α-carotene, μg	0	0	1	0	0	0	3	0	57	0
Lutein-Zeaxanthin, μg	0	0	0	138	75	32	559	50	148	0
Vitamin A, IU	0	3604	73	46	10	10	2163	3	781	0
Total phenols, mg GAE/100g [e]	324	248	NA	NA	661	960	283	679	938	1065

Data is for traditional dried fruits which is defined as those with no added sugars, typically sun-dried or dried with minimal processing. Nutrient information is taken from the United States Department of Agriculture (USDA) Nutrient Database Standard Reference, Release 28 [9]. CHO, carbohydrates; GAE, gallic acid equivalents; IU, international unit; NA, not available. [a] Sulfured; [b] sweetened; [c] Deglet noor is the common variety; [d] seedless; [e] Total phenol content was obtained from Alasalvar and Shahidi [8].

1.3. Diet Quality in the Context of Nut and Dried Fruit Consumption

Epidemiological studies conducted in children and adults have demonstrated a significant positive association between nut consumption and diet quality [17,18]. Furthermore, the results of a clinical trial conducted in obese (Ob) subjects (n = 124) showed that the nutritional dietary quality of nut consumers (reporting to eat 42 g hazelnuts/day for 12 weeks) was remarkably higher than among other groups consuming chocolate, potato crisps or no additional foods [19]. Moreover, including nuts in energy-restricted diets reduced attrition and increased weight loss, indicating that nuts enhance palatability and compliance with diets without compromising health [20].

Several studies have examined the associations of whole fruit or 100% fruit juice [21] with nutritional or health outcomes such as T2D but there is a lack of studies examining potential links between DF and diet quality. A prospective study conducted in adult participants (n = 13,292) in the 1999–2004 National Health and Nutrition Examination Survey (NHANES) demonstrated an association between DF consumption and diet quality [22]. DF consumption was associated with improved nutrient intakes, a higher overall diet quality score, and lower body weight (BW)/adiposity measures [22]. Moreover, in a cross-sectional study in healthy adults (n = 797) from Hong Kong, an inverse association has been found between the intake of vegetables, legumes, fruits, dried fruits and Vitamin C and the prevalence of metabolic disorders such as non-alcoholic fatty liver disease (NAFLD) [23].

The 2015 Dietary Guidelines for Americans included the following three healthy dietary patterns: a Healthy US-style Pattern, a Healthy Vegetarian Pattern and a Healthy Mediterranean-style pattern. Fruits, nuts, and seeds play a prominent role in all three of these food-based dietary patterns, which recommend 350–440 g/day of fruit, and 16–28 g/day of nuts and seeds [24].

2. In Vivo and In Vitro Studies

Even though much of the research on nuts, dried fruits and T2D is based on observational studies and human trials, some in vitro and in vivo studies also evaluate their modulatory effect on glucose and insulin metabolism. In this regard, the effect of nuts on glucose and insulin metabolism has been investigated by evaluating nut extracts [25,26] or nuts as a whole [27–29] mainly in mice or rats. However, dried fruit has been investigated—like their non-dried counterparts—mainly in in vitro studies [30–33]. Almost all the research has focused on the extracts from non-edible parts, such as the shell [34], leaves [35,36], stems [37] and roots [38], and very little on the nut or fruit kernel [27–29,39]. However, this review focuses on those studies evaluating specific nutrients (e.g., polyphenols) or edible parts in both traditional nuts and dried fruits with outcomes related to glucose metabolism, IR, and the T2D oxidation/inflammation axis [32,40].

2.1. Nuts

The in vivo studies on nuts and T2D-related parameters are summarized in Table 3. These studies were mainly performed using extracts from peanuts or walnuts. Peanut oil supplementation for 42 days in diabetes-induced rats significantly reduced glucose and glycated hemoglobin (HbA_{1c}) concentrations and improved lipid metabolism compared to normal rats [27]. Other researchers have found similar improvements in glycaemia in genotypes of diabetes in rats fed with peanut oil extract [41,42] or peanut aqueous extract [25]. In the case of walnuts, a polyphenol-rich walnut extract (PWE) for 4 weeks significantly decreased urinary 8-hydroxy-2′-deoxyguanosin levels (an in vivo marker of oxidative stress) and improved serum TG in *db/db* mice [26]. Moreover, an HFD with a 21.5% of energy from walnuts tested in mice for 20 weeks significantly reduced TG compared to nut-free HFD and tended to improve glucose and IR [29].

Table 3. Summary of in vivo studies and their characteristics in the context of nut consumption and type 2 diabetes (T2D)-related outcomes.

First Author (Year) [Reference]	Nut (Study Length)	Animal Model Used	Control	Intervention	Glucose and Insulin Metabolism Effects	Other Outcomes
Bilbis, L.S.; et al. (2002) [25]	Aqueous extract of peanut (21 days)	Alloxan-induced diabetic rats (n = 12) and non-diabetic rats (n = 12), divided into 3 equal groups	Non-diabetic with unrestricted standard diet and: (a) water ad libitum; (b) unrestricted access to drinking water and 2 mL of the extract 3 times/day; or (c) free access to the extract as the only drinking water.	Diabetic controls: treated as (a), (b) or (c)	The extract (alone or plus water) decreased FBG in both normal and alloxan-induced diabetic rats.	Significant decrease in serum TG, TC, HDL-C and LDL-C in both normal and alloxan-induced diabetic rats.
Fukuda, T.; et al. (2004) [26]	Polyphenol-rich walnut extract (PWE) (4 weeks)	*db/db* (n = 15) and C57BL/KsJ-*db/db* (n = 6) mice	Control *db/db* mice (n = 8) and C57BL/KsJ-*db*/+ m mice (n = 6, used for the blank group) were given water.	Experimental *db/db* mice (n = 7) received oral PWE (200 mg/kg BW)	Significant decrease in the level of urinary 8-hydroxy-2′-deoxyguanosin (in vivo marker of oxidative stress) in PWE-fed mice	Serum TG level was improved after PWE administration
Ramesh, B.; et al. (2006) [27]	Peanut oil (42 days)	Normal (n = 12) and STZ-diabetes induced (n = 18) Wistar rats	G1: Normal rats G3: Diabetic rats	G2: Normal rats + peanut oil diet (2%) G4: Diabetic rats + peanut oil diet (2%) G5: Diabetic rats + GLI (600 µg/kg BW)	Diabetic rats fed with peanut oil significantly reduce glucose, HbA_{1C}, and G6Pase and FBP activities	Diabetic rats fed with peanut oil showed a small but significant reduction in TC, VLDL-C, LDL-C and TG and an increase in HDL-C.
Vassiliou, E.K.; et al. (2009) [41]	Peanut oil (21 days)	Male KKA^y (n = 24) mice	KKA^y mice fed with normal diet (11.4% fat)	Diabetic KKA^y + HFD. Diabetic KKA^y + HFD with peanut oil (0.70 mL/day). HFD is 58% fat.	Diabetic mice administered peanut oil had lower glucose levels than animals administered HFD alone.	
Choi, Y.; et al. (2016) [29]	Walnuts (20 weeks)	Male C57BL/6J mice (≥6 mice/group)	Regular rodent chow	HFD (45% energy-derived) with or without walnuts (21.5% energy-derived)	Glucose and insulin resistance tended to improve with walnut supplementation.	Walnut supplementation did not change the HFD-induced increase in BW or VFM. However, dietary walnuts significantly decreased the amounts of hepatic TG observed in HFD-fed mice.
Adewale, O.F.; et al. (2016) [42]	Peanut oil Palm oil (3 weeks)	Normal (n = 12) and alloxan-induced diabetic Wistar rats (n = 36)	Non-diabetic	Diabetic non-supplemented. Diabetic supplemented with PeO or PaO (200 mg/kg/day)	Significant reduction in blood glucose of supplemented groups (PeO + PaO) compared to the diabetic non-supplemented group.	Plasma Vitamins C and E and albumin levels were significantly increased in the supplemented groups versus the diabetic non-supplemented group.

BW, body weight; FBG, fasting blood glucose; FBP, fructose-1,6-bisphosphatase; G6Pase, glucose 6-phosphatase; GLI, glibenclamide; HDL-C, high-density lipoprotein cholesterol; HFD, high-fat diet; LDL-C, low-density lipoprotein cholesterol; PaO, palm oil; PeO, peanut oil; PWE, polyphenol-rich walnut extract; STZ, streptozotocin; T2D, type 2 diabetes; TC, total cholesterol; TF, tissue factor; TG, triglycerides; VFM, visceral fat mass; VLDL-C, very low-density lipoprotein.

In vitro assessment of the T2D-related antioxidant and inflammatory capacity of nuts has largely been conducted by examining the ability of extracts to increase the resistance of human plasma or low density lipoprotein (LDL) to oxidation. Extracts of walnut [43], almond and almond skins [44,45], pistachio [46], and hazelnut [47] have been found to increase the lag time oxidation of LDL. However, little research has focused on their in vitro effects on glucose and insulin metabolism. Specifically, a hydro-ethanolic extract of cashew nut and its principal compound, anacardic acid, significantly stimulated glucose uptake in C2C12 muscle cells in a concentration-dependent manner, suggesting that it may be a potential anti-diabetic nutraceutical [48]. Moreover, cytoprotective activity of pistachio extracts (methanolic, water or ethyl acetate) against oxidative (reactive oxygen species formation) and carbonyl stress has also been reported in a T2D model in hepatocytes from rats [49].

2.2. Dried Fruits

Both in vitro and in vivo research has mostly focused on grape. Overman and collaborators showed that a grape powder extract (GPE) significantly attenuated lipopolysaccharide (LPS)-mediated inflammation in macrophages and decreased the capacity of LPS-stimulated human macrophages to inflame adipocytes and cause IR [30]. Moreover, GPE further attenuated tumor necrosis factor-α (TNF-α) mediated inflammation and IR in primary cultures of human adipocytes [31]. Grape polyphenol extract modulated in vitro membrane phospholipid fatty acid (FA) composition but also decreased muscle TG content and increased muscle glucose transporter type 4 (GLUT4) expression in high-fat-high-sucrose diet-fed rats. Overall, it improved insulin resistance status (i.e., HOMA-IR parameter) [50]. This is of considerable importance because the accumulation of muscle TG content and the modification of the muscle phospholipid fatty acid pattern may have an impact on lipid metabolism and increase the risk of developing T2D [51]. Mice fed with grape skin extract showed hypoglycaemic and anti-hyperglycaemic effects (independent of an increase in insulin release) but are probably dependent on an increase in insulin sensitivity resulting from the activation of the insulin-signaling cascade in skeletal muscle [52]. Furthermore, grape seed aqueous extract protected the pancreas against oxidative stress, inflammation and apoptosis-induced damage while preserving pancreatic function at near normal levels in diabetic rats [53].

Other DF extracts have also been evaluated. Treatment with a date fruit extract was effective at decreasing behavioral, neurophysiological, and pathological alterations induced by diabetes in the peripheral nerves of streptozotocin (STZ)-induced diabetic rats (well-characterized animal model of type 1 diabetes) [33]. Moreover, daily consumption of a low- or high-fat diet supplemented with 1% black currant powder extract (with 32% of anthocyanins) for 8 weeks reduced body weight gain and improved glucose metabolism [54].

The beneficial effect of fruit juices and fermented grape juice (i.e., wine) have also been an important focus of research. Schmatz and collaborators investigated the ex vivo effects of a moderate consumption of red wine (RW) and grape juice (GJ), and the in vitro effects of various substances (resveratrol, caffeic acid, gallic acid, quercetin and rutin) on STZ-induced diabetic rats. They demonstrated decreased platelet aggregation in diabetic-induced rats after moderate RW and GJ consumption for 45 days [55]. Similarly, resveratrol increased the hydrolysis of adenosine triphosphate (ATP), while quercetin decreased it in platelets [55]. These results were extended using a wine grape powder supplementation, which prevented hyperglycemia and IR, and reduced oxidative stress in a rat model of metabolic syndrome (MetS) [56].

Specific compounds found in both nuts and DFs were also further investigated. Quercetin and trans-resveratrol are plant polyphenols which have showed a significant reduction of IR and inflammation associated with obesity. Eid et al. showed that quercetin (isolated from lingonberry) exerted an anti-diabetic activity by stimulating adenosine monophosphate-activated protein kinase (AMPK) [40]. Moreover, quercetin also enhanced basal glucose uptake in mouse myoblast C2C12 muscle cells in the absence of insulin [40] via a mechanism which is highly analogous to metformin. Importantly, quercetin seems to be as effective as or more effective than resveratrol in attenuating TNF-α-mediated inflammation and IR in primary human adipocytes and macrophages [32,57].

3. Epidemiological Studies on Nuts

The relationship between the consumption of different food categories and the incidence or prevalence of metabolic disorders has been explored all over the world. As is shown in Table 4, numerous epidemiological studies have assessed the associations between nut consumption and T2D. However, no studies have been published on the link between DF consumption and risk of T2D.

As far as nuts are concerned, several studies have found an inverse association between the frequency of consumption and the development of this metabolic pathology [58–64]. In the Nurses' Health Study (NHS) and NHS II cohort, the intake of different types of nut was explored [61,64]. Total nut, walnut and peanut butter intake were associated with a lower risk of T2D in women. In the NHS (n = 83,818 female subjects), those with the highest nut consumption (28 g/day; ≥5 days a week) had a lower relative risk (RR) of developing T2D (0.73 [95% confidence interval (CI), 0.60–0.89]) than those who never/almost never consume (0.92 [95% CI, 0.85–1.00]) [61]. Results were similar for peanut butter: the RR was 0.79 (95% CI, 0.68–0.91) in those women who had a higher intake (5 times or more a week) than those who never/almost never ate peanut butter [61]. After combining NHS and NHS II cohorts, in a total of 137,953 female subjects, Pan and collaborators found that walnut consumption was inversely associated with risk of T2D [64].

These results are in line with those of a cross-sectional study of 7,210 subjects at high CV risk within the context of the PREvención con DIeta MEDiterránea (PREDIMED) study, where the upper category of nut consumption had a lower prevalence of T2D than the lower category [63]. A recent prospective study also associated the consumption of nuts—higher than 4 times a week—with a lower risk of T2D [60]. A cross-sectional study performed in the context of the National Health and Nutrition Examination Survey (NHANES) established a relation between the homeostatic model assessment of insulin resistance (HOMA-IR) and tree nut consumption. Decreased insulin resistance and lower levels of β-cell function markers were found in the nut consumers than the non-consumers [59]. In a large cohort of the Netherlands Cohort Study (NLCS), the total nut intake was associated to lower T2D cause-specific mortality in men and women [65].

Even though current evidence shows that nuts have a strong protective effect against the progress of T2D, especially in women, some epidemiological studies have not identified this relation [66,67]. The latest systematic review and meta-analysis designed to assess the relation between nut consumption and risk of cancer and T2D was published in 2015. It included five studies that were linked to T2D. After pooling data from studies conducted in both genders, it was found that there was no statistically significant association between nut consumption and risk of developing T2D (RR = 0.98 [95% CI, 0.84–1.14]), even though the heterogeneity was significant [68].

Table 4. Summary of epidemiological studies evaluating nut consumption.

First Author (Year) [Reference]	Study Name (Design)	Number of Subjects	Years of Follow-Up	Exposure	Findings
Jiang, R.; et al. (2002) [61]	NHS (Prospective)	83,818 women	16	≥5 times/week vs. never/almost never	Nut and peanut butter consumption was inversely associated with the risk of incident T2D.
Nettleton, J.A.; et al. (2008) [58]	MESA (Prospective)	5011 men and women	5	Quintiles of low-risk food pattern	High intake of whole grains, fruit, nuts/seeds, and green leafy vegetables was inversely associated to the risk of incident T2D.
Villegas, R.; et al. (2008) [62]	SWHS (Prospective)	64,227 women	4.6	Quintiles of peanut consumption	Consumption of peanuts was associated with a decreased risk of incident T2D.
Kochar, J.; et al. (2010) [67]	PHS I (Prospective)	20,224 men	19.2	≥7 servings of nuts/week vs. rarely or never consumers	No statistically significant association was found between nut consumption and T2D in either lean or overweight/obese subjects.
Ibarrola-Jurado, N.; et al. (2013) [63]	PREDIMED (Cross-sectional)	7210 at high cardiovascular risk	Baseline	<1 serving/week, 1–3 servings/week and >3 servings/week	The upper category of nut consumption had a lower prevalence of T2D than the lowest category.
Pan, A.; et al. (2013) [64]	NHS, NHS II (Prospective)	137,953 women	10	1–3 servings/month, 1 serving/week, and ≥2 servings/week of walnuts vs. never/rarely	Higher walnut consumption is associated with a significantly lower risk of T2D incidence.
O'Neil, C.E.; et al. (2015) [59]	NHANES (Cross-sectional)	14,386 men and women	6	Tree nut consumption compared with no consumption	Tree nut consumption was associated with lower HOMA-IR
Buijsse, B.; et al. (2015) [66]	EPIC-InterAct Study (Case-cohort)	16,154 men and women	12.3 Incident cases of T2D at 6.8	Non-consumers vs. the middle tertile of consumption.	Consumption of nuts and seeds does not modify T2D risk under isocaloric conditions and independent from BMI.
Asghari, G.; et al. (2017) [60]	TLGS (prospective)	1984 men and women	6.2 ± 0.7	≥4 servings/week vs. 1 or <1 serving/week	Nut consumption was associated with a lower risk of T2D incidence.

BMI, body mass index; CVD, cardiovascular disease; HOMA-IR, homeostatic model assessment of insulin resistance; MI, myocardial infarction; T2D, type 2 diabetes. Study name acronyms: EPIC, European Prospective Investigation into Cancer; HPFS, Health Professionals Follow-Up Study; MESA, Multi-Ethnic Study of Atherosclerosis; NHANES, National Health and Nutrition Examination Survey; NHS, Nurses' Health Study; NLCS, Netherlands Cohort Study; PHS, Physicians' Health Study; PREDIMED, PREvención con DIeta MEDiterránea; SCCS, Southern Community Cohort Study; SMHS, Shanghai Men's Health Study; SWHS, Shanghai Women's Health Study; TLGS, Tehran Lipid and Glucose Study.

4. Human Clinical Trials

The effect of nut consumption on glucose and insulin metabolism has also been researched in acute and chronic clinical trials. Acute studies mostly demonstrate a decrease in postprandial glycaemia and hyperinsulinemia after nut consumption. In contrast, chronic randomized clinical trials designed to analyze the effects on glucose metabolism provided controversial results.

4.1. Nuts

4.1.1. Acute Clinical Trials on Nuts

Table 5 summarizes various acute clinical studies of nut consumption, most of which focus on almonds [69–73]. In a randomized crossover trial in healthy subjects, almond intake decreased postprandial glycaemia and insulinaemia [69]. In a dose-response study conducted in healthy individuals, almond intake attenuated the postprandial glycaemic response of white bread [70]. In impaired glucose-tolerant subjects, it was observed that the consumption of almonds with a meal also decreased blood glucose in plasma [71]. In a recent crossover study performed in pre-diabetic subjects, a preload of almonds decreased postprandial glycaemia [73]. In healthy and diabetic individuals, Cohen et al. also showed a 30% reduction in postprandial glycaemia after almond consumption compared with a starchy meal [72].

The effect of pistachio intake on postprandial glycaemia was investigated by Kendall et al. in two randomized studies. In overweight (Ow) healthy subjects, pistachio consumption was reported to have a minimal effect on postprandial glycaemia. When pistachios were included in a carbohydrate meal, the relative glycaemic response (RGR) was attenuated [74]. In a crossover trial with 20 subjects with MetS, postprandial glycaemia decreased after the consumption of pistachios (85 g) compared to white bread. In the same study, a peripheral increase in the glucagon-like peptide-1 (GLP-1) concentrations was also observed after pistachio consumption compared with the consumption of white bread [75].

For peanuts, a randomized crossover trial conducted in 13 healthy subjects reported a decreased postprandial glycaemic response after the consumption of a breakfast containing 63 g of one of the following types of peanuts: raw with skin, roasted without skin and ground-roasted without skin [76]. Similarly, in a parallel study conducted in 65 overweight and obese men, peanut consumption reduced postprandial insulinaemia levels compared to high-oleic peanut consumption [77].

Nut consumption was observed to have similar beneficial effects on glucose and insulin metabolism in the only study to analyze the effect of a mix of nuts (almonds, macadamias, walnuts, pistachios, hazelnuts and pecans). In this study conducted in 10 diabetic and 14 non-diabetic subjects, nut consumption decreased the RGR compared to white bread. Importantly, this study also reported that nut consumption improved short-term glycaemic control in patients with T2D [74].

In summary, nuts seem to have beneficial postprandial glycaemic effects when consumed alone or in combination with high carbohydrate foods, and so may potentially help to prevent and manage impaired glucose states.

Table 5. Summary of acute clinical studies analyzing the effect of nut consumption on postprandial response.

First Author (Year) [Reference]	N° of Subjects (M/F) Type of Subject (Age in Years)	Type of Nut (Study Design)	Control Group	Intervention Group	Glucose and Insulin Metabolism Outcomes	Other Outcomes
Jenkins, D.J.; et al. (2006) [69]	15 (7/8) Healthy subjects (26.3 ± 8.6)	Almonds (crossover)	97 g of white bread	- Almond meal: 60 g almonds +97 g bread - Parboiled rice meal: 68 g cheese and 14 g butter +60 g parboiled rice - Mashed potato meal: 62 g cheese and 16 g butter +68 g mashed potatoes	Almonds decrease postprandial glycaemia and insulinaemia.	Almonds are likely to decrease oxidative damage to serum proteins by decreasing glycaemic excursion and providing antioxidants.
Josse, A.R.; et al. (2007) [70]	9 (7/2) Healthy subjects (27.8±6.9)	Almonds (crossover dose-response study)	White bread	- White bread +30 g almonds - White bread +60 g almonds - White bread +90 g almonds	The 90-g almond meal resulted in a significantly lower GI than the white bread control meal	
Mori, A.M.; et al. (2011) [71]	14 (8/6) IGT (39.3 ± 10.9)	Almonds (crossover)	75 g of available CHO (No almonds)	75 g of available CHO from: - Whole almonds - Almond butter - Defatted almond flour - Almond oil	Whole almonds significantly attenuated second-meal and daylong blood glucose IAUC.	GLP-1 concentrations did not significantly vary between treatments.
Kendall, C.W.; et al. (2011) [74]	10 (3/7) Ow healthy subjects (48.3 ± 6.4)	Pistachios (crossover)	White bread	Study 1: - 28, 56 and 84 g pistachios - 28, 56 and 84 g Study 2: - 56 g of pistachios + different commonly consumed carbohydrate foods (50 g available carbohydrate).	Pistachios consumed alone had a minimal effect on postprandial glycaemia. Pistachios consumed with a carbohydrate meal attenuated the RGR.	
Cohen, A.E. and Johnston, C.S. (2011) [72]	20 (6/14) Healthy subjects ($n = 13$) and T2D subjects ($n = 7$) (Healthy: 53.0 ± 3 and T2D: 66.0 ± 3.3)	Almonds (postprandial: crossover trial)	No almond meal	28 g almonds enriched meal	The ingestion of almonds immediately before a starchy meal significantly reduced postprandial glycaemia by 30%.	
Kendall, C.W.; et al. (2011) [78]	24 (11/13) Healthy ($n = 14$) and T2D subjects ($n = 10$) (Healthy: 36.0 ± 4 and T2D: 68.0 ± 2)	Mixed nuts (i.e., almonds, macadamias, walnuts, pistachios, hazelnuts and pecans) (crossover)	White bread	3 doses of 30, 60 and 90 g of mixed nuts	Nuts improve short-term glycaemic control in patients with T2D.	

Table 5. *Cont.*

First Author (Year) [Reference]	N° of Subjects (M/F) Type of Subject (Age in Years)	Type of Nut (Study Design)	Control Group	Intervention Group	Glucose and Insulin Metabolism Outcomes	Other Outcomes
Reis, C.E.; et al. (2011) [76]	13 (4/9) Healthy subjects (28.5 ± 10)	Peanuts (crossover)	Cheese sandwich	63 g of: - raw peanuts with skin - roasted peanuts without skin - ground-roasted peanuts without skin	The ingestion of ground-roasted peanuts without skin for breakfast leads to a lower CHO intake and reduced postprandial glycaemic response.	
Moreira, A.P.; et al. (2014) [77]	65 men Ow/Ob (Range: 18–50)	Conventional peanuts and high-oleic peanuts (parallel)	56 g biscuit	- 56 g conventional peanuts ($n = 21$) - 56 g high-oleic peanuts ($n = 23$)	Conventional peanut consumption was associated with decreased postprandial insulinaemia, which might be beneficial for saving β-cell function, independently of the influence on LPS concentrations.	
Kendall, C.W.; et al. (2014) [75]	20 (8/12) Subjects with MetS (54.0 ± 8)	Pistachios (crossover)	Control 1: white bread Control 2: (white bread + butter + cheese)	Test meal 1: WB + 85 g of pistachios Test meal 2: 85 g of pistachios	Pistachio consumption reduced postprandial glycaemia compared with white bread.	Pistachio consumption increased GLP-1 levels compared with white bread.
Crouch, M.A. and Slater, R.T. (2016) [73]	20 (13/7) Subjects with pre-diabetes * (Mean: 60.8)	Almonds (crossover)	No almonds	12 units of dry-roasted almonds	A low-calorie almond preload "appetizer" decreased postprandial hyperglycemia.	

Age is shown as mean ± SD unless otherwise stated. BMI, body mass index; CHO, carbohydrate; GLP-1, glucagon-like peptide-1; HbA_{1c}, glycated hemoglobin; IAUC, incremental area under the curve; IGT, impaired glucose tolerance; LPS, lipopolysaccharide; MetS, metabolic syndrome; M/F, male/female; Ob, obese; Ow, overweight; RGR, relative glycaemic responses; T2D, type 2 diabetes; WB, white bread. * also include "isolated 1-h glucose > 160 mg/dL".

4.1.2. Chronic Clinical Trials on Nuts

Most of the RCTs have compared nut-enriched diets with control diets in order to analyze their effects on lipid profile, and blood glucose and insulin concentrations as a secondary outcome. However, some, mainly conducted in subjects with T2D [72,79–84], but also in pre-diabetic [85], hyperlipemic [86], overweight/obese [87] and healthy individuals [88], were specifically designed to assess changes in glucose or insulin metabolism after nut consumption (Table 6).

In 2002, Lovejoy and coworkers evaluated the effect of an almond-enriched diet in 20 healthy and 30 T2D subjects in two different studies [79]. Healthy subjects, supplemented with 100 g almonds/day for 4 weeks and advised to reduce their energy intake by an equivalent amount, did not change their insulin sensitivity, whereas their body weight increased and their lipid profile improved. In a second study, subjects with T2D were randomized following a crossover design to one of 4 diets with different fat contents (25% or 37%) with 10% of fat from almonds or from olive or canola oil, with a minimum washout of 2 weeks between periods. Fat source (almond vs. oil) or fat level (high fat vs. low fat) were not observed to have any significant effect on either the glucose or insulin index. In contrast, in a crossover study conducted in 20 Chinese patients with T2D and mild-hyperlipidemia assigned to either a control diet (National Cholesterol Education Program (NCEP) step II diet) or an almond-enriched diet (with almonds replacing the 20% total daily calorie intake) for 4 weeks, a significant decrease in fasting insulin and glucose concentrations together with an improvement of HOMA-IR were reported during the almond phase [80]. In a similar crossover study conducted in 48 diabetic patients who received 50 g/day of pistachios and a pistachio-free diet (12 weeks each period), with an 8-week washout, a significant improvement in fasting blood glucose (FBG) and HbA_{1c} was observed during the pistachio consumption, while no changes in HOMA-IR were reported [83]. Recently, Gulati and coworkers conducted a pre-post intervention study in a group of 50 Asian Indians who consumed 20% of total energy in the form of whole raw almonds for 24 weeks preceded by a control diet free of nuts. Although no changes in FBG were observed during the almond consumption, the authors found a significant reduction in glycosylated hemoglobin, together with an improvement in other T2D risk factors such as waist circumference or inflammation status [84]. To determine whether the beneficial effect of nut consumption on glucose and insulin metabolism could also be extended to pre-diabetic subjects our group conducted a randomized crossover study in 54 pre-diabetic subjects who consumed a pistachio-supplemented diet (55 g pistachio/day) and a control diet (nut-free diet), each for 4 months with a 2-week washout period. We found a beneficial effect of pistachio intake on fasting glucose, insulin, and HOMA-IR. Other cardiometabolic risk markers such as fibrinogen, oxidized LDL, platelet factor 4 and GLP-1 were also modified appropriately during the consumption of pistachios [85].

Changes in fasting glucose or insulin levels, HOMA-IR and glycosylated hemoglobin have also been assessed as secondary outcomes in several clinical feeding trials with different designs (parallel, crossover) and subject characteristics (i.e., healthy, overweight/obese, TD2, MetS), mainly using walnuts and almonds, and with different intervention lengths (from 2 weeks to 2 years). The results obtained are controversial. Although most studies found no improvement in glucose/insulin metabolism [89–103], others reported a significant reduction in FBG levels [89,92,104,105], fasting insulin or insulin resistance [90,92,106,107] and HbA_{1c} [92]. However, a meta-analysis of RCTs including 25 trials with a total of 1,650 particpants who were otherwise healthy or had dyslipidaemia, metabolic syndrome or type 2 diabetes mellitus showed that the consumption of tree nuts led to modest decreases in fasting blood glucose compared with control diet interventions [108].

Table 6. Summary of chronic clinical trials and their characteristics in the context of nut consumption.

First Author (Year) [Reference]	N° of Subjects (M/F) Type of Subjects (Age in Years)	Nut Study Design (Length of the Intervention)	Control Group	Intervention Group(s)	Glucose and Insulin Metabolism Outcomes	Other Outcomes
Lovejoy, J.C.; et al. (2002) [79]	30 (13/17) T2D subjects (mean ± SEM: 53.8 ± 1.9)	Almonds Crossover (1 month per period)	HF-Control LF-Control	HF-HA LF-HA	No significant changes in glycaemia were observed.	Total cholesterol was lowest after the HF-HA diet. HDL-C was significantly decreased after the almond diet; however, no significant effect of fat source on LDL: HDL was reported.
Jenkins, D.J.A.; et al. (2008) [86]	27 (15/12) Hyperlipidemic subjects (64 ± 9)	Almonds Crossover (1 month per period)	147 ± 6 g/day of muffins	Almonds (73 ± 3 g/day) Half portion of almonds (37 ± 2 g/day) plus muffins (75 ± 3 g/day) Isoenergetic (mean, 423 Kcal/day)	No significant changes were observed in FBG, insulin, C-peptide, or HOMA-IR. The 24-h urinary C-peptide output, as a marker of 24-h insulin secretion, was significantly reduced by the half-and full-dose almonds in comparison to the control muffin diet after adjustment for urinary creatinine output.	There were no significant treatment differences in BW.
Claesson, A.L.; et al. 2009 [88]	25 (11/14) Healthy subjects (range: 19–30)	Peanuts Parallel (2 weeks)	Addition of 20 kcal/kg-BW of candy to the regular caloric intake.	Addition of 20 kcal/kg-BW of roasted peanuts to the regular caloric intake.	Plasma-insulin and C-peptide increased in the candy group, but not in the peanut group. FBG was not modified.	Energy intake increased similarly in both groups. BW and WC increased significantly only in the candy group. At the end of the study LDL-C and ApoB/ApoA-1-ratio were higher in the candy group than in the peanut group.
Cohen, A.E.; et al. (2011) [72]	13 (7/6) T2D subjects (66.0 ± 3.3)	Almonds Parallel (3 months)	Nut- free diet	Diet enriched with almonds (28 g, 5 times/week)	Significant reduction of HbA_{1c} in the almond group compared to the nut-free diet group.	Chronic almond ingestion was associated with a reduction in BMI as compared with no change in the nut–free diet group.
Li, S.C.; et al. (2011) [80]	20 (9/11) T2D subjects (Mean: 58)	Almonds Crossover (1 month per period)	NCEP step II diet (control diet); CHO (56 E%), protein (17 E%), and fat (27 E%).	Almonds were added to the control diet to replace 20% of total daily calorie intake.	Compared with subjects in the control diet, those in the almond diet reduced the levels of fasting insulin, FBG, and HOMA-IR.	Almond intake decreased TC, LDL-C, and LDL-C/HDL-C. The almond diet enhanced plasma α-tocopherol level compared with control diet.
Damavandi, R.D.; et al. (2013) [81]	45 (15/33) Medicated T2D subjects (55.68 ± 7.74)	Hazelnuts Parallel (2 months)	Control diet	10% of total daily calorie intake was replaced with hazelnuts	No significant differences in FBG between groups.	No changes in BMI were reported. Significant HDL-C reduction in control group was observed. Although the hazelnut group achieved a greater reduction in TG concentrations than the control group, these changes were non-significant.
Hernández-Alonso, P.; et al. (2014) [85]	54 (29/25) Subjects with Pre-D Mean: 55 (range: 53.4–56.8)	Crossover (4 months per period)	Nut-free diet: the energy intake of other fatty foods, mostly olive oil, was adjusted to compensate for the energy from pistachios included in the PD.	Pistachio diet was supplemented with 2 ounces of pistachio (57 g/day)	FBG, insulin, and HOMA-IR decreased significantly after the chronic pistachio period compared with the nut-free period.	Fibrinogen, oxidized-LDL, and PF-4 significantly decreased under the pistachio period compared to the nut-free period, whereas GLP-1 increased.

Table 6. *Cont.*

First Author (Year) [Reference]	N° of Subjects (M/F) Type of Subjects (Age in Years)	Nut Study Design (Length of the Intervention)	Control Group	Intervention Group(s)	Glucose and Insulin Metabolism Outcomes	Other Outcomes
Lasa, A.; et al. (2014) [82]	191 (77/114) T2D subjects (Mean: 67)	Mixed nuts Parallel (1 year)	LFD	Mediterranean diets supplemented with either virgin olive oil or mixed nuts	Increased values of the adiponectin/leptin ratio and adiponectin/HOMA-IR ratio and decreased values of WC were observed in the three groups.	In both Mediterranean diet groups, but not in the LFD group, this was associated with a significant reduction in BW.
Parham, M.; et al. (2014) [83]	44 (11/33) T2D subjects (Mean: 51)	Pistachios Crossover (3 months per period)	Previous diet without pistachios	Two snacks of 25 g pistachios/day	Marked decrease in HbA_{1c} and FBG concentrations in the pistachio diet group compared with the control group.	There were no overall significant changes in BMI, blood pressure, HOMA-IR, or CRP concentrations.
Le, T.; et al. (2016) [87]	213 women Ow/Ob subjects (Mean: 50)	Walnuts Parallel (1 year)	Control 1: a lower fat (20 E%), higher CHO (65 E%) diet. Control 2: lower CHO (45 E%), higher fat (35 E%) diet	Walnut-enriched diet: high fat (35 E%), lower CHO (45 E%) diet.	Insulin sensitivity and CRP levels improved after walnut-rich diet	TG decreased in all study arms at 6 months. The walnut-rich diet increased HDL-C more than either the lower fat or lower CHO diet. The walnut-rich diet also reduced LDL-C.

Age is shown as mean ± SD unless otherwise stated. Apo, apolipoprotein; BMI, Body mass index; BW, body weight; CHO, carbohydrate; CRP, C-reactive protein; E%, energy percentage; FBG, fasting blood glucose; GLP-1, glucagon-like peptide-1; HA: high almond; HbA_{1c}, glycated hemoglobin; HDL-C, high-density lipoprotein cholesterol; HF, high fat; HOMA-IR, homeostatic model assessment of insulin resistance; LDL-C, low-density lipoprotein cholesterol; LF: low fat; LFD, LF diet; M/F, male/female; NCEP, National Cholesterol Education Program; NS, non-significant; Ob, obese; Ow, overweight; PF-4, platelet factor-4; PM, post-menopausal; Pre-D, pre-diabetes; T2D, type 2 diabetes; TC, total cholesterol; TG, triglycerides; WC, waist circumference; WHtR, waist-to-height ratio.

4.2. Dried Fruits

4.2.1. Acute Clinical Trials on Dried Fruits

Less research has been carried out into DFs than into nuts. However, the findings to date point to a beneficial effect of DFs on postprandial glucose regulation and glycaemic control in T2D subjects.

The putative effect of DFs on postprandial glycaemia and insulinaemia has been studied mainly using raisins (Table 7). However, some research into dried plums has also been published.

First, in 1989 Rasmussen and coworkers evaluated in healthy and T2D subjects the postprandial effects of three meals: raw rolled oats, oatmeal porridge, or a mixture of raw rolled oats with raisins, compared to a control glucose ingestion [109]. The substitution of 25% of the starch meal with raisins (i.e., simple sugars) did not affect blood glucose or insulin responses. In addition, a similar glucose and insulin response in both normal and T2D subjects were reported [109].

Other researchers investigated the postprandial effect of raisins consumed alone. When the GI was investigated in three different groups (sedentary, aerobically trained or pre-diabetic subjects), no significant differences were found among groups, even though the GI (55–69) it seemed moderate for aerobically trained adults, and low (GI, $\leq$55) for the other groups [110]. Kanellos and collaborators found a moderate GI of raisins in healthy and T2D subjects [111], whereas Esfahani et al. found that raisins were low-GI and glycaemic load (GL) foods in healthy subjects [112]. Recently, researchers have found that even though the same available CHO content from raisins and glucose generated a similar postprandial response, raisins significantly modulated the levels of GIP, ghrelin and ghrelin/obestatin ratio, with important implications in terms of appetite regulation and overall insulin secretion [113]. In overweight women, researchers determined that dried plums had a lower plasma glucose and insulin incremental area under the curve (IAUC) than an isoenergetic low-fat cookie meal [114].

Overall, results suggest that raisins have a beneficial postprandial glucose and insulin effect, which may cautiously be extrapolated to other DFs considering their overall macronutrient composition.

Table 7. Summary of acute clinical studies analyzing the effect of dried fruit consumption on postprandial response.

First Author (Year) [Reference]	N° of Subjects (M/F) Type of Subject (Age in Years)	Dried Fruit (Study Design)	Control Group	Intervention Group(s)	Glucose and Insulin Metabolism Outcomes	Other Outcomes
Rasmussen, O.; et al. (1989) [109]	20 (9/11) Healthy (n = 11) and T2D subjects (n = 9) (Healthy: 30 ± 2; T2D subjects: 67 ± 2)	Raisins (crossover)	75 g (healthy) or 50 g (T2D) of CHO	Raw rolled oats; oatmeal porridge or a mixture of raw rolled oats with raisins	Substitution of 25% of the starch meal with raisins (simple sugars) did not affect blood glucose or insulin responses	In normal and T2D subjects, the three meals produce similar glucose and insulin response curves.
Kim, Y.; et al. (2008) [110]	10 S; 11 AT and 10 Pre-D (S (25.7 ± 1.3), AT (23.1 ± 1.0), Pre-D (50.0 ± 2.6))	Raisins (crossover)	50 g of available CHO from glucose	50 g of available CHO from raisins	NS differences among groups. The GI of raisins seemed lower (≤55) in the S and P groups compared to moderate (GI, 56–69) in the A group. The insulinaemic index of raisins was not different among groups.	
Furchner-Evanson, A.; et al. (2010) [114]	19 women ow subjects (39.2 ± 0.7)	Dried plums (crossover)	White bread (238 Kcal)	Dried plums (238 Kcal) Low-fat cookies (238 Kcal)	Dried plums elicited lower plasma glucose and insulin IAUC than low-fat cookies.	The satiety index IAUC was greater for the dried plums than low-fat cookies, and tended to promote a greater plasma ghrelin AOC
Kanellos, P.T.; et al. (2013) [111]	30 (17/13) Healthy and T2D subjects (n = 15 each) (Healthy: 25.9 ± 0.8; T2D: 63.2 ± 1.7)	Corinthian raisins (crossover)	50 g of glucose	74 g of Corinthian raisins; 50 g of available CHO	Significantly different glucose peaks between raisins and glucose in healthy and in diabetic subjects. Glycaemic and insulinaemic responses were decreased after raisin consumption compared to glucose ingestion.	
Esfahani, A.; et al. (2014) [112]	10 (4/6) Healthy subjects (39 ± 11)	Raisins (crossover)	108 g of white bread; 50 g available CHO (consumed on two separate occasions)	R50: 69 g raisins; 50 g available CHO R20: 28 g raisins; 20 g available CHO	The raisin meals, R50 and R20, resulted in significantly reduced postprandial glucose and insulin responses compared with white bread	Raisins were determined to be low in GI, GL and insulinaemic index.
Kaliora, A.C.; et al. (2017) [113]	10 Healthy normo-weight subjects (26.3 ± 0.8)	Raisins (crossover)	50 g of glucose	74 g of raisins; 50 g of available CHO	At 60 min, glucose and insulin levels were maximum in both groups.	GIP was lower after raising intake compared to glucose intake at 60 and 120 min postprandially. Ghrelin was lower after raisin compared to glucose intake at 120 and at 180 min post-ingestion. No differences were reported for GLP-1, apelin or obestatin in either trial.

Age is shown as mean ± SD unless otherwise stated. AT, aerobically trained; AOC, area over the curve; CHO, carbohydrates; GI, glycaemic index; GL, glycaemic load; GLP-1, glucagon-like peptide-1; IAUC, incremental area under the curve; M/F, male/female; NS, non-significant; ow, overweight; Pre-D, pre-diabetic; S, sedentary; T2D, type 2 diabetes; WB, white bread.

4.2.2. Chronic Clinical Trials on Dried Fruits

The study of the beneficial effects of chronic DF consumption also focuses on raisins (Table 8). Randomized clinical trials have been conducted in healthy [115], overweight or obese [116,117], T2D subjects [118,119], or a combination of the three [120]. In a 6-week parallel trial in healthy subjects, Puglisi et al. included 150 g/day of raisins into subjects' habitual diet or increased their physical activity (or combined them both). Neither FPG nor insulin levels were different among groups or compared to baseline. However, the inflammation status reported by plasma TNF-α significantly decreased in the raisin intervention [115].

The results for overweight or obese subjects do not show a significant improvement in glucose or insulin levels after the consumption of raisins [116] or dried plums [117]. However, these studies are only short (2 weeks) which makes it impossible to analyze the chronic effect. In fact, in a parallel study conducted in Ow/Ob subjects, comparing raisin consumption (270 Kcal/day) with a snack (300 Kcal/day) for 12 weeks, researchers [120] found that even though FGP or insulin were not affected by either intervention, HbA_{1c} levels and postprandial glucose levels had been reduced by raisin consumption by the end of the trial. This suggests a beneficial effect of raisin consumption on glycaemic control in Ow/Ob subjects with pre-D. Importantly, raisin intake also improved systolic blood pressure (SBP) and diastolic blood pressure (DBP) and had a null effect on body weight [120].

Two studies have been conducted in individuals with T2D. A parallel study comparing the consumption of 36 g of raisins versus the habitual diet free of raisins or grapes for 24 weeks did not find any change in either body weight or in glycaemic control and lipid profile, but the total antioxidant capacity increased and the DBP decreased after raisin consumption [118]. Likewise, the consumption of raisins as a snack (84 g/day, 270 Kcal/day) for 12 weeks significantly reduced the postprandial glucose response in T2D subjects compared to an alternative snack (300 Kcal/day) for 12 weeks. A non-significant trend to a reduction in fasting glucose and HbA_{1c} was also observed in the same group of raisin consumers [119].

The results of DF consumption on glycaemia/insulinaemia point to a beneficial effect. However, novel acute and long-term RCTs assessing other types of DF should be carried out in order to corroborate and expand what is known about raisins.

Table 8. Summary of chronic clinical trials and their characteristics in the context of dried fruit consumption.

First Author (Year) [Reference]	N° of Subjects (M/F) Type of Subject (Age in Years)	Study Design (Length of the Intervention)	Control Group	Intervention Group(s)	Glucose and Insulin Metabolism Outcomes	Other Outcomes
Puglisi, M.J.; et al. (2008) [115]	34 (17/17 PM) Healthy (range: 50–70)	Raisin Parallel (6 weeks)	Walk (increase in the steps taken per day)	150 g/day of raisins. Walk + 150 g/day of raisins	Changes in FBG and insulin values did not differ among intervention groups or from baseline. Plasma TNF-α decreased in the raisin group but no differences were reported between groups.	Plasma TC and LDL-C decreased in all the intervention groups.
Rankin, J.W.; et al. (2008) [116]	17 (8/9) Ow (26.5 ± 7.6)	Raisin Crossover (2 weeks per period)	Jelly candy (264 Kcal/day)	90 g/day raisins (264 Kcal/day)	NS changes in FBG or markers of inflammation or endothelial dysfunction after the raisin intervention.	Fasting protein-free ORAC was modestly higher after the raisin intervention than the jelly candy intervention.
Howarth, L.; et al. (2010) [117]	26 women Ow/Ob (range: 25–54)	Dried plums Crossover (2 weeks per period)	Low-fat cookies (200 Kcal/day)	Dried plums (200 Kcal/day)	No changes were found in plasma glucose or insulin levels in any intervention.	Plasma TG concentration was unchanged by dried plum consumption and was higher after the consumption of low-fat cookies. Incorporation of dried plums or low-fat cookies into the diet did not alter energy intake or BW.
Anderson, J.W.; et al. (2014) [120]	46 (21/25) Ow/Ob with Pre-D or at T2D risk. (snack (mean: 61.1), raisins (mean: 60.3))	Raisins Parallel (12 weeks)	Snacks (300 Kcal/day)	84 g/day of raisins (270 Kcal/day)	Fasting HbA_{1c} levels were significantly reduced after raisin intake, whereas FBG and insulin levels were not significantly affected by the intake of raisins or snacks. Postprandial glucose levels were significantly reduced by raisin intake vs. snacks.	Raisin intake was associated with reductions in SBP and DBP. BW did not significantly change within or between groups.
Kanellos, P.T.; et al. (2014) [118]	48 (25/23) T2D (raisins (63.7 ± 6.3), control (63 ± 8.5))	Corinthian raisins Parallel (24 weeks)	Usual diet avoiding grapes and raisins	36 g/day of Corinthian raisins	BW, glycaemic control, and lipid profile were not changed in either arm of the intervention. Patients in the CR arm reduced their DBP and increased their total antioxidant potential compared with baseline values and the control group.	No change in CRP was observed. A significant difference in plasma circulating p-hydroxybenzoic acid was observed between groups at the end of the trial.
Bays, H.; et al. (2015) [119]	46 (19/27) T2D (mean: 58)	Dark raisins Parallel (12 weeks)	Snack group (300 Kcal/day)	84 g/day of dark raisins group (270 Kcal/day)	Compared to the snack group, those who consumed raisins reduced their postprandial glucose levels, and an NS trend to a reduction in fasting glucose and HbA_{1c}. NS changes in BW, fasting insulin, HOMA-IR or lipid profile between intervention groups.	Compared to alternative processed snacks, those who consumed raisins had a significant reduction in SBP but not a significant reduction in DBP.

Age is shown as mean ± SD unless otherwise stated. BW, body weight; CRP, C-reactive protein; DBP, diastolic blood pressure; FBG, fasting blood glucose; HbA_{1c}, glycated hemoglobin; HOMA-IR, homeostatic model assessment of insulin resistance; LDL-C, low-density lipoprotein cholesterol; M/F, male/female; NS, non-significant; Ob, obese; ORAC, oxygen radical absorbance capacity; Ow, overweight; pre-D, pre-diabetes; PM, postmenopausal women; SBP, systolic blood pressure; T2D, type 2 diabetes; TC, total cholesterol; TG, triglycerides; TNF-α, tumor necrosis factor-α.

5. Potential Mechanisms Linking Nut and Dried Fruit Consumption to Glucose and Insulin Metabolism

5.1. Nut- and Dried Fruit-Related Nutrients and Their Role in Glucose and Insulin Metabolism

Fiber Content in Nuts and Dried Fruits

Both nuts and DFs are high in dietary fiber [9]. Diets rich in complex CHO and fiber are associated with increased insulin sensitivity and reduced plasma insulin levels, promoting better glycaemic control in diabetic patients [121]. Soluble fiber increases gastric distension, viscosity in the gastrointestinal tract, and slower absorption of macronutrients [122]. As a consequence, the speed of CHO absorption and the concentration of postprandial glucose tend to be lower after the ingestion of fiber-rich foods than foods or meals poor in fibers [123].

Fiber is resistant to enzymatic digestion in the small intestine and thus susceptible to fermentation by bacteria in the colon. It produces short chain fatty acids (SCFA, e.g., acetate, propionate and butyrate) which reduce the production of hepatic glucose and stimulate the secretion of GLP-1 [124,125]. Incretins such as GLP-1 and gastric inhibitory polypeptide (GIP) stimulate the secretion of insulin by β-cells and promote the proliferation of these cells, favoring the maintenance of normal blood glucose levels [125]. The secretion of GLP-1—which is mainly performed by enteroendocrine L-cells of the gastrointestinal tract -is partly mediated by monosaccharides, peptides and amino-acids, MUFA and PUFA as well as by SCFA. Therefore, the positive influence of GLP-1 on blood glucose homeostasis, appetite sensations, and food intake provides a strong rationale for its therapeutic potential in the nutritional management of T2D and obesity [126].

Overall fiber contained in nuts and DFs is also able to decrease postprandial glycaemic levels and this could be a strategy for increasing insulin sensitivity which improves T2D and several other CV risk factors for chronic diseases [74,127].

Carbohydrate Content—Glycaemic Index of Nuts and Dried Fruits

It should be noted that nuts are relatively low in CHO (approximately 15% of the total energy) whereas DFs have a high amount of CHO (60–80%). Nuts have a low glycaemic index and therefore increase the blood glucose level less and require less insulin secretion, thus favoring the control of T2D. However, because DFs are high in carbohydrates and fiber, their specific GI has been the object of considerable study. The GI of raisins was first evaluated in three heterogeneous groups of subjects (aerobically trained, sedentary or pre-diabetic) and was described between 49 and 69, therefore corresponding to the low-to-moderate GI foods [110]. However, later studies have reported that raisins are in the low GI category in healthy subjects (a GI of 49.4 and an insulinemic index of 47.1) [15]. This suggests a favorable postprandial glucose and insulin response [112], that could be explained by the high proportion of fructose that DFs contain.

Overall, the inclusion of both nuts and DFs in a balanced diet may reduce the overall glycaemic index of the diet, with benefits to glycaemic and insulinemic control in both healthy and T2D subjects [128].

Fat Content in Nuts

The high content of MUFA and PUFA in nuts seems to enhance the reduction of IR, thus consequently reducing the risk of developing T2D [129–131]. However, the mechanisms by which these fatty acids (FA) affect insulin sensitivity are not yet fully understood [132]. It is believed, however, that the FAs present in the phospholipids of different cell membranes are affected by the type of fatty acid intake, thus affecting insulin sensitivity. The different unsaturated FAs that are part of the cell membrane influence the action of insulin via affecting the binding or affinity of insulin to its cellular receptor [133]. It is hypothesized that a higher unsaturation of FA in the cell membrane facilitates the movement of the glucose receptor to the cell surface, thus increasing insulin sensitivity [134].

In addition, as we have seen, unsaturated fatty acids act through the stimulation of GLP-1 secretion, thus improving the efficiency of β-cells. SFA and MUFA act on the lipogenic gene expression, while PUFA inhibit the expression of these genes, partly by binding and activating nuclear receptors, such as those activated by peroxisome proliferators (PPAR) [131]. It has been suggested that the activation of PPAR has a therapeutic role in the treatment of T2D, because it induces fatty acid clearance by the adipose tissue, decreasing its plasma levels and thus increasing insulin sensitivity in the muscle [135].

Mineral Content in Nuts and Dried Fruits

Nuts contain relatively high quantities of different minerals such as potassium, magnesium and calcium, whereas DF contains more moderate quantities (mainly potassium, magnesium and boron). Magnesium has been associated with beneficial effects on glycaemic control [136]. Low magnesium levels have been implicated in IR development [124]. In fact, kidneys lose the ability to retain magnesium in periods of acute hyperglycemia. It is excreted in the urine, leading to low mineral blood levels. It has been shown that correcting this depletion improves response and insulin action. Magnesium deficiency also interferes with the reactions that use or produce ATP, thus altering the enzyme cascade involved in the CHO metabolism and favoring the development of T2D [137].

Therefore, the minerals present in nuts and DF could explain the relationship observed between magnesium intake and the lower risk of developing T2D and other chronic diseases [138,139].

Other Bioactive Compounds in Nuts and Dried Fruits

The other bioactive compounds contained in nuts and DF could partially explain their protective anti-oxidant and anti-inflammatory properties [2] and their implication in glucose and insulin metabolism (and therefore in T2D). Significant evidence suggests that polyphenol-rich diets have the ability to protect against diabetes [140]. It appears that anthocyanins (or anthocyanin-rich foods) are inversely associated to the risk of T2D, but there is no association for other polyphenol subclasses [141,142]. Dietary polyphenols have some benefits for T2D: they protect pancreatic β-cells against glucose toxicity and they have anti-inflammatory and anti-oxidant effects, among other things. Quercetin is a member of the flavonoid class of polyphenols which is abundant in such foods as fruits, vegetables, nuts and seeds [143]. Several in vitro studies have sought to elucidate the mechanisms behind the antidiabetic properties of quercetin: for example the inhibition of the α-amylase and α-glucosidase activities, and the prevention of the lipid peroxidation of pancreatic tissue homogenates [144]. Moreover, ellagic acid (EA) is another polyphenol which naturally occurs in some fruits, such as berries (strawberries and red and black raspberries), nuts, and pomegranates [145]. There is emerging in vitro evidence that EA may ameliorate symptoms of chronic metabolic diseases—by decreasing chronic inflammation at the expression level—which include dyslipidemia, IR and T2D [146–148]. Despite the growing amount of information on EA, a definitive mechanism of action has not been established. This may be attributed to the complexity of EA metabolism, which is governed by various factors [145].

A growing body of evidence suggests that dietary agents and the non-nutrient components of fruits, vegetables and nuts can affect epigenetic processes related to T2D [149,150]. Epigenetics generally refers to heritable and reversible changes affecting gene expression and chromatin organization that are not due to alterations in the DNA sequence [151,152]. No specific data is available on the role of nuts and DFs in T2D epigenetics. However, dietary polyphenol resveratrol—most abundant in the skin of grapes and raisins, but also found in peanuts and cranberries [153]—and other phytochemicals (e.g., curcumin) have proved to be effective agents against cancer and to act through epigenetic mechanisms that affect the global epigenome [154,155]. However, future studies are needed to determine the biological importance of the altered tissue-specific DNA methylation in T2D resulting from nutritional modifications [152].

5.2. Cellular and Molecular Mechanisms Linking Nut and Dried Fruit Consumption and the Prevention and/or Management of T2D/IR

Gene Expression

Some studies have analyzed the effect of nut and DF consumption on changes in the gene expression of particular cells and/or tissues and its relationship with glucose and insulin metabolism or T2D. In particular, a crossover study conducted in pre-diabetic subjects consuming pistachio for 4 months reported a downregulation of interleukin-6 (*IL-6*) and resistin (*RETN*) genes in leukocytes, whereas the pistachio diet led to a lower significant increase of solute carrier family 2 member 4 (*SLC2A4*, codifying GLUT4) [85]. Consistent with this attenuation in the expression of glucose transporters, leukocytes significantly reduced the uptake of glucose following pistachio consumption, suggesting a decrease in the cell hyperactivity described in T2D.

To our knowledge no published studies have evaluated gene expression after the consumption of DF. However, a translational study conducted in 120 healthy young subjects has shown that individuals in the highest tertile of fruit and vegetable consumption had statistically lower values of the expression of some pro-inflammatory marker genes such as intercellular adhesion molecule-1 (ICAM-1), IL-6 and TNF-α, in peripheral blood mononuclear cells (PBMC) [156].

Therefore, these results shed new light on the nutrient-gene interactions in nuts and DFs. However, further research is needed.

MicroRNAs

The modulatory role of nuts and DF on the expression of genes related to inflammation, oxidative stress and glucose metabolism can also be mediated by the effect of nutrients on microRNAs. MicroRNAs (miRNAs) are RNA molecules that belong to a family of small non-coding RNAs with 20 to 25 nucleotides [157,158] that post-transcriptionally and negatively regulate gene expression.

Research into the nutritional modulation of miRNA is still in its infancy and few studies have assessed whether a specific dietary pattern, food, supplements or a particular nutrient can influence miRNA levels [159]. In humans, consumption of grape extract rich in resveratrol, and Vitamin supplementation modulated specific miRNAs towards a healthier status [160]. Similarly, a PUFA-enriched diet including almonds and walnuts was effective at modifying several miRNAs [161]. More recently, pistachio consumption in pre-diabetic subjects significantly diminished the levels of miR-375 and miR-192, both related to the glucose and insulin metabolism [162]. However, there is still much to discover about the exact mechanisms linking miRNAs with the glucose and insulin metabolism and the dietary modulation of miRNA expression.

Microbiota and Metabolomic Modulation

In recent years, many studies have pointed out that the gut microbiome might make an important contribution to the development of insulin resistance and T2D. Several mechanisms related to the composition of gut microbes—including changes in bowel permeability, endotoxemia and interaction with bile acids—may contribute to the onset of insulin resistance. On the other hand, it is well established that long-term dietary patterns and shorter-term dietary variation influence gut microbiota composition [163]. Many potential prebiotic components can be present in a particular food. For example, the fermentation of fiber from nuts and DF to beneficial end-products (e.g., butyric acid) and the biotransformation of phytochemicals (i.e., tocopherols, phytosterols, and phenolic compounds) are associated with the transition to a healthier microbiota composition [2,164].

There is little information on the putative effect of nuts and DF on microbiota modulation. In fact, only two publications have evaluated the effect of nut consumption (almonds and pistachios) on changes in microbiota. Mandalari et al. conducted an in vitro study with almond skins and they found that almond fiber significantly altered the composition of gut bacteria, specifically *Bifidobacteria*, thus showing that almond skins had a potential prebiotic use [165]. Some years later, Ukhanova and collaborators carried out two separate crossover feeding trials with nuts and pistachios, and showed that they both significantly affected microbiota modulation [166]. However, a greater prebiotic effect was found after pistachio intake. In fact, pistachio increased the number of butyrate-producing bacteria, which are potentially beneficial, whereas the numbers of *Bifidobacteria* were not affected by the consumption of either nut [166].

Recently, dietary polyphenols have been found to be involved in gut microbiota dysbiosis processes which may lead to a reduction of fat storage, inflammation and IR (reviewed in [167]). In fact, a cranberry extract also altered the gut microbiome of mice by increasing mucin-degrading bacteria, a potential link to reverse the dysbiosis and metabolic inflammation underlying T2D [168].

Very few studies have been made on metabolomic modulation after nut and DF intake. Of the studies that have been made, some have evaluated changes in metabolites after a chronic consumption of nuts. They showed a modulation in the levels of metabolites such as raffinose, (12Z)-9,10-dihydroxyoctadec-12-enoate, sucrose, together with some modulations of plasma amino acids and fatty acids [169], and a modulation of gut-related metabolites and cis-aconitate, an intermediate of tricarboxylic acid [170], after pistachio consumption.

Therefore, several specific nutrients—together with their synergic effects—in both nuts and DFs may explain their beneficial role in glucose and insulin metabolism, which helps to prevent or maintain T2D (Figure 1).

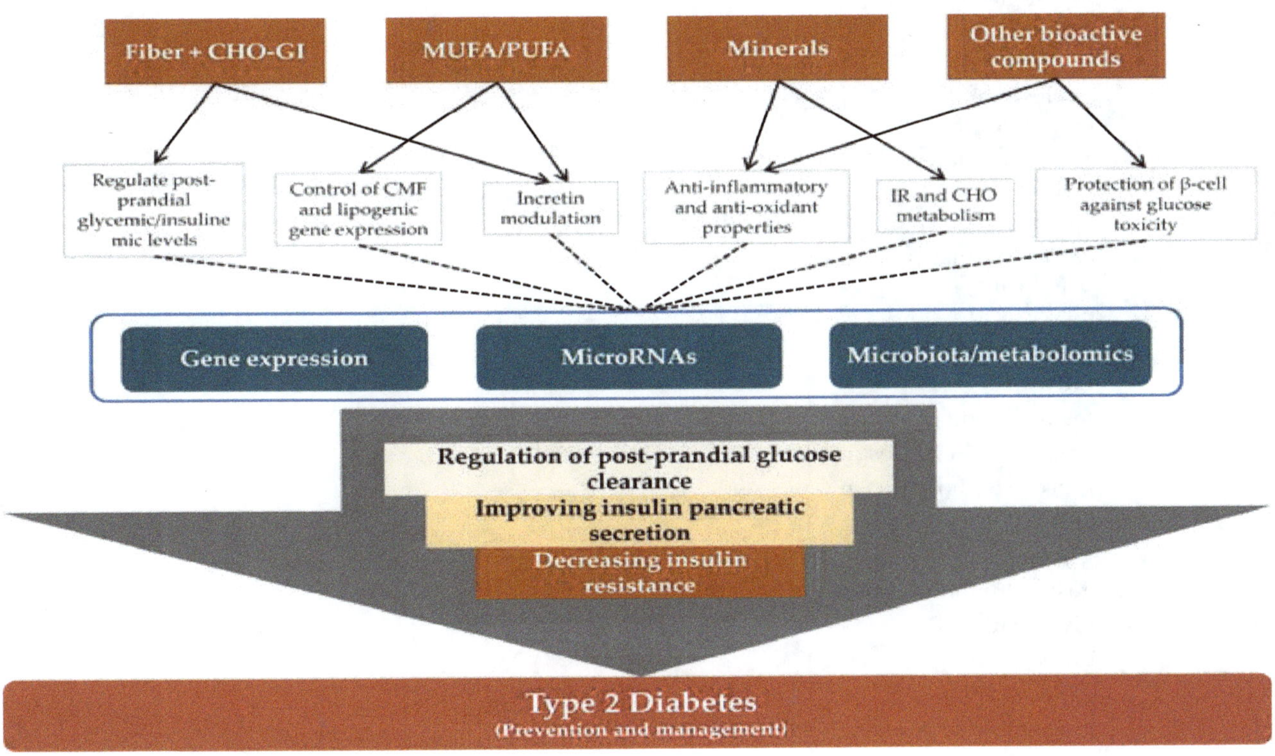

Figure 1. Role of nutrients from nuts and dried fruits in glucose and insulin metabolism, and cellular and molecular mechanisms related to T2D/IR. CHO, carbohydrate; CMF, cellular membrane fluidity; GI, glycaemic index; IR, insulin resistance; MUFA, monounsaturated fatty acid; PUFA, polyunsaturated fatty acid; T2D, type 2 diabetes.

6. Concluding Remarks

Undoubtedly, the specific composition of nuts and dried fruits means that they can be used to efficiently counteract metabolic diseases such as type 2 diabetes. Their unique profile of macronutrients, micronutrients and other bioactive compounds may explain the beneficial effects observed in clinical and epidemiological studies. However, the exact mechanisms by which they modulate glucose and insulin metabolism and influence T2D have yet to be fully discovered. They contain fiber, fat, minerals and other bioactive molecules that modulate several gene mechanisms at the cellular and molecular level. This may explain some of their beneficial effects. However, further basic and translational research is needed in order to extend their positive health benefits and to find novel mechanisms and targets to explain their contribution to the management of type 2 diabetes.

Acknowledgments: We thank Carles Munné and Susana Segura (Universitat Rovira i Virgili) for their help as editor assistance. Lucía Camacho-Barcia is the recipient of a pre-doctoral fellowship from the Generalitat de Catalunya's Department of Universities (FI-DGR 2017).

Author Contributions: Pablo Hernández-Alonso, Lucía Camacho-Barcia, Mònica Bulló and Jordi Salas-Salvadó designed the review. Pablo Hernández-Alonso, Lucía Camacho-Barcia and Mònica Bulló performed the bibliographical search. Pablo Hernández-Alonso, Lucía Camacho-Barcia, Mònica Bulló and Jordi Salas-Salvadó wrote the first draft of the manuscript, and all authors contributed to the editing of the manuscript. All authors approved the final manuscript.

Abbreviations

AMPK	adenosine monophosphate-activated protein kinase
AT	aerobically trained
ATP	adenosine triphosphate
AOC	area over the curve
Apo	apolipoprotein
BMI	body mass index
BW	body weight
C	cholesterol
CHO	carbohydrate
CI	confidence interval
CMF	cellular membrane fluidity
CRP	C-reactive protein
CVD	cardiovascular disease
DF	dried fruit
EA	ellagic acid
EPIC	European Prospective Investigation into Cancer
FA	fatty acid
FBG	fasting blood glucose
FBP	fructose-1,6-bisphosphatase
G6Pase	glucose 6-phosphatase
GAE	gallic acid equivalents
GI	glycaemic index
GIP	gastric inhibitory polypeptide
GL	glycaemic load
GJ	grape juice
GLI	glibenclamide
GLP-1	glucagon-like peptide-1
GLUT	glucose transporter type
GPE	grape powder extract
HA	high almond
HbA_{1c}	glycated hemoglobin
HDL	high-density lipoprotein
HF	high fat
HFD	high-fat diet
HOMA-IR	homeostatic model assessment of insulin resistance
HPFS	Health Professionals Follow-Up Study
IAUC	incremental area under the curve
ICAM-1	intercellular adhesion molecule-1

IGT	impaired glucose tolerance
IL-6	interleukin-6
IR	insulin resistance
LDL	low-density lipoprotein
LF	low-fat
LPS	lipopolysaccharide
MedDiet	Mediterranean diet
MESA	Multi-Ethnic Study of Atherosclerosis
MetS	metabolic syndrome
MI	myocardial infarction
miRNA and miR	microRNA
M/F	male/female
MUFA	monounsaturated fatty acids
NA	not available
NAFLD	non-alcoholic fatty liver disease
NCEP	National Cholesterol Education Program
NHANES	National Health and Nutrition Examination Survey
NHS	Nurses' Health Study
NLCS	Netherlands Cohort Study
NS	non-significant
Ob	obese
ORAC	oxygen radical absorbance capacity
Ow	overweight
PBMC	peripheral blood mononuclear cell
PF-4	platelet factor-4
PHS	Physicians' Health Study
PM	post-menopausal
PPAR	peroxisome proliferator-activated receptors
pre-D	pre-diabetes
PREDIMED	PREvención con DIeta MEDiterránea
PUFA	polyunsaturated fatty acids
PWE	polyphenol-rich walnut extract
Re	range
RETN	resistin
RCT	randomized clinical trial
RGR	relative glycaemic responses
RR	relative risk
RW	red wine
ROS	reactive oxygen species
S	sedentary
SBP	systolic blood pressure
SCCS	Southern Community Cohort Study
SCFA	short chain fatty acids
SFA	saturated fatty acids
SLC2A4	solute carrier family 2 member 4
SMHS	Shanghai Men's Health Study
STZ	streptozotocin
SWHS	Shanghai Women's Health Study
T2D	type 2 diabetes
TC	total cholesterol
TF	tissue factor
TG	triglycerides
TLGS	Tehran Lipid and Glucose Study
TNF-α	tumor necrosis factor-α
USDA	United States Department of Agriculture
VFM	visceral fat mass
WB	white bread
WC	waist circumference
WHtR	*waist-to-height ratio*

References

1. Widmer, R.J.; Flammer, A.J.; Lerman, L.O.; Lerman, A. The Mediterranean diet, its components, and cardiovascular disease. *Am. J. Med.* **2015**, *128*, 229–238. [CrossRef] [PubMed]
2. Ros, E. Health Benefits of Nut Consumption. *Nutrients* **2010**, *2*, 652–682. [CrossRef] [PubMed]
3. Chang, S.K.; Alasalvar, C.; Shahidi, F. Review of dried fruits: Phytochemicals, antioxidant efficacies, and health benefits. *J. Funct. Foods* **2016**, *21*, 113–132. [CrossRef]
4. Ros, E. Nuts and CVD. *Br. J. Nutr.* **2015**, *113* (Suppl.), S111–S120. [CrossRef] [PubMed]
5. Casas-Agustench, P.; Salas-Huetos, A.; Salas-Salvadó, J. Mediterranean nuts: Origins, ancient medicinal benefits and symbolism. *Public Health Nutr.* **2011**, *14*, 2296–2301. [CrossRef] [PubMed]
6. Salas-Salvadó, J.; Casas-Agustench, P.; Salas-Huetos, A. Cultural and historical aspects of Mediterranean nuts with emphasis on their attributed healthy and nutritional properties. *Nutr. Metab. Cardiovasc. Dis.* **2011**, *21* (Suppl. 1), S1–S6. [CrossRef] [PubMed]
7. Sofi, F. The Mediterranean diet revisited: Evidence of its effectiveness grows. *Curr. Opin. Cardiol.* **2009**, *24*, 442–446. [CrossRef] [PubMed]
8. Alasalvar, C.; Shahidi, F. Composition, phytochemicals, and beneficial health effects of dried fruits: An overview. In *Dried Fruits: Phytochemicals and Health Effects*; Wiley-Blackwell: Oxford, UK, 2013; pp. 372–392.
9. US Department of Agriculture, Agricultural Research Service, Nutrient Data Laboratory. USDA National Nutrient Database for Standard Reference, Release 28 (revised), Version Current: May 2015. Available online: http://www.ars.usda.gov/ba/bhnrc/ndl (accessed on 3 March 2017).
10. Halvorsen, B.L.; Carlsen, M.H.; Phillips, K.M.; Bøhn, S.K.; Holte, K.; Jacobs, D.R.; Blomhoff, R. Content of redox-active compounds (ie, antioxidants) in foods consumed in the United States. *Am. J. Clin. Nutr.* **2006**, *84*, 95–135. [PubMed]
11. Phillips, K.M.; Ruggio, D.M.; Ashraf-Khorassani, M. Phytosterol composition of nuts and seeds commonly consumed in the United States. *J. Agric. Food Chem.* **2005**, *53*, 9436–9445. [CrossRef] [PubMed]
12. Montonen, J.; Knekt, P.; Jarvinen, R.; Reunanen, A. Dietary Antioxidant Intake and Risk of Type 2 Diabetes. *Diabetes Care* **2004**, *27*, 362–366. [CrossRef] [PubMed]
13. Sluijs, I.; Cadier, E.; Beulens, J.W.J.; van der A, D.L.; Spijkerman, A.M.W.; van der Schouw, Y.T. Dietary intake of carotenoids and risk of type 2 diabetes. *Nutr. Metab. Cardiovasc. Dis.* **2015**, *25*, 376–381. [CrossRef] [PubMed]
14. Zhao, B.; Hall, C.A. Composition and antioxidant activity of raisin extracts obtained from various solvents. *Food Chem.* **2008**, *108*, 511–518. [CrossRef] [PubMed]
15. Anderson, J.W.; Waters, A.R. Raisin consumption by humans: Effects on glycemia and insulinemia and cardiovascular risk factors. *J. Food Sci.* **2013**, *78*, A11–A17. [CrossRef] [PubMed]
16. Mandalari, G.; Bisignano, C.; Filocamo, A.; Chessa, S.; Sarò, M.; Torre, G.; Faulks, R.M.; Dugo, P. Bioaccessibility of pistachio polyphenols, xanthophylls, and tocopherols during simulated human digestion. *Nutrition* **2013**, *29*, 338–344. [CrossRef] [PubMed]
17. O'Neil, C.E.; Keast, D.R.; Fulgoni, V.L.; Nicklas, T.A. Tree nut consumption improves nutrient intake and diet quality in US adults: An analysis of national health and nutrition examination survey (NHANES) 1999–2004. *Asia Pac. J. Clin. Nutr.* **2010**, *19*, 142–150. [PubMed]
18. O'Neil, C.E.; Keast, D.R.; Nicklas, T.A.; Fulgoni, V.L. Out-of-hand nut consumption is associated with improved nutrient intake and health risk markers in US children and adults: National Health and Nutrition Examination Survey 1999–2004. *Nutr. Res.* **2012**, *32*, 185–194. [CrossRef] [PubMed]
19. Tey, S.L.; Brown, R.; Gray, A.; Chisholm, A.; Delahunty, C. Nuts improve diet quality compared to other energy-dense snacks while maintaining body weight. *J. Nutr. Metab.* **2011**, *2011*, 357350. [CrossRef] [PubMed]
20. McManus, K.; Antinoro, L.; Sacks, F. A randomized controlled trial of a moderate-fat, low-energy diet compared with a low fat, low-energy diet for weight loss in overweight adults. *Int. J. Obes. Relat. Metab. Disord.* **2001**, *25*, 1503–1511. [CrossRef] [PubMed]
21. Bazzano, L.A.; Li, T.Y.; Joshipura, K.J.; Hu, F.B. Intake of fruit, vegetables, and fruit juices and risk of diabetes in women. *Diabetes Care* **2008**, *31*, 1311–1317. [CrossRef] [PubMed]

22. Keast, D.R.; O'Neil, C.E.; Jones, J.M. Dried fruit consumption is associated with improved diet quality and reduced obesity in US adults: National Health and Nutrition Examination Survey, 1999–2004. *Nutr. Res.* **2011**, *31*, 460–467. [CrossRef] [PubMed]
23. Chan, R.; Wong, V.W.-S.; Chu, W.C.-W.; Wong, G.L.-H.; Li, L.S.; Leung, J.; Chim, A.M.-L.; Yeung, D.K.-W.; Sea, M.M.-M.; Woo, J.; et al. Diet-Quality Scores and Prevalence of Nonalcoholic Fatty Liver Disease: A Population Study Using Proton-Magnetic Resonance Spectroscopy. *PLoS ONE* **2015**, *10*, e0139310. [CrossRef] [PubMed]
24. U.S. Department of Health and Human Services and U.S. Department of Agriculture. 2015–2020 Dietary Guidelines for Americans, 8th Edition edDecember 2015. Available online: http://health.gov/dietaryguidelines/2015/guidelines/ (accessed on 10 March 2017).
25. Bilbis, L.S.; Shehu, R.A.; Abubakar, M.G. Hypoglycemic and hypolipidemic effects of aqueous extract of Arachis hypogaea in normal and alloxan-induced diabetic rats. *Phytomedicine* **2002**, *9*, 553–555. [CrossRef] [PubMed]
26. Fukuda, T.; Ito, H.; Yoshida, T. Effect of the walnut polyphenol fraction on oxidative stress in type 2 diabetes mice. *Biofactors* **2004**, *21*, 251–253. [CrossRef] [PubMed]
27. Ramesh, B.; Saravanan, R.; Pugalendi, K. V Effect of dietary substitution of groundnut oil on blood glucose, lipid profile, and redox status in streptozotocin-diabetic rats. *Yale J. Biol. Med.* **2006**, *79*, 9–17. [PubMed]
28. Emekli-Alturfan, E.; Kasikci, E.; Yarat, A. Tissue factor activities of streptozotocin induced diabetic rat tissues and the effect of peanut consumption. *Diabetes Metab. Res. Rev.* **2007**, *23*, 653–658. [CrossRef] [PubMed]
29. Choi, Y.; Abdelmegeed, M.A.; Akbar, M.; Song, B.-J.J. Dietary walnut reduces hepatic triglyceride content in high-fat-fed mice via modulation of hepatic fatty acid metabolism and adipose tissue inflammation. *J. Nutr. Biochem.* **2016**, *30*, 116–125. [CrossRef] [PubMed]
30. Overman, A.; Bumrungpert, A.; Kennedy, A.; Martinez, K.; Chuang, C.-C.; West, T.; Dawson, B.; Jia, W.; McIntosh, M. Polyphenol-rich grape powder extract (GPE) attenuates inflammation in human macrophages and in human adipocytes exposed to macrophage-conditioned media. *Int. J. Obes. (Lond.)* **2010**, *34*, 800–808. [CrossRef] [PubMed]
31. Chuang, C.-C.; Bumrungpert, A.; Kennedy, A.; Overman, A.; West, T.; Dawson, B.; McIntosh, M.K. Grape powder extract attenuates tumor necrosis factor α-mediated inflammation and insulin resistance in primary cultures of human adipocytes. *J. Nutr. Biochem.* **2011**, *22*, 89–94. [CrossRef] [PubMed]
32. Chuang, C.-C.; Martinez, K.; Xie, G.; Kennedy, A.; Bumrungpert, A.; Overman, A.; Jia, W.; McIntosh, M.K. Quercetin is equally or more effective than resveratrol in attenuating tumor necrosis factor—Mediated inflammation and insulin resistance in primary human adipocytes. *Am. J. Clin. Nutr.* **2010**, *92*, 1511–1521. [CrossRef] [PubMed]
33. Zangiabadi, N.; Asadi-Shekaari, M.; Sheibani, V.; Jafari, M.; Shabani, M.; Asadi, A.R.; Tajadini, H.; Jarahi, M. Date fruit extract is a neuroprotective agent in diabetic peripheral neuropathy in streptozotocin-induced diabetic rats: A multimodal analysis. *Oxid. Med. Cell. Longev.* **2011**, *2011*, 976948. [CrossRef] [PubMed]
34. Porto, L.C.S.; da Silva, J.; Ferraz, A.B.F.; Ethur, E.M.; Porto, C.D.L.; Marroni, N.P.; Picada, J.N. The Antidiabetic and Antihypercholesterolemic Effects of an Aqueous Extract from Pecan Shells in Wistar Rats. *Plant Foods Hum. Nutr.* **2015**, *70*, 414–419. [CrossRef] [PubMed]
35. Tédong, L.; Dzeufiet, P.D.D.; Dimo, T.; Asongalem, E.A.; Sokeng, S.N.; Flejou, J.-F.; Callard, P.; Kamtchouing, P. Acute and subchronic toxicity of Anacardium occidentale Linn (Anacardiaceae) leaves hexane extract in mice. *Afr. J. Tradit. Complement. Altern. Med. AJTCAM* **2006**, *4*, 140–147. [CrossRef] [PubMed]
36. Asgary, S.; Parkhideh, S.; Solhpour, A.; Madani, H.; Mahzouni, P.; Rahimi, P. Effect of ethanolic extract of *Juglans regia* L. on blood sugar in diabetes-induced rats. *J. Med. Food* **2008**, *11*, 533–538. [CrossRef] [PubMed]
37. Ojewole, J.A.O. Laboratory evaluation of the hypoglycemic effect of Anacardium occidentale Linn (Anacardiaceae) stem-bark extracts in rats. *Methods Find. Exp. Clin. Pharmacol.* **2003**, *25*, 199–204. [CrossRef] [PubMed]
38. Egwim, E. Hypoglycemic potencies of crude ethanolic extracts of cashew roots and unripe pawpaw fruits in guinea pigs and rats. *J. Herb. Pharmacother.* **2005**, *5*, 27–34. [CrossRef] [PubMed]
39. Jelodar, G.; Mohsen, M.; Shahram, S. Effect of walnut leaf, coriander and pomegranate on blood glucose and histopathology of pancreas of alloxan induced diabetic rats. *Afr. J. Tradit. Complement. Altern. Med. AJTCAM* **2007**, *4*, 299–305. [CrossRef] [PubMed]

40. Eid, H.M.; Martineau, L.C.; Saleem, A.; Muhammad, A.; Vallerand, D.; Benhaddou-Andaloussi, A.; Nistor, L.; Afshar, A.; Arnason, J.T.; Haddad, P.S. Stimulation of AMP-activated protein kinase and enhancement of basal glucose uptake in muscle cells by quercetin and quercetin glycosides, active principles of the antidiabetic medicinal plant Vaccinium vitis-idaea. *Mol. Nutr. Food Res.* **2010**, *54*, 991–1003. [CrossRef] [PubMed]
41. Vassiliou, E.K.; Gonzalez, A.; Garcia, C.; Tadros, J.H.; Chakraborty, G.; Toney, J.H. Oleic acid and peanut oil high in oleic acid reverse the inhibitory effect of insulin production of the inflammatory cytokine TNF-alpha both in vitro and in vivo systems. *Lipids Health Dis.* **2009**, *8*, 25. [CrossRef] [PubMed]
42. Adewale, O.F.; Isaac, O.; Tunmise, M.T.; Omoniyi, O. Palm oil and ground nut oil supplementation effects on blood glucose and antioxidant status in alloxan-induced diabetic rats. *Pak. J. Pharm. Sci.* **2016**, *29*, 83–87. [PubMed]
43. Anderson, K.J.; Teuber, S.S.; Gobeille, A.; Cremin, P.; Waterhouse, A.L.; Steinberg, F.M. Walnut polyphenolics inhibit in vitro human plasma and LDL oxidation. *J. Nutr.* **2001**, *131*, 2837–2842. [PubMed]
44. Chen, C.-Y.; Milbury, P.E.; Lapsley, K.; Blumberg, J.B. Flavonoids from almond skins are bioavailable and act synergistically with vitamins C and E to enhance hamster and human LDL resistance to oxidation. *J. Nutr.* **2005**, *135*, 1366–1373. [PubMed]
45. Wijeratne, S.S.K.; Abou-Zaid, M.M.; Shahidi, F. Antioxidant polyphenols in almond and its coproducts. *J. Agric. Food Chem.* **2006**, *54*, 312–318. [CrossRef] [PubMed]
46. Gentile, C.; Tesoriere, L.; Butera, D.; Fazzari, M.; Monastero, M.; Allegra, M.; Livrea, M.A. Antioxidant activity of Sicilian pistachio (Pistacia vera L Var. Bronte) nut extract and its bioactive components. *J. Agric. Food Chem.* **2007**, *55*, 643–648. [CrossRef] [PubMed]
47. Shahidi, F.; Alasalvar, C.; Liyana-Pathirana, C.M. Antioxidant phytochemicals in hazelnut kernel (Corylus avellana L) and hazelnut byproducts. *J. Agric. Food Chem.* **2007**, *55*, 1212–1220. [CrossRef] [PubMed]
48. Tedong, L.; Madiraju, P.; Martineau, L.C.; Vallerand, D.; Arnason, J.T.; Desire, D.D.P.; Lavoie, L.; Kamtchouing, P.; Haddad, P.S. Hydro-ethanolic extract of cashew tree (Anacardium occidentale) nut and its principal compound, anacardic acid, stimulate glucose uptake in C2C12 muscle cells. *Mol. Nutr. Food Res.* **2010**, *54*, 1753–1762. [CrossRef] [PubMed]
49. Shahraki, J.; Zareh, M.; Kamalinejad, M.; Pourahmad, J. Cytoprotective Effects of Hydrophilic and Lipophilic Extracts of Pistacia vera against Oxidative Versus Carbonyl Stress in Rat Hepatocytes. *Iran. J. Pharm. Res. IJPR* **2014**, *13*, 1263–1277. [PubMed]
50. Aoun, M.; Michel, F.; Fouret, G.; Schlernitzauer, A.; Ollendorff, V.; Wrutniak-Cabello, C.; Cristol, J.-P.; Carbonneau, M.-A.; Coudray, C.; Feillet-Coudray, C. A grape polyphenol extract modulates muscle membrane fatty acid composition and lipid metabolism in high-fat–high-sucrose diet-fed rats. *Br. J. Nutr.* **2011**, *106*, 491–501. [CrossRef] [PubMed]
51. Weijers, R.N.M. Lipid composition of cell membranes and its relevance in type 2 diabetes mellitus. *Curr. Diabetes Rev.* **2012**, *8*, 390–400. [CrossRef] [PubMed]
52. Soares de Moura, R.; da Costa, G.F.; Moreira, A.S.B.; Queiroz, E.F.; Moreira, D.D.C.; Garcia-Souza, E.P.; Resende, A.C.; Moura, A.S.; Teixeira, M.T. Vitis vinifera L. grape skin extract activates the insulin-signalling cascade and reduces hyperglycaemia in alloxan-induced diabetic mice. *J. Pharm. Pharmacol.* **2012**, *64*, 268–276. [CrossRef] [PubMed]
53. Adam, S.H.; Giribabu, N.; Kassim, N.; Kumar, K.E.; Brahmayya, M.; Arya, A.; Salleh, N. Protective effect of aqueous seed extract of Vitis Vinifera against oxidative stress, inflammation and apoptosis in the pancreas of adult male rats with diabetes mellitus. *Biomed. Pharmacother.* **2016**, *81*, 439–452. [CrossRef] [PubMed]
54. Esposito, D.; Damsud, T.; Wilson, M.; Grace, M.H.; Strauch, R.; Li, X.; Lila, M.A.; Komarnytsky, S. Black Currant Anthocyanins Attenuate Weight Gain and Improve Glucose Metabolism in Diet-Induced Obese Mice with Intact, but Not Disrupted, Gut Microbiome. *J. Agric. Food Chem.* **2015**, *63*, 6172–6180. [CrossRef] [PubMed]
55. Schmatz, R.; Mann, T.R.; Spanevello, R.; Machado, M.M.; Zanini, D.; Pimentel, V.C.; Stefanello, N.; Martins, C.C.; Cardoso, A.M.; Bagatini, M.; et al. Moderate red wine and grape juice consumption modulates the hydrolysis of the adenine nucleotides and decreases platelet aggregation in streptozotocin-induced diabetic rats. *Cell Biochem. Biophys.* **2013**, *65*, 129–143. [CrossRef] [PubMed]

56. Hernández-Salinas, R.; Decap, V.; Leguina, A.; Cáceres, P.; Perez, D.; Urquiaga, I.; Iturriaga, R.; Velarde, V. Antioxidant and anti hyperglycemic role of wine grape powder in rats fed with a high fructose diet. *Biol. Res.* **2015**, *48*, 53. [CrossRef] [PubMed]
57. Overman, A.; Chuang, C.-C.; McIntosh, M. Quercetin attenuates inflammation in human macrophages and adipocytes exposed to macrophage-conditioned media. *Int. J. Obes. (Lond.)* **2011**, *35*, 1165–1172. [CrossRef] [PubMed]
58. Nettleton, J.A.; Steffen, L.M.; Ni, H.; Liu, K.; Jacobs, D.R. Dietary patterns and risk of incident type 2 diabetes in the Multi-Ethnic Study of Atherosclerosis (MESA). *Diabetes Care* **2008**, *31*, 1777–1782. [CrossRef] [PubMed]
59. O'Neil, C.E.; Fulgoni, V.L.; Nicklas, T.A. Tree Nut consumption is associated with better adiposity measures and cardiovascular and metabolic syndrome health risk factors in U.S. Adults: NHANES 2005–2010. *Nutr. J.* **2015**, *14*, 64. [CrossRef] [PubMed]
60. Asghari, G.; Ghorbani, Z.; Mirmiran, P.; Azizi, F. Nut consumption is associated with lower incidence of type 2 diabetes: The Tehran Lipid and Glucose Study. *Diabetes Metab.* **2017**, *43*, 18–24. [CrossRef] [PubMed]
61. Jiang, R.; Manson, J.E.; Stampfer, M.J.; Liu, S.; Willett, W.C.; Hu, F.B. Nut and peanut butter consumption and risk of type 2 diabetes in women. *JAMA* **2002**, *288*, 2554–2560. [CrossRef] [PubMed]
62. Villegas, R.; Gao, Y.-T.T.; Yang, G.; Li, H.-L.L.; Elasy, T.A.; Zheng, W.; Shu, X.O. Legume and soy food intake and the incidence of type 2 diabetes in the Shanghai Women's Health Study. *Am. J. Clin. Nutr.* **2008**, *87*, 162–167. [PubMed]
63. Ibarrola-Jurado, N.; Bulló, M.; Guasch-Ferré, M.; Ros, E.; Martínez-González, M.A.; Corella, D.; Fiol, M.; Wärnberg, J.; Estruch, R.; Román, P.; et al. Cross-sectional assessment of nut consumption and obesity, metabolic syndrome and other cardiometabolic risk factors: The PREDIMED study. *PLoS ONE* **2013**, *8*, e57367. [CrossRef] [PubMed]
64. Pan, A.; Sun, Q.; Manson, J.E.; Willett, W.C.; Hu, F.B. Walnut consumption is associated with lower risk of type 2 diabetes in women. *J. Nutr.* **2013**, *143*, 512–518. [CrossRef] [PubMed]
65. van den Brandt, P.A.; Schouten, L.J. Relationship of tree nut, peanut and peanut butter intake with total and cause-specific mortality: A cohort study and meta-analysis. *Int. J. Epidemiol.* **2015**, *44*, 1038–1049. [CrossRef] [PubMed]
66. Buijsse, B.; Boeing, H.; Drogan, D.; Schulze, M.B.; Feskens, E.J.; Amiano, P.; Barricarte, A.; Clavel-Chapelon, F.; de Lauzon-Guillain, B.; Fagherazzi, G.; et al. Consumption of fatty foods and incident type 2 diabetes in populations from eight European countries. *Eur. J. Clin. Nutr.* **2015**, *69*, 455–461. [CrossRef] [PubMed]
67. Kochar, J.; Gaziano, J.M.; Djoussé, L. Nut consumption and risk of type II diabetes in the Physicians' Health Study. *Eur. J. Clin. Nutr.* **2010**, *64*, 75–79. [CrossRef] [PubMed]
68. Pimpin, L.; Wu, J.H.Y.; Haskelberg, H.; Del Gobbo, L.; Mozaffarian, D. Is Butter Back? A Systematic Review and Meta-Analysis of Butter Consumption and Risk of Cardiovascular Disease, Diabetes, and Total Mortality. *PLoS ONE* **2016**, *11*, e0158118. [CrossRef] [PubMed]
69. Jenkins, D.J.A.; Kendall, C.W.C.; Josse, A.R.; Salvatore, S.; Brighenti, F.; Augustin, L.S.A.; Ellis, P.R.; Vidgen, E.; Rao, A.V. Almonds Decrease Postprandial Glycemia, Insulinemia, and Oxidative Damage in Healthy Individuals. *J. Nutr.* **2006**, *136*, 2987–2992. [PubMed]
70. Josse, A.R.; Kendall, C.W.C.; Augustin, L.S.A.; Ellis, P.R.; Jenkins, D.J.A. Almonds and postprandial glycemia—A dose-response study. *Metabolism.* **2007**, *56*, 400–404. [CrossRef] [PubMed]
71. Mori, A.M.; Considine, R.V.; Mattes, R.D.; Wong, J.; Jenkins, D.; Jiang, R.; Manson, J.; Stampfer, M.; Liu, S.; Willett, W.; et al. Acute and second-meal effects of almond form in impaired glucose tolerant adults: A randomized crossover trial. *Nutr. Metab. (Lond.)* **2011**, *8*, 6. [CrossRef] [PubMed]
72. Cohen, A.E.; Johnston, C.S. Almond ingestion at mealtime reduces postprandial glycemia and chronic ingestion reduces hemoglobin A1c in individuals with well-controlled type 2 diabetes mellitus. *Metabolism* **2011**, *60*, 1312–1317. [CrossRef] [PubMed]
73. Crouch, M.A.; Slater, R.T. Almond "Appetizer" Effect on Glucose Tolerance Test (GTT) Results. *J. Am. Board Fam. Med.* **2016**, *29*, 759–766. [CrossRef] [PubMed]
74. Kendall, C.W.C.; Josse, A.R.; Esfahani, A.; Jenkins, D.J.A. The impact of pistachio intake alone or in combination with high-carbohydrate foods on post-prandial glycemia. *Eur. J. Clin. Nutr.* **2011**, *65*, 696–702. [CrossRef] [PubMed]

75. Kendall, C.W.C.; West, S.G.; Augustin, L.S.; Esfahani, A.; Vidgen, E.; Bashyam, B.; Sauder, K.A.; Campbell, J.; Chiavaroli, L.; Jenkins, A.L.; et al. Acute effects of pistachio consumption on glucose and insulin, satiety hormones and endothelial function in the metabolic syndrome. *Eur. J. Clin. Nutr.* **2014**, *68*, 370–375. [CrossRef] [PubMed]
76. Reis, C.E.G.; Bordalo, L.A.; Rocha, A.L.C.; Freitas, D.M.O.; da Silva, M.V.L.; de Faria, V.C.; Martino, H.S.D.; Costa, N.M.B.; Alfenas, R.C. Ground roasted peanuts leads to a lower post-prandial glycemic response than raw peanuts. *Nutr. Hosp.* **2011**, *26*, 745–751. [PubMed]
77. Moreira, A.P.B.; Teixeira, T.F.S.; Alves, R.D.M.; Peluzio, M.C.G.; Costa, N.M.B.; Bressan, J.; Mattes, R.; Alfenas, R.C.G. Effect of a high-fat meal containing conventional or high-oleic peanuts on post-prandial lipopolysaccharide concentrations in overweight/obese men. *J. Hum. Nutr. Diet.* **2016**, *29*, 95–104. [CrossRef] [PubMed]
78. Kendall, C.W.C.; Esfahani, A.; Josse, A.R.; Augustin, L.S.A.; Vidgen, E.; Jenkins, D.J.A. The glycemic effect of nut-enriched meals in healthy and diabetic subjects. *Nutr. Metab. Cardiovasc. Dis.* **2011**, *21* (Suppl. 1), S34–S39. [CrossRef] [PubMed]
79. Lovejoy, J.C.; Most, M.M.; Lefevre, M.; Greenway, F.L.; Rood, J.C. Effect of diets enriched in almonds on insulin action and serum lipids in adults with normal glucose tolerance or type 2 diabetes. *Am. J. Clin. Nutr.* **2002**, *76*, 1000–1006. [PubMed]
80. Li, S.-C.; Liu, Y.-H.; Liu, J.-F.; Chang, W.-H.; Chen, C.-M.; Chen, C.-Y.O. Almond consumption improved glycemic control and lipid profiles in patients with type 2 diabetes mellitus. *Metabolism* **2011**, *60*, 474–479. [CrossRef] [PubMed]
81. Damavandi, R.D.; Eghtesadi, S.; Shidfar, F.; Heydari, I.; Foroushani, A.R. Effects of hazelnuts consumption on fasting blood sugar and lipoproteins in patients with type 2 diabetes. *J. Res. Med. Sci.* **2013**, *18*, 314–321. [PubMed]
82. Lasa, A.; Miranda, J.; Bulló, M.; Casas, R.; Salas-Salvadó, J.; Larretxi, I.; Estruch, R.; Ruiz-Gutiérrez, V.; Portillo, M.P. Comparative effect of two Mediterranean diets versus a low-fat diet on glycaemic control in individuals with type 2 diabetes. *Eur. J. Clin. Nutr.* **2014**, *68*, 767–772. [CrossRef] [PubMed]
83. Parham, M.; Heidari, S.; Khorramirad, A.; Hozoori, M.; Hosseinzadeh, F.; Bakhtyari, L.; Vafaeimanesh, J. Effects of pistachio nut supplementation on blood glucose in patients with type 2 diabetes: A randomized crossover trial. *Rev. Diabet. Stud.* **2014**, *11*, 190–196. [CrossRef] [PubMed]
84. Gulati, S.; Misra, A.; Pandey, R.M. Effect of Almond Supplementation on Glycemia and Cardiovascular Risk Factors in Asian Indians in North India with Type 2 Diabetes Mellitus: A 24–Week Study. *Metab. Syndr. Relat. Disord.* **2017**, *15*, 98–105. [CrossRef] [PubMed]
85. Hernández-Alonso, P.; Salas-Salvadó, J.; Baldrich-Mora, M.; Juanola-Falgarona, M.; Bulló, M. Beneficial Effect of Pistachio Consumption on Glucose Metabolism, Insulin Resistance, Inflammation, and Related Metabolic Risk Markers: A Randomized Clinical Trial. *Diabetes Care* **2014**, *37*, 3098–3105. [CrossRef] [PubMed]
86. Jenkins, D.J.A.; Kendall, C.W.C.; Marchie, A.; Josse, A.R.; Nguyen, T.H.; Faulkner, D.A.; Lapsley, K.G.; Singer, W. Effect of almonds on insulin secretion and insulin resistance in nondiabetic hyperlipidemic subjects: A randomized controlled crossover trial. *Metabolism* **2008**, *57*, 882–887. [CrossRef] [PubMed]
87. Le, T.; Flatt, S.W.; Natarajan, L.; Pakiz, B.; Quintana, E.L.; Heath, D.D.; Rana, B.K.; Rock, C.L. Effects of Diet Composition and Insulin Resistance Status on Plasma Lipid Levels in a Weight Loss Intervention in Women. *J. Am. Heart Assoc.* **2016**, *5*, e002771. [CrossRef] [PubMed]
88. Claesson, A.-L.; Holm, G.; Ernersson, A.; Lindström, T.; Nystrom, F.H. Two weeks of overfeeding with candy, but not peanuts, increases insulin levels and body weight. *Scand. J. Clin. Lab. Invest.* **2009**, *69*, 598–605. [CrossRef] [PubMed]
89. Wien, M.A.; Sabaté, J.M.; Iklé, D.N.; Cole, S.E.; Kandeel, F.R. Almonds vs. complex carbohydrates in a weight reduction program. *Int. J. Obes. Relat. Metab. Disord.* **2003**, *27*, 1365–1372. [CrossRef] [PubMed]
90. Esposito, K.; Marfella, R.; Ciotola, M.; Di Palo, C.; Giugliano, F.; Giugliano, G.; D'Armiento, M.; D'Andrea, F.; Giugliano, D. Effect of a mediterranean-style diet on endothelial dysfunction and markers of vascular inflammation in the metabolic syndrome: A randomized trial. *JAMA* **2004**, *292*, 1440–1446. [CrossRef] [PubMed]
91. Tapsell, L.C.; Gillen, L.J.; Patch, C.S.; Batterham, M.; Owen, A.; Baré, M.; Kennedy, M. Including walnuts in a low-fat/modified-fat diet improves HDL cholesterol-to-total cholesterol ratios in patients with type 2 diabetes. *Diabetes Care* **2004**, *27*, 2777–2783. [CrossRef] [PubMed]

92. Tapsell, L.C.; Batterham, M.J.; Teuss, G.; Tan, S.-Y.; Dalton, S.; Quick, C.J.; Gillen, L.J.; Charlton, K.E. Long-term effects of increased dietary polyunsaturated fat from walnuts on metabolic parameters in type II diabetes. *Eur. J. Clin. Nutr.* **2009**, *63*, 1008–1015. [CrossRef] [PubMed]
93. Ma, Y.; Njike, V.Y.; Millet, J.; Dutta, S.; Doughty, K.; Treu, J.A.; Katz, D.L. Effects of walnut consumption on endothelial function in type 2 diabetic subjects: A randomized controlled crossover trial. *Diabetes Care* **2010**, *33*, 227–232. [CrossRef] [PubMed]
94. Brennan, A.M.; Sweeney, L.L.; Liu, X.; Mantzoros, C.S. Walnut consumption increases satiation but has no effect on insulin resistance or the metabolic profile over a 4-day period. *Obesity (Silver Spring)* **2010**, *18*, 1176–1182. [CrossRef] [PubMed]
95. Wang, X.; Li, Z.; Liu, Y.; Lv, X.; Yang, W. Effects of pistachios on body weight in Chinese subjects with metabolic syndrome. *Nutr. J.* **2012**, *11*, 20. [CrossRef] [PubMed]
96. Katz, D.L.; Davidhi, A.; Ma, Y.; Kavak, Y.; Bifulco, L.; Njike, V.Y. Effects of walnuts on endothelial function in overweight adults with visceral obesity: A randomized, controlled, crossover trial. *J. Am. Coll. Nutr.* **2012**, *31*, 415–423. [CrossRef] [PubMed]
97. Richmond, K.; Williams, S.; Mann, J.; Brown, R.; Chisholm, A. Markers of Cardiovascular Risk in Postmenopausal Women with Type 2 Diabetes Are Improved by the Daily Consumption of Almonds or Sunflower Kernels: A Feeding Study. *ISRN Nutr.* **2013**, *2013*, 1–9. [CrossRef] [PubMed]
98. Tan, S.Y.; Mattes, R.D. Appetitive, dietary and health effects of almonds consumed with meals or as snacks: A randomized, controlled trial. *Eur. J. Clin. Nutr.* **2013**, *67*, 1205–1214. [CrossRef] [PubMed]
99. Liu, J.-F.; Liu, Y.-H.; Chen, C.-M.; Chang, W.-H.; Chen, C.-Y.O. The effect of almonds on inflammation and oxidative stress in Chinese patients with type 2 diabetes mellitus: A randomized crossover controlled feeding trial. *Eur. J. Nutr.* **2013**, *52*, 927–935. [CrossRef] [PubMed]
100. Wu, L.; Piotrowski, K.; Rau, T.; Waldmann, E.; Broedl, U.C.; Demmelmair, H.; Koletzko, B.; Stark, R.G.; Nagel, J.M.; Mantzoros, C.S.; et al. Walnut-enriched diet reduces fasting non-HDL-cholesterol and apolipoprotein B in healthy Caucasian subjects: A randomized controlled cross-over clinical trial. *Metabolism* **2014**, *63*, 382–391. [CrossRef] [PubMed]
101. Wien, M.; Oda, K.; Sabaté, J. A randomized controlled trial to evaluate the effect of incorporating peanuts into an American Diabetes Association meal plan on the nutrient profile of the total diet and cardiometabolic parameters of adults with type 2 diabetes. *Nutr. J.* **2014**, *13*, 10. [CrossRef] [PubMed]
102. Sauder, K.A.; McCrea, C.E.; Ulbrecht, J.S.; Kris-Etherton, P.M.; West, S.G. Effects of pistachios on the lipid/lipoprotein profile, glycemic control, inflammation, and endothelial function in type 2 diabetes: A randomized trial. *Metabolism* **2015**, *64*, 1521–1529. [CrossRef] [PubMed]
103. Njike, V.Y.; Ayettey, R.; Petraro, P.; Treu, J.A.; Katz, D.L. Walnut ingestion in adults at risk for diabetes: Effects on body composition, diet quality, and cardiac risk measures. *BMJ Open Diabetes Res. Care* **2015**, *3*, e000115. [CrossRef] [PubMed]
104. Sari, I.; Baltaci, Y.; Bagci, C.; Davutoglu, V.; Erel, O.; Celik, H.; Ozer, O.; Aksoy, N.; Aksoy, M. Effect of pistachio diet on lipid parameters, endothelial function, inflammation, and oxidative status: A prospective study. *Nutrition* **2010**, *26*, 399–404. [CrossRef] [PubMed]
105. Gulati, S.; Misra, A.; Pandey, R.M.; Bhatt, S.P.; Saluja, S. Effects of pistachio nuts on body composition, metabolic, inflammatory and oxidative stress parameters in Asian Indians with metabolic syndrome: A 24-week, randomized control trial. *Nutrition* **2014**, *30*, 192–197. [CrossRef] [PubMed]
106. Wien, M.; Bleich, D.; Raghuwanshi, M.; Gould-Forgerite, S.; Gomes, J.; Monahan-Couch, L.; Oda, K. Almond consumption and cardiovascular risk factors in adults with prediabetes. *J. Am. Coll. Nutr.* **2010**, *29*, 189–197. [CrossRef] [PubMed]
107. Casas-Agustench, P.; López-Uriarte, P.; Bulló, M.; Ros, E.; Cabré-Vila, J.J.; Salas-Salvadó, J. Effects of one serving of mixed nuts on serum lipids, insulin resistance and inflammatory markers in patients with the metabolic syndrome. *Nutr. Metab. Cardiovasc. Dis.* **2011**, *21*, 126–135. [CrossRef] [PubMed]
108. Mejia, S.B.; Kendall, C.W.C.; Viguiliouk, E.; Augustin, L.S.; Ha, V.; Cozma, A.I.; Mirrahimi, A.; Maroleanu, A.; Chiavaroli, L.; Leiter, L.A.; et al. Effect of tree nuts on metabolic syndrome criteria: A systematic review and meta-analysis of randomised controlled trials. *BMJ Open* **2014**, *4*, e004660. [CrossRef] [PubMed]
109. Rasmussen, O.; Winther, E.; Hermansen, K. Postprandial glucose and insulin responses to rolled oats ingested raw, cooked or as a mixture with raisins in normal subjects and type 2 diabetic patients. *Diabet. Med.* **1989**, *6*, 337–341. [CrossRef] [PubMed]

110. Kim, Y.; Hertzler, S.R.; Byrne, H.K.; Mattern, C.O. Raisins are a low to moderate glycemic index food with a correspondingly low insulin index. *Nutr. Res.* **2008**, *28*, 304–308. [CrossRef] [PubMed]
111. Kanellos, P.T.; Kaliora, A.C.; Liaskos, C.; Tentolouris, N.K.; Perrea, D.; Karathanos, V.T. A study of glycemic response to Corinthian raisins in healthy subjects and in type 2 diabetes mellitus patients. *Plant Foods Hum. Nutr.* **2013**, *68*, 145–148. [CrossRef] [PubMed]
112. Esfahani, A.; Lam, J.; Kendall, C.W.C. Acute effects of raisin consumption on glucose and insulin reponses in healthy individuals. *J. Nutr. Sci.* **2014**, *3*, e1. [CrossRef] [PubMed]
113. Kaliora, A.C.; Kanellos, P.T.; Gioxari, A.; Karathanos, V.T. Regulation of GIP and Ghrelin in Healthy Subjects Fed on Sun-Dried Raisins: A Pilot Study with a Crossover Trial Design. *J. Med. Food* **2017**, *20*, 301–308. [CrossRef] [PubMed]
114. Furchner-Evanson, A.; Petrisko, Y.; Howarth, L.; Nemoseck, T.; Kern, M. Type of snack influences satiety responses in adult women. *Appetite* **2010**, *54*, 564–569. [CrossRef] [PubMed]
115. Puglisi, M.J.; Vaishnav, U.; Shrestha, S.; Torres-Gonzalez, M.; Wood, R.J.; Volek, J.S.; Fernandez, M.L. Raisins and additional walking have distinct effects on plasma lipids and inflammatory cytokines. *Lipids Health Dis.* **2008**, *7*, 14. [CrossRef] [PubMed]
116. Rankin, J.W.; Andreae, M.C.; Oliver Chen, C.-Y.; O'Keefe, S.F. Effect of raisin consumption on oxidative stress and inflammation in obesity. *Diabetes Obes. Metab.* **2008**, *10*, 1086–1096. [CrossRef] [PubMed]
117. Howarth, L.; Petrisko, Y.; Furchner-Evanson, A.; Nemoseck, T.; Kern, M. Snack Selection Influences Nutrient Intake, Triglycerides, and Bowel Habits of Adult Women: A Pilot Study. *J. Am. Diet. Assoc.* **2010**, *110*, 1322–1327. [CrossRef] [PubMed]
118. Kanellos, P.T.; Kaliora, A.C.; Tentolouris, N.K.; Argiana, V.; Perrea, D.; Kalogeropoulos, N.; Kountouri, A.M.; Karathanos, V.T. A pilot, randomized controlled trial to examine the health outcomes of raisin consumption in patients with diabetes. *Nutrition* **2014**, *30*, 358–364. [CrossRef] [PubMed]
119. Bays, H.; Weiter, K.; Anderson, J. A randomized study of raisins versus alternative snacks on glycemic control and other cardiovascular risk factors in patients with type 2 diabetes mellitus. *Phys. Sportsmed.* **2015**, *43*, 37–43. [CrossRef] [PubMed]
120. Anderson, J.W.; Weiter, K.M.; Christian, A.L.; Ritchey, M.B.; Bays, H.E. Raisins Compared with Other Snack Effects on Glycemia and Blood Pressure: A Randomized, Controlled Trial. *Postgrad. Med.* **2014**, *126*, 37–43. [CrossRef] [PubMed]
121. Chandalia, M.; Garg, A.; Lutjohann, D.; von Bergmann, K.; Grundy, S.M.; Brinkley, L.J. Beneficial effects of high dietary fiber intake in patients with type 2 diabetes mellitus. *N. Engl. J. Med.* **2000**, *342*, 1392–1398. [CrossRef] [PubMed]
122. Dikeman, C.L.; Fahey, G.C. Viscosity as Related to Dietary Fiber: A Review. *Crit. Rev. Food Sci. Nutr.* **2006**, *46*, 649–663. [CrossRef] [PubMed]
123. Hopping, B.N.; Erber, E.; Grandinetti, A.; Verheus, M.; Kolonel, L.N.; Maskarinec, G. Dietary fiber, magnesium, and glycemic load alter risk of type 2 diabetes in a multiethnic cohort in Hawaii. *J. Nutr.* **2010**, *140*, 68–74. [CrossRef] [PubMed]
124. Lovejoy, J.C. The impact of nuts on diabetes and diabetes risk. *Curr. Diab. Rep.* **2005**, *5*, 379–384. [CrossRef] [PubMed]
125. Heppner, K.M.; Perez-Tilve, D. GLP-1 based therapeutics: Simultaneously combating T2DM and obesity. *Front. Neurosci.* **2015**, *9*, 92. [CrossRef] [PubMed]
126. Bodnaruc, A.M.; Prud'homme, D.; Blanchet, R.; Giroux, I. Nutritional modulation of endogenous glucagon-like peptide-1 secretion: A review. *Nutr. Metab. (Lond.)* **2016**, *13*, 92. [CrossRef] [PubMed]
127. Brand-Miller, J.; Hayne, S.; Petocz, P.; Colagiuri, S. Low-glycemic index diets in the management of diabetes: A meta-analysis of randomized controlled trials. *Diabetes Care* **2003**, *26*, 2261–2267. [CrossRef] [PubMed]
128. Mirrahimi, A.; Chiavaroli, L.; Srichaikul, K.; Augustin, L.S.A.; Sievenpiper, J.L.; Kendall, C.W.C.; Jenkins, D.J.A. The role of glycemic index and glycemic load in cardiovascular disease and its risk factors: A review of the recent literature. *Curr. Atheroscler. Rep.* **2014**, *16*, 381. [CrossRef] [PubMed]
129. Storlien, L.H.; Baur, L.A.; Kriketos, A.D.; Pan, D.A.; Cooney, G.J.; Jenkins, A.B.; Calvert, G.D.; Campbell, L. V Dietary fats and insulin action. *Diabetologia* **1996**, *39*, 621–631. [CrossRef] [PubMed]
130. Haag, M.; Dippenaar, N.G. Dietary fats, fatty acids and insulin resistance: Short review of a multifaceted connection. *Med. Sci. Monit.* **2005**, *11*, RA359–RA367. [PubMed]

131. Risérus, U.; Willett, W.C.; Hu, F.B. Dietary fats and prevention of type 2 diabetes. *Prog. Lipid Res.* **2009**, *48*, 44–51. [CrossRef] [PubMed]
132. Segal-Isaacson, C.J.; Carello, E.; Wylie-Rosett, J. Dietary fats and diabetes mellitus: Is there a good fat? *Curr. Diabetes Rep.* **2001**, *1*, 161–169. [CrossRef]
133. Rajaram, S.; Sabaté, J. Nuts, body weight and insulin resistance. *Br. J. Nutr.* **2006**, *96* (Suppl. 2), S79–S86. [CrossRef] [PubMed]
134. Kien, C.L. Dietary interventions for metabolic syndrome: Role of modifying dietary fats. *Curr. Diabetes Rep.* **2009**, *9*, 43–50. [CrossRef]
135. Grygiel-Górniak, B. Peroxisome proliferator-activated receptors and their ligands: Nutritional and clinical implications - a review. *Nutr. J.* **2014**, *13*, 17. [CrossRef] [PubMed]
136. Martini, L.A.; Catania, A.S.; Ferreira, S.R. Role of vitamins and minerals in prevention and management of type 2 diabetes mellitus. *Nutr. Rev.* **2010**, *68*, 341–354. [CrossRef] [PubMed]
137. Chaudhary, D.P.; Sharma, R.; Bansal, D.D. Implications of magnesium deficiency in type 2 diabetes: A review. *Biol. Trace Elem. Res.* **2010**, *134*, 119–129. [CrossRef] [PubMed]
138. Lopez-Ridaura, R.; Willett, W.C.; Rimm, E.B.; Liu, S.; Stampfer, M.J.; Manson, J.E.; Hu, F.B. Magnesium intake and risk of type 2 diabetes in men and women. *Diabetes Care* **2004**, *27*, 134–140. [CrossRef] [PubMed]
139. Guasch-Ferré, M.; Bulló, M.; Estruch, R.; Corella, D.; Martínez-González, M.A.; Ros, E.; Covas, M.; Arós, F.; Gómez-Gracia, E.; Fiol, M.; et al. Dietary magnesium intake is inversely associated with mortality in adults at high cardiovascular disease risk. *J. Nutr.* **2014**, *144*, 55–60. [CrossRef] [PubMed]
140. Pandey, K.B.; Rizvi, S.I. Current Understanding of Dietary Polyphenols and their Role in Health and Disease. *Curr. Nutr. Food Sci.* **2009**, *5*, 249–263. [CrossRef]
141. Xiao, J.B.; Högger, P. Dietary polyphenols and type 2 diabetes: Current insights and future perspectives. *Curr. Med. Chem.* **2015**, *22*, 23–38. [CrossRef] [PubMed]
142. Guo, X.; Yang, B.; Tan, J.; Jiang, J.; Li, D. Associations of dietary intakes of anthocyanins and berry fruits with risk of type 2 diabetes mellitus: A systematic review and meta-analysis of prospective cohort studies. *Eur. J. Clin. Nutr.* **2016**, *70*, 1360–1367. [CrossRef] [PubMed]
143. Oboh, G.; Ademosun, A.O.; Ogunsuyi, O.B. Quercetin and Its Role in Chronic Diseases. In *Advances in Experimental Medicine and Biology*; Springer Science+Business Media: Berlin/Heidelberg, Germany, 2016; Volume 929, pp. 377–387.
144. Meng, Y.; Su, A.; Yuan, S.; Zhao, H.; Tan, S.; Hu, C.; Deng, H.; Guo, Y. Evaluation of Total Flavonoids, Myricetin, and Quercetin from Hovenia dulcis Thunb. As Inhibitors of α-Amylase and α-Glucosidase. *Plant Foods Hum. Nutr.* **2016**, *71*, 444–449. [CrossRef] [PubMed]
145. Kang, I.; Buckner, T.; Shay, N.F.; Gu, L.; Chung, S. Improvements in Metabolic Health with Consumption of Ellagic Acid and Subsequent Conversion into Urolithins: Evidence and Mechanisms. *Adv. Nutr.* **2016**, *7*, 961–972. [CrossRef] [PubMed]
146. Yoshimura, Y.; Nishii, S.; Zaima, N.; Moriyama, T.; Kawamura, Y. Ellagic acid improves hepatic steatosis and serum lipid composition through reduction of serum resistin levels and transcriptional activation of hepatic ppara in obese, diabetic KK-Ay mice. *Biochem. Biophys. Res. Commun.* **2013**, *434*, 486–491. [CrossRef] [PubMed]
147. Panchal, S.K.; Ward, L.; Brown, L. Ellagic acid attenuates high-carbohydrate, high-fat diet-induced metabolic syndrome in rats. *Eur. J. Nutr.* **2013**, *52*, 559–568. [CrossRef] [PubMed]
148. Ahad, A.; Ganai, A.A.; Mujeeb, M.; Siddiqui, W.A. Ellagic acid, an NF-κB inhibitor, ameliorates renal function in experimental diabetic nephropathy. *Chem. Biol. Interact.* **2014**, *219*, 64–75. [CrossRef] [PubMed]
149. Karachanak-Yankova, S.; Dimova, R.; Nikolova, D.; Nesheva, D.; Koprinarova, M.; Maslyankov, S.; Tafradjiska, R.; Gateva, P.; Velizarova, M.; Hammoudeh, Z.; et al. Epigenetic alterations in patients with type 2 diabetes mellitus. *Balkan J. Med. Genet.* **2015**, *18*, 15–24. [CrossRef] [PubMed]
150. Paluszczak, J.; Krajka-Kuźniak, V.; Baer-Dubowska, W. The effect of dietary polyphenols on the epigenetic regulation of gene expression in MCF7 breast cancer cells. *Toxicol. Lett.* **2010**, *192*, 119–125. [CrossRef] [PubMed]
151. Holliday, R. Mechanisms for the control of gene activity during development. *Biol. Rev. Camb. Philos. Soc.* **1990**, *65*, 431–471. [CrossRef] [PubMed]
152. Choi, S.-W.; Claycombe, K.J.; Martinez, J.A.; Friso, S.; Schalinske, K.L. Nutritional Epigenomics: A Portal to Disease Prevention. *Adv. Nutr. Int. Rev. J.* **2013**, *4*, 530–532. [CrossRef] [PubMed]
153. Das, D.K.; Mukherjee, S.; Ray, D. Resveratrol and red wine, healthy heart and longevity. *Heart Fail. Rev.* **2010**, *15*, 467–477. [CrossRef] [PubMed]

154. Lee, K.W.; Lee, H.J.; Lee, C.Y. Vitamins, phytochemicals, diets, and their implementation in cancer chemoprevention. *Crit. Rev. Food Sci. Nutr.* **2004**, *44*, 437–452. [CrossRef] [PubMed]
155. Link, A.; Balaguer, F.; Goel, A. Cancer chemoprevention by dietary polyphenols: Promising role for epigenetics. *Biochem. Pharmacol.* **2010**, *80*, 1771–1792. [CrossRef] [PubMed]
156. Hermsdorff, H.H.M.; Zulet, M.Á.; Puchau, B.; Martínez, J.A. Fruit and vegetable consumption and proinflammatory gene expression from peripheral blood mononuclear cells in young adults: A translational study. *Nutr. Metab. (Lond.)* **2010**, *7*, 42. [CrossRef] [PubMed]
157. Ambros, V. The functions of animal microRNAs. *Nature* **2004**, *431*, 350–355. [CrossRef] [PubMed]
158. Ambros, V.; Bartel, B.; Bartel, D.P.; Burge, C.B.; Carrington, J.C.; Chen, X.; Dreyfuss, G.; Eddy, S.R.; Griffiths-Jones, S.; Marshall, M.; et al. A uniform system for microRNA annotation. *RNA* **2003**, *9*, 277–279. [CrossRef] [PubMed]
159. Ross, S.A.; Davis, C.D. The emerging role of microRNAs and nutrition in modulating health and disease. *Annu. Rev. Nutr.* **2014**, *34*, 305–336. [CrossRef] [PubMed]
160. Tomé-Carneiro, J.; Larrosa, M.; Yáñez-Gascón, M.J.; Dávalos, A.; Gil-Zamorano, J.; Gonzálvez, M.; García-Almagro, F.J.; Ruiz Ros, J.A.; Tomás-Barberán, F.A.; Espín, J.C.; et al. One-year supplementation with a grape extract containing resveratrol modulates inflammatory-related microRNAs and cytokines expression in peripheral blood mononuclear cells of type 2 diabetes and hypertensive patients with coronary artery disease. *Pharmacol. Res.* **2013**, *72*, 69–82. [CrossRef] [PubMed]
161. Ortega, F.J.; Cardona-Alvarado, M.I.; Mercader, J.M.; Moreno-Navarrete, J.M.; Moreno, M.; Sabater, M.; Fuentes-Batllevell, N.; Ramírez-Chávez, E.; Ricart, W.; Molina-Torres, J.; et al. Circulating profiling reveals the effect of a polyunsaturated fatty acid-enriched diet on common microRNAs. *J. Nutr. Biochem.* **2015**, *26*, 1095–1101. [CrossRef] [PubMed]
162. Hernández-Alonso, P.; Giardina, S.; Salas-Salvadó, J.; Arcelin, P.; Bulló, M. Chronic pistachio intake modulates circulating microRNAs related to glucose metabolism and insulin resistance in prediabetic subjects. *Eur. J. Nutr.* **2016**. [CrossRef] [PubMed]
163. Conlon, M.A.; Bird, A.R. The Impact of Diet and Lifestyle on Gut Microbiota and Human Health. *Nutrients* **2014**, *7*, 17–44. [CrossRef] [PubMed]
164. Ansell, J.; Parkar, S.; Paturi, G.; Rosendale, D.; Blatchford, P. Modification of the Colonic Microbiota. *Adv. Food Nutr. Res.* **2013**, *68*, 205–217. [PubMed]
165. Mandalari, G.; Faulks, R.M.; Bisignano, C.; Waldron, K.W.; Narbad, A.; Wickham, M.S.J. In vitro evaluation of the prebiotic properties of almond skins (Amygdalus communis L.). *FEMS Microbiol. Lett.* **2010**, *304*, 116–122. [CrossRef] [PubMed]
166. Ukhanova, M.; Wang, X.; Baer, D.J.; Novotny, J.A.; Fredborg, M.; Mai, V. Effects of almond and pistachio consumption on gut microbiota composition in a randomised cross-over human feeding study. *Br. J. Nutr.* **2014**, *111*, 2146–2152. [CrossRef] [PubMed]
167. Anhê, F.F.; Varin, T.V.; Le Barz, M.; Desjardins, Y.; Levy, E.; Roy, D.; Marette, A. Gut Microbiota Dysbiosis in Obesity-Linked Metabolic Diseases and Prebiotic Potential of Polyphenol-Rich Extracts. *Curr. Obes. Rep.* **2015**, *4*, 389–400. [CrossRef] [PubMed]
168. Anhê, F.F.; Roy, D.; Pilon, G.; Dudonné, S.; Matamoros, S.; Varin, T.V.; Garofalo, C.; Moine, Q.; Desjardins, Y.; Levy, E.; et al. A polyphenol-rich cranberry extract protects from diet-induced obesity, insulin resistance and intestinal inflammation in association with increased *Akkermansia* spp. population in the gut microbiota of mice. *Gut* **2015**, *64*, 872–883. [PubMed]
169. Nieman, D.C.; Scherr, J.; Luo, B.; Meaney, M.P.; Dréau, D.; Sha, W.; Dew, D.A.; Henson, D.A.; Pappan, K.L. Influence of pistachios on performance and exercise-induced inflammation, oxidative stress, immune dysfunction, and metabolite shifts in cyclists: A randomized, crossover trial. *PLoS ONE* **2014**, *9*, e113725. [CrossRef] [PubMed]
170. Hernández-Alonso, P.; Cañueto, D.; Giardina, S.; Salas-Salvadó, J.; Cañellas, N.; Correig, X.; Bulló, M. Effect of pistachio consumption on the modulation of urinary gut microbiota-related metabolites in pre-diabetic subjects. *J. Nutr. Biochem.* **2017**, *45*, 48–53. [CrossRef] [PubMed]

Permissions

All chapters in this book were first published by MDPI; hereby published with permission under the Creative Commons Attribution License or equivalent. Every chapter published in this book has been scrutinized by our experts. Their significance has been extensively debated. The topics covered herein carry significant findings which will fuel the growth of the discipline. They may even be implemented as practical applications or may be referred to as a beginning point for another development.

The contributors of this book come from diverse backgrounds, making this book a truly international effort. This book will bring forth new frontiers with its revolutionizing research information and detailed analysis of the nascent developments around the world.

We would like to thank all the contributing authors for lending their expertise to make the book truly unique. They have played a crucial role in the development of this book. Without their invaluable contributions this book wouldn't have been possible. They have made vital efforts to compile up to date information on the varied aspects of this subject to make this book a valuable addition to the collection of many professionals and students.

This book was conceptualized with the vision of imparting up-to-date information and advanced data in this field. To ensure the same, a matchless editorial board was set up. Every individual on the board went through rigorous rounds of assessment to prove their worth. After which they invested a large part of their time researching and compiling the most relevant data for our readers.

The editorial board has been involved in producing this book since its inception. They have spent rigorous hours researching and exploring the diverse topics which have resulted in the successful publishing of this book. They have passed on their knowledge of decades through this book. To expedite this challenging task, the publisher supported the team at every step. A small team of assistant editors was also appointed to further simplify the editing procedure and attain best results for the readers.

Apart from the editorial board, the designing team has also invested a significant amount of their time in understanding the subject and creating the most relevant covers. They scrutinized every image to scout for the most suitable representation of the subject and create an appropriate cover for the book.

The publishing team has been an ardent support to the editorial, designing and production team. Their endless efforts to recruit the best for this project, has resulted in the accomplishment of this book. They are a veteran in the field of academics and their pool of knowledge is as vast as their experience in printing. Their expertise and guidance has proved useful at every step. Their uncompromising quality standards have made this book an exceptional effort. Their encouragement from time to time has been an inspiration for everyone.

The publisher and the editorial board hope that this book will prove to be a valuable piece of knowledge for researchers, students, practitioners and scholars across the globe.

List of Contributors

Nicole L. Stott and Joseph S. Marino
Laboratory of Systems Physiology, Department of Kinesiology, The University of North Carolina at Charlotte, Charlotte, NC 28223, USA

Savvas Katsaridis
Department of Nutritional Sciences & Dietetics, Faculty of Health Sciences, Alexander Campus, International Hellenic University, Sindos, GR-57400 Thessaloniki, Greece

Maria G. Grammatikopoulou
Department of Nutritional Sciences & Dietetics, Faculty of Health Sciences, Alexander Campus, International Hellenic University, Sindos, GR-57400 Thessaloniki, Greece
Unit of Reproductive Endocrinology, 1st Department of Obstetrics and Gynecology, Medical School, Aristotle University of Thessaloniki, Papageorgiou General Hospital, GR-56429 Thessaloniki, Greece

Dimitrios G. Goulis
Unit of Reproductive Endocrinology, 1st Department of Obstetrics and Gynecology, Medical School, Aristotle University of Thessaloniki, Papageorgiou General Hospital, GR-56429 Thessaloniki, Greece

Konstantinos Gkiouras
Laboratory of Clinical Pharmacology, Faculty of Health Sciences, Medical School, Aristotle University of Thessaloniki, GR-54124 Thessaloniki, Greece

Christos Tzimos
Northern Greece Statistics Directorate, Hellenic Statistical Authority, 218 Delfon Str, GR-54646 Thessaloniki, Greece

Stefanos T. Papageorgiou
Faculty of Health Sciences, Medical School, Aristotle University of Thessaloniki, GR-54124 Thessaloniki, Greece

Satoru Yamada
Diabetes Center, Kitasato Institute Hospital, 5-9-1 Shirokane, Minato-ku, Tokyo 108-8642, Japan

Triada Exiara
Department of Internal Medicine, Sismanoglio General Hospital, 45 Sismanogliou Str, GR-69133 Komotini, Greece

Anastasia G. Markaki
Department of Nutrition and Dietetics, Faculty of Health Sciences, Hellenic Mediterranean University, Trypitos, GR-72300 Sitia, Greece

Theodora Papamitsou
Laboratory of Histology and Embryology, Medical School, Aristotle University of Thessaloniki, GR-54124 Thessaloniki, Greece

Alexander M. Vaiserman
D.F. Chebotarev Institute of Gerontology, Kiev 04114, NAMS, Ukraine

Araceli Muñoz-Garach
Department of Endocrinology and Nutrition, Virgen de la Victoria University Hospital, Institute of Biomedical Research in Malaga (IBIMA), 29010 Malaga, Spain
Instituto de Salud Carlos III, 28029 Madrid, Spain

Beatriz García-Fontana
Instituto de Investigación Biosanitaria (Ibs. GRANADA), 18106 Granada, Spain
Centro de Investigación Biomédica en Red sobre Fragilidad y Envejecimiento Saludable (CIBERFES), Instituto de Salud Carlos III, 28029 Madrid, Spain

Manuel Muñoz-Torres
Instituto de Investigación Biosanitaria (Ibs. GRANADA), 18106 Granada, Spain
Centro de Investigación Biomédica en Red sobre Fragilidad y Envejecimiento Saludable (CIBERFES), Instituto de Salud Carlos III, 28029 Madrid, Spain
Unidad de Gestión Clínica Endocrinología y Nutrición, Hospital Universitario San Cecilio de Granada, Avenida de la Innovacion, 18016 Granada, Spain
Department of Medicine, University of Granada, 18016 Granada, Spain

Yusuke Kabeya
Department of Home Care Medicine, Saiyu Clinic, 3-217-1 Sagamicho, Koshigaya-shi, Saitama 343-0823, Japan

Hiroshi Noto
Endocrinology Department, St. Luke's International Hospital, 9-1 Akashicho, Chuo-ku, Tokyo 104-8560, Japan

Rui Liu, Hui Li, Wenjuan Fan, Qiu Jin, Tingting Chao, Yuanjue Wu, Junmei Huang, Liping Hao and Xuefeng Yang
Department of Nutrition and Food Hygiene, Hubei Key Laboratory of Food Nutrition and Safety, MOE Key Laboratory of Environment and Health, School of Public Health, Tongji Medical College, Huazhong University of Science and Technology, Wuhan 430030, Hubei, China

Ling-Shan Tse and Yu-Wen Cheng
School of Pharmacy, College of Pharmacy, Taipei Medical University, Taipei 110, Taiwan

Po-Lin Liao and Jaw-Jou Kang
Institute of Food Safety and Health Risk Assessment, School of Pharmaceutical Sciences, National Yang-Ming University, Taipei 112, Taiwan

Chi-Hao Tsai
School of Pharmacy, College of Pharmacy, Taipei Medical University, Taipei 110, Taiwan
Institute of Toxicology, College of Medicine, National Taiwan University, Taipei 100, Taiwan

Ching-Hao Li
Department of Physiology, School of Medicine, Graduate Institute of Medical Sciences, College of Medicine, Taipei Medical University, Taipei 110, Taiwan

Jiunn-Wang Liao
Graduate Institute of Veterinary Pathobiology, National Chung Hsing University, Taichung 402, Taiwan

Charlotte E. Pelgrim, Bart A. A. Franx, Ilse A. C. Arnoldussen and Amanda J. Kiliaan
Donders Institute for Brain, Cognition and Behaviour, Preclinical Imaging Centre, Department of Anatomy, Radboud University Medical Center, 6525 EZ Nijmegen, The Netherlands

Jessica Snabel and Robert Kleemann
Department of Metabolic Health Research, Netherlands Organisation for Applied Scientific Research (TNO), 2301 CE Leiden, The Netherlands

Sara Nunes, Frederico C. Pereira, Flávio Reis, Ana Burgeiro, Manuela G. Cerqueira and Bárbara M. Varela-Rodríguez
Center of Neuroscience and Cell Biology (CNC) and CNC.IBILI Research Consortium, University of Coimbra, 3004-504 Coimbra, Portugal
Laboratory of Pharmacology and Experimental Therapeutics, Institute for Biomedical Imaging and Life Sciences (IBILI), Faculty of Medicine, University of Coimbra, 3000-548 Coimbra, Portugal

Paula Neto
Service of Anatomical Pathology, Coimbra University Hospital Centre (CHUC), 3000-075 Coimbra, Portugal

Eugénia Carvalho
Center of Neuroscience and Cell Biology (CNC) and CNC.IBILI Research Consortium, University of Coimbra, 3004-504 Coimbra, Portugal
The Portuguese Diabetes Association (APDP), 1250-203 Lisbon, Portugal
Department of Geriatrics, University of Arkansas for Medical Sciences, Little Rock, AR 72202, USA
Arkansas Children's Hospital Research Institute, Little Rock, AR 72202, USA

Christina M. Gant, S. Heleen Binnenmars and Gozewijn D. Laverman
Department of Internal Medicine/Nephrology, Ziekenhuisgroep Twente, Zilvermeeuw 1, 7609 PP Almelo, The Netherlands
Department of Internal Medicine, Division of Nephrology, University of Groningen, University Medical Center Groningen, Hanzeplein 1, 9713 GZ Groningen, The Netherlands

Else van den Berg, Stephan J. L. Bakker and Gerjan Navis
Department of Internal Medicine, Division of Nephrology, University of Groningen, University Medical Center Groningen, Hanzeplein 1, 9713 GZ Groningen, The Netherlands

Tanja Diederichs, Sarah Roßbach, Ute Nöthlings and Ute Alexy
IEL-Nutritional Epidemiology, DONALD Study, Rheinische Friedrich-Wilhelms-University Bonn, Heinstueck 11, 44225 Dortmund, Germany

Christian Herder
Institute for Clinical Diabetology, German Diabetes Center, Leibniz Center for Diabetes Research at Heinrich Heine University Düsseldorf, Düsseldorf, Auf'm Hennekamp 65, 40225 Düsseldorf, Germany
German Center for Diabetes Research (DZD), Ingolstädter Landstr. 1, 85764 München-Neuherberg, Germany

Rosa-Virgen Pardo-Morales
Instlituto Materno-Infantil del Estado de México, Paseo Colón s/n, Col. Villa Hogar, Toluca 50170, Mexico

Michael Roden
Institute for Clinical Diabetology, German Diabetes Center, Leibniz Center for Diabetes Research at Heinrich Heine University Düsseldorf, Düsseldorf, Auf'm Hennekamp 65, 40225 Düsseldorf, Germany
German Center for Diabetes Research (DZD), Ingolstädter Landstr. 1, 85764 München-Neuherberg, Germany
Department of Endocrinology and Diabetology, Medical Faculty, Heinrich Heine University Düsseldorf, Moorenstraße 5, 40225 Düsseldorf, Germany

Stefan A. Wudy
Pediatric Endocrinology and Diabetology, Laboratory for Translational Hormone Analytics, Peptide Hormone Research Unit, Center of Child and Adolescent Medicine, Justus Liebig University Giessen, Feulgenstraße 10-12, 35392 Gießen, Germany

Anette E. Buyken
IEL-Nutritional Epidemiology, DONALD Study, Rheinische Friedrich-Wilhelms-University Bonn, Heinstueck 11, 44225 Dortmund, Germany
Institute of Nutrition, Consumption and Health, Faculty of Natural Sciences, University Paderborn, Warburger Straße 100, 33098 Paderborn, Germany

M. Gorety Jacobo-Cejudo, Roxana Valdés-Ramos, Ana L. Guadarrama-López and Beatriz E. Martínez-Carrillo
Faculty of Medicine, Universidad Autónoma del Estado de México, Paseo Tollocan esq. Jesús Carranza, Col. Moderna de la Cruz, Toluca 50180, Mexico

Laurence S. Harbige
Faculty of Life Sciences and Computing, London Metropolitan University, 166-220 Holloway Road, London N7 8DB, UK

Mikael Fogelholm and Elli Jalo
Department of Food and Environmental Sciences, University of Helsinki, 00014 Helsinki, Finland

Thomas Meinert Larsen, Pia Christensen, Laura Pastor-Sanz and Anne Raben
Department of Nutrition, Exercise and Sports, Faculty of Science, University of Copenhagen, Rolighedsvej 30, Frederiksberg C, DK-1958 Copenhagen, Denmark

Mathijs Drummen and Margriet Westerterp-Plantenga
Department of Human Biology, Maastricht University, 6200 MD Maastricht, The Netherlands

Elizabeth Simpson and Ian Macdonald
School of Life Sciences, Faculty of Medicine and Health Sciences, University of Nottingham, Nottingham NG7 2UH, UK

Santiago Navas-Carretero and J. Alfredo Martinez
Center for Nutrition Research, University of Navarra, 31008 Pamplona, Spain
CIBERobn, Instituto de Salud Carlos III, 28029 Madrid, Spain

Teodora Handjieva-Darlenska and Nadka Boyadjieva
Department of pharmacology and toxicology, Medical University of Sofia, 1431 Sofia, Bulgaria

Marta P. Silvestre and Sally Poppitt
Human Nutrition Unit, School of Biological Sciences, University of Auckland, Auckland 1024, New Zealand

Wolfgang Schlicht
Department of Exercise and Health Sciences, University of Stuttgart, 70569 Stuttgart, Germany

Gareth Stratton
School of Sport and Exercise Sciences, A.STEM Research Centre, Swansea University, Swansea SA1 8EN, UK

Jouko Sundvall
National Institute for Health and Welfare THL, 00300 Helsinki, Finland

Tony Lam
NetUnion sarl, Ave des Figuires 20, 1007 Lausanne, Switzerland

Jennie Brand-Miller and Roslyn Muirhead
Charles Perkins Centre, University of Sydney, Sydney 2006, Australia

Daniela Kahlert
Department of Health Science, University of Education Schwäbisch Gmünd, 73525 Gmünd, Germany

Pablo Hernández-Alonso, Lucía Camacho-Barcia, Mònica Bulló and Jordi Salas-Salvadó
Human Nutrition Unit, Biochemistry and Biotechnology Department, Faculty of Medicine and Health Sciences, University Hospital of Sant Joan de Reus, IISPV, Universitat Rovira i Virgili, St/Sant Llorenç 21, 43201 Reus, Spain
CIBERobn Physiopathology of Obesity and Nutrition, Instituto de Salud Carlos III, 28029 Madrid, Spain

Index

A

Adipocyte, 4, 6, 15, 41, 111-112, 114-122, 124, 129, 133, 181

Adipose Tissue, 4, 6, 12, 14-19, 38, 49, 55, 65, 89-90, 92, 96, 111-115, 118, 120-129, 133-134, 136-137, 139-141, 174-175, 180, 182, 221, 227

Adiposity, 6, 65, 119-120, 122-125, 136-137, 141, 205, 229

Alanine, 80-81, 84-86, 93, 128, 131, 160, 189

Aldosterone, 99, 102, 105-107, 109-110, 149

Animal Models, 1-2, 13-14, 39-40, 92, 99-100, 103, 107, 175

Antibodies, 82, 114-115, 129

Aspartic Acid, 81, 85-86

Autophagy, 6, 14, 16, 100

B

Birth Weight, 38-39, 43-44, 46, 48, 51, 161-163, 166

Blood Pressure, 22, 25, 27, 38, 43-44, 46, 50-51, 56, 60, 106, 111, 142-143, 145-156, 187-188, 192, 195, 218, 225, 232

Body Mass Index, 22, 26-27, 41, 55, 67, 71, 76, 123, 142-143, 161, 164, 176, 178, 187, 195, 224

Branched-chain Amino Acids, 79, 85, 95-97

Butyrate, 111-114, 118-124, 220, 223

C

Calcitriol, 54-55

Calcium Flux, 54-55

Caloric Intake, 1, 13, 128-130, 136

Carbohydrate Restricted Diet, 70-73, 75-76

Cholecalciferol, 54, 56-57

Co-morbidities, 1, 15, 125, 139, 198

Cytokine, 2, 14, 55, 59, 175, 228

D

Diabetes Mellitus, 14, 20-21, 32-34, 36, 48, 50-52, 64-67, 76-78, 80, 96, 98-99, 107-111, 122-124, 126, 140, 142, 146, 148, 154-156, 158-160, 167, 174-175, 180, 182-184, 199-200, 213, 228-233

Dietary Habits, 1, 186

Dietary Supplements, 21, 26, 35, 98

E

Energy Restricted Diet, 70-72, 75-76

F

Fasting Glucose, 6, 9, 81, 84, 101, 127, 132, 137, 162, 176, 179, 183, 188, 194, 213, 218

Fatty Acids, 1-2, 4, 6, 14, 29, 32, 55, 112, 121, 123-124, 127, 134, 139, 162, 164-166, 172, 175, 177-178, 180-184, 192, 202-203, 220-221, 223, 225, 232

Folk Medicine, 99-100, 106

G

Gene Expression, 4, 14, 18, 37, 39, 49, 91, 133, 141, 221-222, 233-234

Glucagon, 6, 210, 224, 232

Glucose Intolerance, 1-2, 6, 17, 39-40, 43-44, 57, 96, 124, 132, 137, 141

Glucose Metabolism, 11, 18, 38-39, 46, 54, 59, 63-64, 66, 79, 91, 96, 127, 139-141, 167, 179-180, 184, 197, 205, 207, 210, 222, 228, 230, 234

Glucose Tolerance, 1, 6, 9, 17, 32, 52, 54, 57, 64-66, 77, 81, 84, 92, 99, 101-104, 106-108, 126-128, 132, 137-138, 140-141, 179, 183, 187-188, 192, 194, 196, 198-200, 225, 229-230

Glucotoxicity, 126-127

Glycemic Control, 27-30, 35-36, 57, 71-72, 75-78, 96, 143, 152, 170, 179, 230-232

H

Hedychium Coronarium, 99-101, 108-109

Hepatic Glucose, 4, 6, 38, 127, 137-138, 220

High-density Lipoprotein, 22, 99, 104, 224

High-fat Diet, 1, 11-18, 39, 79-80, 85-87, 94, 96-97, 111-113, 123-124, 207, 224, 233

Hippocampus, 9, 16-17, 123

Histidine, 81, 85-86

Homeostasis, 1, 6, 11, 13, 15-16, 18, 53-57, 59, 63-67, 79, 92, 106, 137-138, 164, 175, 183, 220

Hydrogenated Coconut Oil, 1-2

Hyperglycemia, 2, 4, 6, 11, 51, 68, 101, 122, 126-127, 136-138, 141, 175, 179, 207, 221

Hyperinsulinemia, 2, 6, 11, 96, 123, 126, 137-138, 210

Hyperplasia, 4, 6, 13

Hypertension, 43-44, 50-51, 67, 70-71, 100, 106-107, 140, 147, 149-152, 154-156, 175, 201

I

Insulin Resistance, 1-2, 4, 6, 9, 11, 14-15, 17-18, 37-41, 46, 48, 51, 53-55, 59-62, 64-68, 79-80, 86, 91-98, 107, 111, 120-122, 124-125, 127-128, 132, 137-141, 159, 167, 170-172, 174, 179, 181-184, 201, 207-208, 213, 222-225, 227, 230-234

Insulin Sensitivity, 4, 9, 16-18, 38, 53-55, 57, 59, 65-67, 79-81, 83-84, 91-98, 106, 112, 118, 120-121, 123-124, 126, 136-138, 140, 158-160, 162-164, 167-169, 171, 175, 179-181, 183-184, 186-187, 199, 207, 213, 220-221

Insulin Signaling, 4, 80, 92, 96, 98, 111-112, 120-121

Insulin Therapy, 20, 22, 26-27

L

Leucine, 79-81, 83-87, 89-98

Lipid Accumulation, 2, 4, 6, 9, 11, 14, 18

Lipogenesis, 4, 60, 112, 120, 124, 136-139, 167, 172, 175
Lipotoxicity, 126-127, 139
Low-density Lipoprotein, 22, 99, 104, 107, 110, 120, 138, 225

M

Macronutrient, 1-2, 11-12, 34, 67, 171, 181, 186, 189, 202, 216
Macrophages, 4, 6, 15, 111-112, 115, 118, 121-122, 175, 207-208, 227, 229
Malnutrition, 37-38, 41, 43, 49-50, 94, 137
Metabolic Health, 79, 111-112, 159, 168, 233
Metabolic Syndrome, 14, 34, 46, 54-55, 61-62, 64-65, 68, 71, 76, 99, 104, 110, 122, 140-141, 182, 184, 201, 207, 213, 225, 229-231, 233
Metabolites, 54, 56, 66, 80, 83, 86-90, 92-93, 95, 127, 167, 223, 234
Methionine, 81, 85-86, 89
Micronutrient, 2, 26
Mitochondrial Biogenesis, 4, 67, 79-80, 91, 93-96, 98

N

Neuroinflammation, 112
Neurons, 96
Nutrition Therapy, 21, 28, 34-35, 70, 75-76

O

Obesity, 1, 4, 6, 9, 11, 13-19, 23, 34, 37-39, 41, 43, 46-49, 51-55, 60-62, 65, 67-68, 76, 80, 91, 94-97, 101, 107, 111-112, 119-127, 138, 140-141, 152, 161, 164, 167, 170-172, 174-175, 179-183, 186, 198-199, 201, 207, 220, 227, 229, 231-232, 234
Oxidative Stress, 2, 6, 11, 14-15, 65, 110, 168, 172, 205, 207, 222, 227-228, 231-232, 234

P

Palmitic Acid, 1, 4, 86-89
Pancreas, 6, 38, 40, 49, 67, 102, 104-105, 109, 207, 227-228
Pancreatic Beta Cells, 53-55, 59-60
Pathogenesis, 2, 9, 15, 39, 47, 55, 96, 110, 139, 141
Peripheral Insulin, 38, 59-60, 137
Peroxisome, 9, 40, 55, 67, 91, 120, 221, 225, 233
Phenotype, 1, 4, 6, 9, 11-12, 38-40, 43, 46, 48-49, 93, 95, 140
Polyunsaturated Fats, 1, 4, 12
Prediabetes, 16, 23, 34-35, 54-57, 59, 62-63, 66-67, 126-127, 137-141, 167, 170, 183, 231

R

Randomized Controlled Trials, 28, 54, 62, 67, 70, 72-73, 182, 232
Renin, 55, 105, 109, 149, 154
Resistin, 111-113, 118-119, 174-184, 222, 225, 233

S

Saturated Fat, 1-2, 4, 9, 11-13, 30, 60
Streptozotocin, 99, 101-102, 109, 207, 225, 227-228

T

Threonine, 81, 85-86
Type 2 Diabetes, 1, 12, 14-16, 20-21, 32-38, 40, 46-54, 64-68, 70-73, 76-78, 80, 98-99, 101-102, 104, 107-109, 111, 122-126, 139-142, 148, 151, 154-159, 161-162, 164, 167-172, 174-175, 180, 182-184, 198-199, 201, 213, 223-234

V

Valine, 79-81, 84-86, 90
Vitamin D Deficiency, 53-54, 63, 65

W

Weight Gain, 2, 14, 83, 92, 119, 123, 125, 136, 162-163, 166, 186, 189, 198, 207, 228
Western Blot Analysis, 81, 129

www.ingramcontent.com/pod-product-compliance
Lightning Source LLC
LaVergne TN
LVHW081029210926
848485LV00004B/984